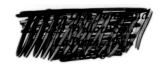

Second Edition
Clinical Electrotherapy

Edited by

Roger M. Nelson, PhD, PT
Professor and Chairman
Department of Physical Therapy
College of Allied Health Sciences
Thomas Jefferson University
Philadelphia, Pennsylvania

and

Dean P. Currier, PhD, PT
Professor and Director
Division of Physical Therapy
College of Allied Health Professions
University of Kentucky
Lexington, Kentucky

APPLETON & LANGE
Norwalk, Connecticut/San Mateo, California

0-8385-1334-4

Notice: Our knowledge in clinical sciences is constantly changing. As new information becomes available, changes in treatment and in the use of drugs become necessary. The authors and the publisher of this volume have taken care to make certain that the doses of drugs and schedules of treatment are correct and compatible with the standards generally accepted at the time of publication. The reader is advised to consult carefully the instruction and information material included in the package insert of each drug or therapeutic agent before administration. This advice is especially important when using new or infrequently used drugs.

91 92 93 94 95 / 10 9 8 7 6 5 4 3 2 1

Prentice Hall International (UK) Limited, *London*
Prentice Hall of Australia Pty. Limited, *Sydney*
Prentice Hall Canada, Inc., *Toronto*
Prentice Hall Hispanoamericana, S.A., *Mexico*
Prentice Hall of India Private Limited, *New Delhi*
Prentice Hall of Japan, Inc., *Tokyo*
Simon & Schuster Asia Pte. Ltd., *Singapore*
Editora Prentice Hall do Brasil Ltda., *Rio de Janeiro*
Prentice Hall, *Englewood Cliffs*, *New Jersey*

Library of Congress Cataloging-in-Publication Data

Clinical electrotherapy / [edited] by Roger M. Nelson and Dean P. Currier.—2nd ed.
   p. cm.
   Includes bibliographical references.
   Includes index.
   ISBN 0-8385-1334-4
   1. Neuromuscular diseases—Treatment. 2. Electric stimulation.
I. Nelson, Roger M. II. Currier, Dean P.
   [DNLM: 1. Electric Stimulation Therapy. WB 495 C6411]
RC925.5.C58 1991
616.7'40645—dc20
DNLM/DLC   90–1127
for Library of Congress   CIP

Acquisitions Editor: Stephany S. Scott
Production Editor: Charles F. Evans
Cover Designer: Janice Barsevich

PRINTED IN THE UNITED STATES OF AMERICA

Contributors

Gad Alon, PhD, PT
Department of Physical Therapy, University of Maryland
School of Medicine, Baltimore, Maryland

Lucinda L. Baker, PhD, PT
Department of Physical Therapy, University of Southern
California, Los Angeles, California

John O. Barr, PhD, PT
Physical Therapy Graduate Program, University of Iowa,
Iowa City, Iowa

Thomas M. Cook, PhD, PT
Physical Therapy Graduate Program, University of Iowa,
Iowa City, Iowa

John Cummings, PhD, PT
Program in Physical Therapy, State University of New York,
Syracuse, New York

Dean P. Currier, PhD, PT
Division of Physical Therapy, University of Kentucky,
Lexington, Kentucky

Robert Kellogg, MS, PT, ECS
Division of Physical Therapy, University of Kentucky,
Lexington, Kentucky

Luther C. Kloth, MS, PT
Program in Physical Therapy, Marquette University,
Milwaukee, Wisconsin

Roger M. Nelson, PhD, PT
Department of Physical Therapy, Thomas Jefferson University,
Philadelphia, Pennsylvania

David Nestor, MS, PT
Division of Physical Therapy, West Virginia University,
Morgantown, West Virginia

Roberta Newton, PhD, PT
Department of Physical Therapy, Temple University,
Philadelphia, Pennsylvania

Neil I. Spielholz, PhD, PT
Department of Rehabilitation Medicine, New York
University, New York, New York

Nancy L. Urbscheit, PhD, PT
Physical Therapy Program, University of Louisville,
Louisville, Kentucky

Steven L. Wolf, PhD, PT
Department of Rehabilitation Medicine, Emory University,
Atlanta, Georgia

Contents

Preface

The purpose of this second edition of *Clinical Electrotherapy* is to update the electrotherapy nomenclature into the standardized format developed by the Section on Clinical Electrotherapy, American Physical Therapy Association. The standardized electrotherapy nomenclature was developed to improve communication among all professional groups who use and manufacture electrotherapy equipment.

The chapters have been revised to reflect the standard terminology used in electrotherapy. Each chapter contributor has been diligent in updating the scientific information that has been published in the past several years. Great care was taken by the chapter contributors to improve the content of each area. The student and clinician will find this edition both informative and current.

Research related to microcurrent electrical neuromuscular stimulation (MENS) is slow in developing despite increasing clinical interest. Chapter 3 offers an introduction to MENS as a therapeutic modality. The reader should be aware that MENS electrical characteristics do not significantly differ from those of existing electrostimulators. The singular difference between MENS and existing equipment is the pulse durations. Existing stimulators are capable of producing subthreshold stimuli as are the MENS-specific equipment. Randomized, controlled clinical studies are desperately needed to critically examine the stated therapeutic claims of MENS.

The reader may experience some overlap of electrophysics throughout the text. The editors have made a conscious effort to leave some of the overlap in the second edition. Repetition in some content is not necessarily a bad idea. One author may present the information in a slightly different manner, which may make all the difference for a student or clinician. The reader is offered different approaches and sometimes different opinions for neuromuscular electrical stimulation (NMES). The different opinions result because electrotherapy remains, to some extent, a science based on the clinical model. The chapter authors are all authorities in their area and as such provide a valuable useful introduction for the variety of uses for NMES.

We have added a new chapter to the second edition. Magnetic stimulation of skeletal muscle may be a breakthrough in electrotherapy. Magnetic stimulation for chronic inflammation is also presented. These magnetic stimulation devices are currently available. For the results of ongoing clinical investigations, please review current peer-reviewed journals. This edition will serve to introduce the emerging technology of magnetically induced neuromuscular stimulation for the clinician.

The chapter on NMES for pain suppression is completely new, while chapters on biofeedback and electrophysiologic evaluation have had major revisions. We have also added wound healing by NMES to this edition. The remaining chapters have been revised to reflect recent scientific information, but with little structural change from the first edition.

This book is more than just a guide for students and clinicians. We have made every attempt to provide the scientific basis for electrotherapy. This edition offers theory, detailed review of state-of-the-art subject matter, and an immediate reference for the practitioner who seeks an answer to his or her problems on patient management techniques in clinical electrotherapy. This book is inclusive of electrotherapy as presently understood, although much research is needed to support its efficacy. Clinical electrotherapy also offers considerable potential in the successful management of patients and healthy subjects in athletic training.

Roger M. Nelson, PhD, PT
Dean P. Currier, PhD, PT

CHAPTER 1

Review of Physiology

Nancy L. Urbscheit

The use of electrical stimulation by a physical therapist is effective in treating various disorders. It is essential, however, that the therapist possess intimate knowledge, not only of the disorder to be treated, but also of the mechanism by which electrical stimulation affects tissues in the path of the current. If such knowledge is either absent or ignored, the physical therapist will be unable to select effective, safe, and comfortable procedures of electrical stimulation.

This chapter discusses the properties of muscle and nerve cell membranes and their response to electrical stimulation. The purpose of the chapter is to provide the therapist with the knowledge necessary to understand the phenomena of both natural and invoked discharge of excitable membranes.

PROPERTIES OF EXCITABLE CELL MEMBRANES

Resting Membrane Potentials

Before the manner in which nerve and muscle cells respond to electrical stimulation can be considered, it is necessary to understand the normal properties of the cells. Both nerve and muscle cells are enveloped by a membrane that separates a charge across the membrane. This charge is maintained as long as the cell is healthy and undisturbed. This resting charge can be measured experimentally and is typically between 60 and 90 millivolts (mV), the inside of the cell being negative with respect to the outside. The charge on the membrane is a result of an unequal concentration of ions on either side of the membrane. In a normal muscle or nerve cell, the sodium (Na^+) concentration is higher outside the cell whereas the potassium (K$^+$) concentration is higher inside the cell. These concentration differences are maintained by an active pump that expels Na$^+$ and takes in K$^+$ on a one-to-one exchange (Fig. 1-1A). Each ion, however, will attempt to diffuse across the membrane passively in an attempt to equalize its concentration (Fig. 1–1B). This diffusion process is much more successful for K$^+$ than for Na$^+$, because the membrane has a greater permeability to K$^+$ than to Na$^+$. As the passive diffusion of the ions continues, a charge develops on the membrane. As positively charged K$^+$ ions leave the cell, a net negativity develops inside the cell. The diffusion of K$^+$ ions out of the cell is eventually retarded as the negative charge inside the cell increases. The force acting on K$^+$ ions to move out of the cell to equalize the concentration is eventually matched by an opposing force to return the ions to the cell, due to the negative charge. When these forces are equal, K$^+$ ions will be in equilibrium, with one K$^+$ ion leaving the cell for every one that enters. When K$^+$ is at equilibrium in its passive movement in and out of the cell, the cell membrane will be charged at -100 mV.

As was mentioned earlier, however, the resting membrane potential is -60

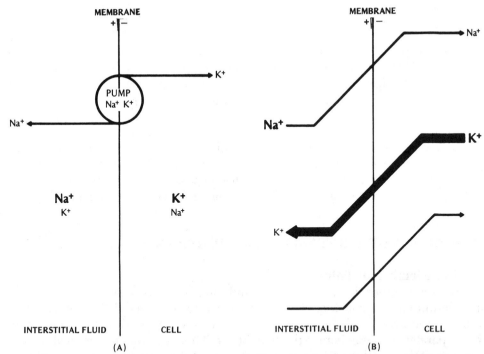

Figure 1–1. A. Active movement of Na$^+$–K$^+$ ions across an excitable membrane via an active Na$^+$–K$^+$ pump. **B.** Passive movement of Na$^+$ and K$^+$ ions. Each arrow represents the direction of movement of an ion. The width of an arrow is proportional to the number of ions moving and the slope of the arrow is proportional to the driving force.

mV. Therefore, in the typical resting excitable cell, K$^+$ ions are not at equilibrium, and more potassium will be passively leaving the cell than entering it.

Why does the resting membrane fail to remain at -90 mV, the equilibrium potential for potassium? Sodium ions will also be passively moving across the membrane in an attempt to equalize the concentration difference (Fig. 1–2). In the case of the Na$^+$ ions, the passive diffusion will be into the cell. The passive movement of Na$^+$ into the cell will not be as large as the passive movement of K$^+$ out of the cell because of the lower membrane permeability to Na$^+$. The inward movement of the Na$^+$ ions will reduce the negative charge developed by the outward leak of the K$^+$ ions. The movement of the Na$^+$ and K$^+$ ions reaches a steady state at approximately the resting membrane potential of -60 mV. At this potential, however, Na$^+$ has not equalized its concentration, and forces still exist to passively move it into the cell. In order for Na$^+$ to be at equilibrium (one Na$^+$ ion passively entering per every one that leaves), the membrane would have to be charged at $+50$ mV inside with respect to the outside. The reason the resting membrane potential normally lies much closer to the equilibrium potential of K$^+$ is that the excitable membrane is much more permeable to K$^+$.

In summary, the resting membrane potential of an excitable membrane is the consequence of both the concentration differences across the membrane and the different permeabilities of the resting excitable membrane to Na$^+$ and K$^+$.

Discharge of an Action Potential

Most excitable cells in the body spend little time at their resting membrane potential because excitable cells are continuously subjected to events that change the membrane's permeability to Na$^+$ and K$^+$ ions. If a cell membrane is exposed to a neural transmitter or a sensory stimulus, the cell may undergo a slight increase in its permeability to Na$^+$. As the number of Na$^+$ ions moving into the cell increases, the cell membrane will undergo a reduction of its negative charge (depolarization). If this depolarization reaches a certain critical level (threshold), Na$^+$ permeability will increase explosively, and Na$^+$ ions will rush into the cell (Fig. 1–2). The membrane potential will rapidly change to $+25$ to $+35$ mV because of the influx of these positive ions. Yet, this increase in permeability to Na$^+$ ions lasts only very briefly.

The initial depolarization of the membrane also increases the membrane's permeability to K$^+$. This increase in permeability to K$^+$ occurs a little more slowly than the increase to Na$^+$ and will reach a peak soon after the membrane has closed down again to Na$^+$ ions (Fig. 1–2). This latter change in the membrane's permeability to K$^+$ causes the membrane potential to become negative, reaching the equilibrium potential of -100 mV for potassium (hyperpolarization). The increase in permeability to K$^+$ ions is also very brief. The active Na$^+$–K$^+$ pump will return the ions to their original concentrations, and the resting membrane potential will be restored quickly. This sudden, rapid alteration in the membrane's potential is known as an *action potential*. The

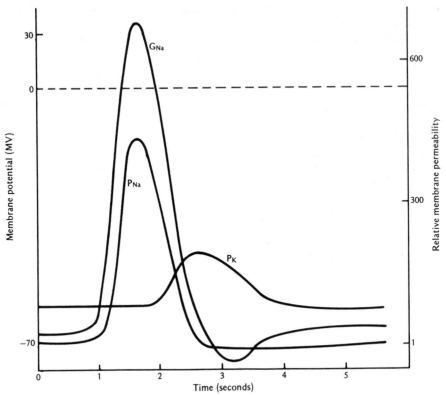

Figure 1-2. Changes in the permeability of K+ (P$_K$) and Na+ (P$_{Na}$) during an action potential.

ability of a membrane to generate an action potential is the property that defines an excitable membrane.

Although normal excitable cells undergo action potentials very frequently, there do exist conditions that will cause an excitable membrane to fail. If a membrane has been depolarized at a subthreshold level for a period of time, an action potential will not be evoked, even if the normal threshold depolarization occurs. The membrane can discharge an action potential, however, if depolarization reaches a level that is much higher than the normal firing threshold. The excitable membrane in these circumstances is said to have *accommodated.* The subthreshold, prolonged depolarization apparently raises the threshold level of depolarization at which the sudden explosive increase in permeability to Na+ occurs. A strong, slowly rising depolarization may also prevent the initiation of an action potential by blocking the increase in permeability to Na+.

If a membrane becomes sufficiently hyperpolarized, it may also be unable to discharge an action potential, because the firing threshold cannot be easily reached.

Propagation of an Action Potential

An action potential occurring in one region of an excitable membrane can trigger an action potential in a neighboring region of the membrane. The depolarization occurring in the beginning of an action potential causes a localized flow of current around the site of the action potential. This current may cause a threshold depolarization of the neighboring membrane, which may evoke an action potential. If the excitable membrane is very large, such as in a nerve axon or a muscle fiber, the action potential can be propagated over the entire membrane. If propagation is occurring in the normal direction (for example, progressing in a proximal direction for a sensory fiber), it is called *orthodromic conduction. Antidromic conduction* occurs in the direction opposite to normal and can be evoked by electrical stimulation.

The speed at which an action potential is propagated varies from one excitable membrane to another. In nerve cell fibers that are unmyelinated, action potentials create localized eddy currents that cross the membrane (Fig. 1–3A). The span of membrane encompassed by the eddy currents is small because of the high resistance of the membrane. In nerve membranes that are myelinated, the local current generated by an action potential travels inside the fiber, because the myelin prevents the eddy currents from crossing the membrane. The next action potential will occur only where a break in the myelin exists. Conduction in a myelinated fiber is much faster than in an unmyelinated fiber. In the unmyelinated fibers, numerous small areas of the membrane must sequentially undergo an action potential to propagate the length of an excitable membrane. In myelinated fibers, the action potential skips from node to node; thus, fewer action potentials will be propagated along the length of the membrane. Each action potential lasts approximately 1.0 milliseconds (ms); thus, the fewer action potentials produced during propagation of activity along the length of a nerve fiber, the less time to conduct from one end to the other.

Conduction velocity within a group of either unmyelinated or myelinated

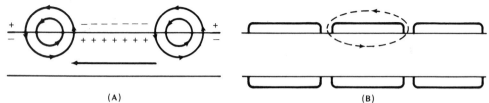

(A)   (B)

Figure 1–3. Local current flow generated by an action potential in nerve axons. **A.** Eddy currents produced by an action potential in an unmyelinated axon. The arrow indicates direction of impulse propagation. Propagated impulses would proceed only in the orthodromic direction, as the membrane would be refractory in the antidromic direction. **B.** Local current flow evoked by an action potential in a myelinated axon. The current crosses the membrane only at a node.

fibers will vary, as well. The larger the diameter of the fiber, the less resistance offered to conduction currents generated by action potentials, and thus, the faster the speed of conduction of an action potential. Nerve fibers also conduct faster if the temperature is raised.

Conduction of an action potential along a nerve fiber can be stopped in a number of ways. If a nerve fiber is exposed to local pressure or to anoxia, that region of the fiber will begin to depolarize slowly. If this occurs, the sudden, explosive increase in permeability to Na^+ ions will not occur; therefore, propagation of an action potential will cease in this area. An injection of a local anesthetic (such as novocaine) will block conduction of an action potential in the region by preventing the sudden increase in permeability to Na^+ ions. Extreme cooling can also stop conduction.

RESPONSE OF AN EXCITABLE MEMBRANE TO ELECTRICAL STIMULATION

The behavior of an excitable membrane can be modified by the application of electrical current through two external electrodes. The membrane will undergo depolarization at the cathode (negative electrode) and hyperpolarization at the anode (positive electrode).

Subthreshold Currents

If the amplitude of the electrical stimulus is too weak to produce a threshold depolarization at the cathode, an action potential will not take place. An understanding of subthreshold current flow is a prerequisite to a discussion of how an action potential is generated by electrical stimulation. A membrane exposed to a subthreshold electrical stimulus does not immediately change its charge. Upon exposure to a maintained electrical stimulus, the excitable membrane will eventually reach a steady state in which the charge on the membrane reaches its peak in response to the externally applied current. The amount of time that it takes an applied current to charge the cell membrane is directly related to the capacitance and resistance of the membrane. The time will be longer for excitable membranes of large capacitance, such as skeletal muscle fibers (35 ms), and much shorter for nerve cell membranes of small capacitance (1 ms).

Threshold for Excitation

If the applied current depolarizes the membrane to threshold, the membrane will fire an action potential. Whether the membrane reaches the threshold depends partially upon the stimulus amplitude. The stimulus amplitude required, however, varies from membrane to membrane, and even from minute to minute in the same membrane. For example, narrow-diameter fibers require a higher stimulus amplitude to reach threshold because of the high internal resistance of such fibers to current flow. In addition, a fiber that has been exposed to a continuous level of depolarization at the cathode may eventually become inexcitable unless the stimulus amplitude is increased (known as *accommodation*, or *depolarization*, *block*).

The duration of the stimulus also affects whether the membrane reaches firing threshold. If a 1.0-ms pulse is applied to a skeletal muscle cell membrane, the membrane will not fire regardless of the amplitude of the stimulus. The amount of time that a skeletal muscle cell needs to reach a maximum charge in response to an externally applied current is approximately 35 ms. To ensure that the membrane responds to the stimulus, a pulse duration closer to 35 ms will be needed. If a moderately shorter stimulus is used, a stronger stimulus amplitude may cause the membrane to fire. The relationship between the threshold stimulus amplitude and the stimulus duration needed to evoke a consistent response is plotted on a strength—duration curve.

Refractory Periods

When an electrical current is applied to a nerve cell membrane, the stimulation may be applied in pulses separated by time. Even if the pulses are of sufficient duration and amplitude, the membrane may not discharge to the second pulse if it occurs too close to the first because the membrane needs approximately 0.5 ms to recover its excitability after an action potential. This recovery time is called the *absolute refractory period*. A higher-amplitude stimulus may be needed before the membrane will again fire for a period between 0.5 and 1 ms after having discharged an action potential. This time of recovery is called the *relative refractory period*. The refractoriness of the membrane limits the maximum frequency of discharge that an excitable membrane can undergo.

Stimulating Nerve Trunks

When therapists apply electrodes for electrical stimulation, the path of current will most likely include nerve fibers of different diameters. Large fibers require the lowest stimulus amplitude and shortest pulse duration to reach threshold because of their lower axonal resistance. Thin fibers require a higher stimulus amplitude and longer duration to reach threshold. Fibers that provide the sensation of cutaneous pain are typically of small diameter. Thus, use of short pulse duration, lower stimulus amplitude, or both, may reduce the painful sensation accompanying electrical stimulation.

When stimulating a nerve to evoke a muscle contraction, not all of the alpha motor axons in the nerve will discharge at the same threshold or stimulus amplitude. Because of differences in both axonal diameter and anatomical orientation to the current, the stimulus amplitude may have to be quite high (sometimes beyond tolerance) to recruit all of the motor axons.

SPECIFIC RESPONSES OF MUSCLE
TO ELECTRICAL STIMULATION

In a normal muscle, electrical stimulation evokes a contraction by excitation of the nerve rather than by excitation of the muscle directly. Nerve fibers need only a short pulse duration to be able to discharge, whereas muscle requires a much longer pulse duration in order to respond. Few of the electrical stimulators in use today have pulse durations long enough to excite a muscle membrane directly.

Critical Fusion Frequency

If a muscle nerve is exposed to a single electrical pulse of adequate duration and amplitude, a single twitch contraction results. The evoked twitch is a synchronous contraction of all of the motor units whose alpha motor axons are excited by the pulse. The tension produced by a group of motor units may be increased if a volley of pulses, rather than a single pulse, is used. When muscle twitches are evoked in rapid succession, there may not be enough time for complete relaxation between twitches. If the tension developed during one twitch fuses with that of the successive twitch, the tension will be cumulative. When the twitches are completely fused (Fig. 1–4), the contraction produced is said to be *tetanic*. The frequency of pulses at which this occurs is called the *critical fusion frequency* (CFF).

The CFF of each muscle depends upon its individual twitch duration. Postural muscles have slow twitch times (approximately 75 ms) and, therefore, undergo a tetanic contraction at around 13 to 15 pulses per second (pps). By contrast, muscles in the hands have faster twitch times (approximately 25 ms), thereby undergoing a tetantic contraction around 40 pps.

Gradation of Tension

The contractions evoked by electrical stimulation are nonphysiologic, in that they do not duplicate the normal recruitment and firing patterns of motor units. During a normal contraction, motor units fire asynchronously. Therefore, a complete tetanic contraction is not possible. Normally, motor units can be recruited to produce very fine, smooth gradations of tensions. With electrical stimulation, however, the motor units participating fire synchronously and are recruited in larger groups; hence, it is difficult to produce small, smooth increments of tension. If a weak, but smooth, contraction of a muscle is desired during electrical stimulation, the CFF of a muscle should be used (to

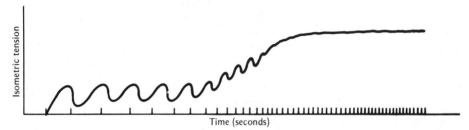

Figure 1–4. Accumulated tension of isometric twitches of skeletal muscle produced by gradually increasing the frequency of electrical stimulation.

avoid the shuddering effect of unfused twitches), as should a low-stimulus amplitude, in order to excite only a fraction of the alpha motor axons. To increase the strength of the fused contraction, stimulus amplitude is increased. The maximal muscle tension possible can be produced by recruiting all motor axons to fire at CFF. The resultant tension will be greater than what a subject can achieve normally, because all motor units cannot fire synchronously in a normal contraction. Very few stimulators can be used to evoke a maximal tetanic contraction, because the stimulus amplitude needed, in combination with the pulse duration available, will evoke strong excitation of pain fibers. Even when using stimulators that do not excite pain fibers, recruitment of all motor axons may still not be possible when stimulating deep, large nerves.

SUMMARY

Nerve and muscle cells are excitable cells because they are able to discharge action potentials. Prior to discharge, an excitable membrane has a resting potential of -60 mV, which is due to differences in concentration and permeability of Na^+ and K^+ ions across the membrane. During an action potential, the permeability to Na^+ and K^+ ions increases momentarily, and there is a sudden reversal in the membrane's charge. An action potential is conducted along an excitable membrane by triggering discharge in adjacent resting zones of the membrane. Conduction speed in a nerve fiber is enhanced by myelinization or by increased diameter of the fiber.

Electrical stimulation of nerve or muscle membranes can evoke action potentials. For an action potential to be evoked, stimulus amplitude and pulse duration must be sufficient to pass the threshold. Muscle membranes require a longer pulse duration, due to their higher capacitance. Threshold amplitude is lowest for large-diameter axons. Threshold stimulus amplitude may increase if the membrane has been depolarized for a period of time. Following an action potential, all excitable membranes pass through a recovery period, which limits maximal frequency of discharge.

Motor units will undergo a twitch contraction in response to electrical stimulation of their motor axons. Fusion of the twitch tension occurs as frequency of electrical stimulation increases. Postural muscles will undergo complete fusion at frequencies lower than for skilled muscles. Contraction evoked by electrical stimulation is not normal, in that motor units are forced to twitch synchronously.

CHAPTER **2**

Instrumentation

Thomas M. Cook and John O. Barr

As was seen in Chapter 1, excitation of nerve and muscle fibers is produced by the transport of ions across the cell membrane. This chapter reviews some fundamental descriptors of electrical phenomena and serves as a basis for understanding the various possible stimulator output characteristics that can be used to cause cell membrane depolarization. Attention will then focus on functional stimulator components, different electrode configurations, methods of monitoring the signal being generated, and, finally, on the safety considerations common to all therapeutic applications of electricity. The terms and concepts presented in this chapter will occur repeatedly throughout subsequent portions of this text.

ELECTRICAL PHENOMENA

Electrons and Ions

Biological matter, like all matter in the universe, is made up of atoms containing positively charged nuclei and negatively charged electrons, held in concentric orbits around them. An atom, therefore, is electrically neutral. When acted upon by an outside force (such as light, heat, electrostatic fields, magnetic fields, and chemical reactions), an atom can lose or gain electrons thus altering its neutral charge and causing it to take on electrical properties. An atom that is no longer in its original neutral state is called an *ion*, and the process of changing the electrical state of an atom is called *ionization*. A *positive ion* is an atom that has lost one or more electrons; a *negative ion* is an atom that has gained one or more electrons. Ions are present in electrolytic solutions of acids, bases, and salts such as those of which biological tissues are composed. Bases, alkaloids, and metals tend to form positive ions, whereas acid radicals tend to form negative ions. An ion has the same nucleus that the atom had prior to adding or losing electrons and thus possesses the basic characteristics of the original atom.

Current

There is a naturally occurring random drift of positive ions, negative ions, and free electrons within all matter. Because of the composition of their orbital shells, some atoms tend to both give up and take on free electrons more readily than do others. Those materials that have their valence shells almost filled tend to be very stable, with very few free electrons (insulators). Materials (principally metals) with only one or two valence electrons tend to give up their electrons very easily (conductors) and readily allow electron movement, or flow, within them. Electrolytic solutions allow the free movement of positive and negative ions, as well as the free movement of electrons. The charge on an object is a measure of the number of free electrons that it has lost or gained. If the atom has lost electrons, its charge is positive; if it has gained electrons, its charge is negative. The unit of electrical charge is called the coulomb; which is equal to the charge of 6.25 times 10^{18} electrons.

Current flow can be defined as the directed flow of free electrons from one place to another. The unit of current is the ampere (A), which is defined as the rate at which electrons move past a given point. An ampere is equal to 1 coulomb (C) per second. Coulombs indicate the number of electrons; amperes indicate the rate of electron flow. A milliampere (mA) is one thousandth of an ampere; a microampere (μA) is one millionth of an ampere. To have current flow, then, there must be a source of free electrons and positive ions, a material that will allow the electrons to "flow," and a force tending to move or concentrate the electrons in one place (electromotive force). In practical application, it should be appreciated that charge represents the electrical threshold for excitation of nerve and muscle. This relationship of charge (Q) as equal to stimulus amplitude (A) multiplied by duration (t) defines the individual points comprising the physiological strength-duration curve.

Voltage

In order to cause a membrane depolarization, large numbers of electrons must be forced to move through the conductive media of the body tissues. This "electron-moving force" is the difference in concentration of free electrons and is referred to as the electromotive force (EMF), electrical potential difference, or voltage. In order for electrical current to "flow," there must be one location where there is a dense concentration of free electrons and another location with a relative absence of free electrons. Since unlike charges attract each other, electron flow will be from the location of high concentration to the location of low concentration. The greater the difference in concentrations, the greater the potential for electron flow. The unit of electromotive force, or potential difference, is the *volt* (V). One volt is the electromotive force required to move one ampere of current through a resistance of one ohm (Ω). In other words, 1 V is the force needed to move 1 C of charge through a resistance of 1 Ω in 1 sec. The relationship between current, voltage, and resistance is expressed by *Ohm's law*:

$$\text{Electromotive force (V)} = \text{Current (A)} \times \text{resistance } (\Omega)$$

or

$$\text{Electromotive force (V)/Resistance } (\Omega) = \text{Current (A)}$$

In describing the electrical potential difference between two points, the concept of a reference is highly important. The planet earth is considered to have zero potential and is the most commonly used voltage reference, being referred to as *ground* (or as *earth* in some countries). Two points may have very little potential difference between them but may still have very great potential compared to the neutral earth. The term *isoelectric point* is often used to describe the condition in which there is no electrical potential difference between two locations or between a given location and some reference point. (This topic is discussed further, when safety considerations are presented, later in this chapter.)

Resistance

Resistance is that property of a substance which opposes current flow. Conductors have very low resistance and insulators have very high resistance. Some materials, such as silicon and germanium, are neither good conductors nor good insulators. The special properties of these *semiconductor materials* form the basis of modern solid-state electronic components. As discussed in the previous section, the unit of resistance is the ohm, and the amount of resistance in a material is given by Ohm's law. If 1 V of potential difference causes 1 A of current to flow in a circuit, then the resistance of the circuit is 1 Ω. Common values for resistance include kilohms (kΩ) and megohms (MΩ)— thousands and millions of ohms, respectively. The term *resistor* often refers to a particular electronic component used to introduce a desired amount of resistance in a circuit.

Sometimes it is more convenient to think in terms of how well a material conducts current rather than how well it opposes it. *Conductance* is the term used to define the ease with which a material allows current flow; it is the inverse of resistance. The unit of conductance is the mho.

Amplitude

There are several different ways to specify the magnitude or amplitude of a voltage or current. If the current flow is unidirectional and constant (i.e., if it is a direct current), the peak (maximum) or the average value can be specified. If the current flow is fluctuating or bidirectional (i.e., biphasic or an alternating current), there are at least three commonly used descriptors (Fig. 2–1). As

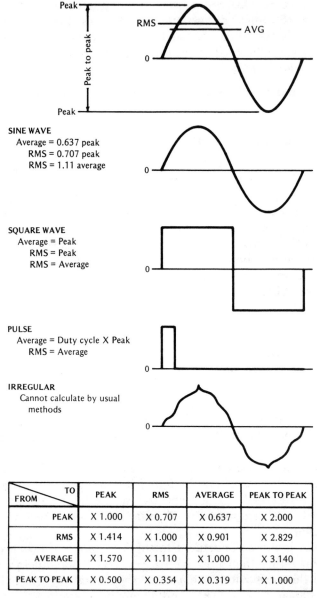

Figure 2–1. Common descriptors of wave form amplitudes.

with the monophasic wave form, the *peak value* is measured from the zero line, or reference, to the maximum positive (or negative) point. The *peak-to-peak value* is measured from the positive-most point to the negative-most point. The third term used to describe a biphasic wave form is the *rms value*. Rms refers to the root-mean-square method of determining the equivalent area contained by the curve. For a pure sine wave, the rms value is 0.707 times the peak value. The rms value is also referred to as the *effective value* because it corresponds to an equivalent amount of direct current or voltage in terms of heating power. The average value has also been used to describe alternating currents. Again, for a pure sine wave, the average current flow is 0.637 times the peak flow. Caution should be exercised so as not to confuse average value with effective (rms) value. Because of its broader applicability, the use of the latter term is usually preferred. (When more complex wave forms are used, the description of current, or voltage amplitude, becomes somewhat more difficult and will be considered in more detail later in subsequent chapters.)

Frequency

The frequency of a wave form is determined by the number of cycles per second that it exhibits. *Hertz* (Hz) is the unit of frequency for alternating current and stands for cycles per second. A thousand cycles per second is a *kilohertz* (kHz). The period of a wave form is the amount of time that it takes to complete one cycle of a signal in seconds, thousandths of a second (ms), or millionths of a second (μs). In pulsed current frequency is the number of pulses per second (pps).

Phase

Two alternating-current sine waves can differ from each other in regard to their amplitude, their frequency, or both. They may also differ in terms of the phase angle between them. There are 360 electrical degrees in one cycle of a sine wave, beginning with the zero reference line and returning to that same point to begin the next cycle. If two wave forms do not begin at this reference line at the same time, the difference can be described as a portion of a cycle or as a number of degrees. The wave form crossing the zero line first is described as exhibiting a *phase lead;* the wave form crossing the zero line later in time shows a *phase lag* of a specified number of degrees.

Impedance

Earlier, when discussing direct-current flow, we defined resistance as the property of a substance that opposes current flow. In alternating-current flow, there are two other properties of circuits (including biological tissues) and devices that can affect the pattern of current flow—impedance and capacitance. The unit of impedance is the ohm, just as for direct-current flow, and the symbol for impedance is Z.

Capacitance is the property of a circuit or device that enables it to store electrical energy by means of an electrostatic field. A specific electronic component, a capacitor, consists of two conductors placed close to each other but separated by some insulating material. A capacitor has the ability to store electrons and to release them at a later time. A capacitor tends to block the flow of direct current while allowing alternating current to pass. Capacitance is a measure of the amount of charge that a capacitor can store when a given voltage is applied. The unit of capacitance is the *farad* (F), the *microfarad* (μF), or the *picofarad* (pF), one millionth or one trillionth of a farad, respectively. One farad is the amount of capacitance that will store a charge of 1 coulomb when 1 volt is applied. In general, the lower the capacitance in a circuit, the higher the frequencies of alternating current that it will allow. Conversely, the larger the capacitance, the greater the opposition to higher-frequency signals.

Inductance is the property of a circuit or device that enables it to store electrical energy by means of an electromagnetic field. As specific electronic components, inductors consist of a coil (or coils) of wire and are most commonly found as transformers. Similarly to a capacitor, an inductor tends to oppose changes in current flow. One *henry* (H) is defined as the amount of inductance that induces an electromotive force of 1 V into a conductor when the current changes at a rate of 1 A per second. The *millihenry* (mH) and *microhenry* (μH) are more common values of inductance. In the case of AC, or biphasic current, flow, these three properties (resistance, capacitance, and inductance) together make up the total opposition to current flow and constitute the total impedance of the circuit or device.

In a complex circuit consisting of resistive, capacitive, and inductive elements (such as the circuit formed by an electrical stimulator and the human body), the total opposition to current flow within the circuit is described by its total impedance. When an electrical potential is applied, the amount of current passing through the circuit is determined by the combined effects of each of the impedance-producing elements of which it is composed, as well as by the frequency and amplitude of the signal generated by the stimulator.

STIMULATOR OUTPUT

Wave Forms
The most fundamental classification of electrotherapeutic wave forms is based on the direction of current flow—namely, *unidirectional* or *bidirectional;* (ie, electrons flow in only one direction or they flow in both directions). Unidirectional currents are also referred to as *monophasic, monopolar, galvanic,* or (in more generic electrical terms) *direct currents* (DC). DC wave forms are often subdivided into continuous DC and pulsed (interrupted DC or AC). Figure 2–2 shows some examples of possible DC or "DC-like" wave forms, although the shape of a DC "pulse" has many more possibilities than those shown in the figure. Bidirectional wave forms are also referred to as *biphasic, bipolar, faradic* or, simply, *alternating currents* (AC). The distinguishing feature of AC wave forms is that the current does indeed change direction, although the electron flow in each direction may not be equal. Figure 2–3 shows some examples of the many possible AC wave forms.

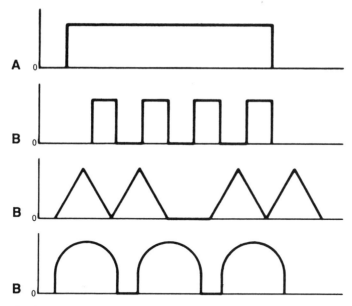

Figure 2–2. Examples of (**A**) DC and (**B**) monophasic pulsed ("DC-like") wave forms.

Amplitude

As was mentioned earlier, there are several different ways to specify the amplitude of a wave form, and the rms (or effective) value was suggested as the most appropriate and universally applicable. Given that the impedance of the biological tissues to be stimulated is constant, the higher the effective voltage applied, the larger the current that will pass through the tissues. Therefore, a low-voltage stimulating source will deliver less current than will a high-voltage stimulating source of the same frequency. The division between low- and high-voltage currents is not precise. High-voltage wave form generators are usually considered those above peak voltages of approximately 150 V. Low-voltage generators tend to be those producing peak voltages of 100 V or less.

Duration

Duration can refer to the total time over which electrical stimulation is applied; for example, from seconds to hours. More commonly in electrotherapy, duration refers to the time for one pulse of stimulation to be delivered and is usually referred to as the *pulse duration*. Pulse durations may vary from several microseconds to several hundred milliseconds in AC. In the case of continuous DC stimulation, the duration is equal to the entire time of stimulation.

Repetition Rate or Frequency

If pulses (or wave forms of any shape) are repeated at regular intervals, we can describe this repetition rate as the *pulse rate, pulse repetition rate,* or *pulse* frequency. Units are pulses per second (pps), [cycles per second (cps), or Hertz (Hz)]. The reciprocal of this pulse rate is the *period*, defined as the time from the beginning of one pulse to the beginning of the subsequent pulse. The period is composed of the pulse duration time and the interpulse interval time. These two times may or may not be equal, depending on the particular wave form being used.

Rise Time

Rise time refers to the time required for the wave form to go from 0 V to its peak amplitude. This parameter is important because of the physiologic "accommodation that can occur with repeated stimulation. Typical rise times range from several nanoseconds (ns), one billionth of a second, up to several hundred milliseconds (ms), thousandths of a second, or longer. The wave forms shown in Figure 2–3 exhibit a variety of rise times.

Decay Time

Analogous to rise time is the *parameter decay time,* defined as the time in which the signal goes from its peak amplitude to 0 V. If the decay time follows

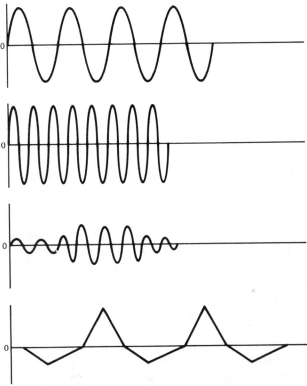

Figure 2–3. Examples of AC wave forms.

an exponential pattern, it is possible to describe the decay in terms of a *time constant*; that is, the time required for the signal to decrease to approximately one third of its amplitude.

Duty Cycle

In many clinical applications, whether using continuous DC or pulsed wave forms, periods of electrical stimulation are alternated with periods of rest (or no stimulation). The terms duty cycle, ON/OFF cycle, or reciprocate are used to refer to the relative proportion of "on" time to "total" cycle time, expressed as a percentage. For example, if pulses are generated for 1 second and then no stimulation is delivered for 2 seconds, the duty cycle would be 1:3, or 33%. Duty cycles can range from much less than 1.0 to much greater than 1.0.

Modulation

The wave forms, or pulses, in the ON portion of the duty cycle may all be identical, or they may vary or be "modulated" in regard to one or more of their characteristics. This modulation, or ordered variation, may occur in any of the wave form, or pulse, parameters, such as amplitude, pulse duration, and frequency. Most commonly, the pulse (or wave form) begins at a very low peak amplitude and progressively increases with each successive pulse until a desired "steady-state" amplitude is achieved. This type of progressive amplitude modulation has been referred to as ramp (surged) buildup, or as amplitude rise time. If a similar progressive decrease occurs at the end of the pulse train, it is described as a ramp (surged) decline.

The other most commonly used form of pulse train, or on-time, modulation is to progressively increase the duration of each pulse from a very brief time (initially) to the eventual desired pulse duration. *Duration rise time* is another term used to refer to this process.

STIMULATOR HARDWARE

Regardless of whether electrotherapeutic stimulators are DC or AC, high- or low-voltage, modulated or not, they all have the common functional components shown in Figure 2–4.

Power Source

The flow of electrons to be delivered to a patient must come from some power source. *Electrical power* is defined as the product of voltage and current, and

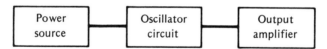

Figure 2–4. Stimulator functional components.

there are two basic power sources used in electrotherapeutics—batteries and conventional "house current." Neither of these power sources is directly usable for electrotherapeutic stimulation, so that transformation or regulation (or both) of each is necessary.

Batteries are a source of chemically stored electrical charge and are capable of producing direct current. Readily available batteries are low-voltage, usually in the range of 1.5 to 9.0 V. In order to deliver higher voltages for purposes of electrical stimulation, the voltages supplied by these batteries must somehow be "multiplied." Such a multiplication is accomplished through the use of special electronic circuits containing either a DC-to-DC converter or a switching regulator, or both. These devices work in conjunction with either a capacitor or an inductor to store charge. Power is drawn from the battery at a given voltage and is delivered to the other components of the stimulator circuit at a higher voltage (but at a lower current). The product of the voltage and current of the output is the same (actually, slightly less) than the product of the voltage and current of the input to the circuit.

In North America, standard "house current," as delivered from the local power company, is 115 V of alternating current with a basic frequency of 60 Hz. Since the electronic components that produce the various stimulating wave forms use DC power, the power line AC must be "converted" to DC. This conversion occurs in a unit called a *power supply*, which usually consists of four major components: a transformer, a rectifier, a filter, and a regulator. The *transformer* consists of two intersecting coils and uses the principle of mutual inductance to "induce" a different voltage in the second coil. For example, the 115-V AC line current can be "stepped down" (using a transformer) to 15-V AC. The *rectifier* portion of the power supply converts an AC sine wave to a pulsating DC voltage. A half-wave rectifier simply discards the negative portion of the AC signal, whereas a full-wave rectifier actually inverts the negative portion of the AC signal so as to make it positive. The rectifier circuit is followed by a *filter* that converts the pulsating DC to a smooth DC voltage, usually through the use of fairly large capacitors. In the example mentioned above, the pulsating 15-V (peak) DC wave form might be filtered to produce a smooth 13.5-V (peak) current. The final stage of the AC power conversion process is the use of a *regulator*, which consists of a prepackaged electronic circuit that further filters and controls the voltage in order to produce a very smooth, precise DC output; for example, 12.0 V. This voltage is then available to power the oscillator and amplifier portions of the stimulator. A particular stimulator may have a dual, triple, or higher-order power supply that delivers several different precisely regulated voltages.

Oscillator Circuit

An *oscillator* is a circuit that generates a repetitive signal. The frequency of the signal could be as low as from 1 Hz or less to as high as several megahertz (MHz) or more. Based on information presented in the previous section, it may seem illogical to use a power supply to convert AC house current into DC in order to power an oscillator that generates AC. As was mentioned earlier, however, house current is supplied at a fixed voltage and frequency. By having its own oscillator, a stimulator can be adjusted to produce a wide range of frequencies at a wide range of voltages, making it possible to produce wave forms that are substantially more complex than the sine waves generated by the local power company. The oscillator circuit may actually contain several oscillators functioning together to produce a complex wave form. For example, there may be one oscillator that controls the basic pulse repetition rate of a wave form. A second oscillator with a much lower frequency may "modulate" the amplitude of the pulse train in order to control both the surge build-up and the surge decline. A third oscillator-like circuit might control the duty cycle or ON/OFF times of the pulse train. This wave form may be combined with a much higher "carrier" frequency, resulting in the final wave form sent on to the amplifier or final output stage of the stimulator. Separate amplitude and frequency controls may or may not be provided for each of these different oscillators. Within the oscillator circuit, there is also likely to be one or more provisions for timing or counting, referred to as a logic circuit. This logic circuit may be used to control such parameters as the number of pulses within a train or the number of pulse trains that are delivered before the unit turns itself off.

Output Amplifier

The final set of functional components in a typical stimulator circuit comprise the *output amplifier.* This amplifier provides the final regulation of the amplitude of the wave form and usually has provisions to deliver "constant current," "constant voltage," or both. These descriptors mean that the output current or voltage should be constant (ie, repeatable and unchanging) regardless of changes in impedance in the remainder of the circuit (namely, the electrodes, skin, and other body tissues being stimulated). For example, in a constant-voltage stimulator, if the impedance increases because the electrode gel begins to dry out, the output amplifier of the stimulator should, theoretically, increase the current flow so as to maintain the same voltage wave form. Constant current generators have important provisions for voltage limitation in order to avoid burning the skin if electrode contact is partially disrupted. Similarly, constant-voltage generators should be current-limited for the same reason. The term *load* is often used to describe the total impedance encountered (or seen) by an amplifier output. As was mentioned earlier, this impedance is composed of the total opposition to current flow from the resistive, capacitive, and inductive elements in the circuit. Different stimulator units—especially portable, battery-powered units—have been shown to vary considerably from their espoused characteristic of being constant-current stimulators. For example, of the ten transcutaneous nerve stimulators evaluated by Campbell,[1] most units displayed changes in current output (ranging from 22 to 31 percent) when different loads were applied to their outputs. Larger (and usually more expensive) AC-powered units would be expected to function better than battery-powered units in this regard.[1]

    With the proliferation of small, portable, battery-powered stimulators, the largest physical components of these devices tend to be the control knobs that determine amplitude, frequency, pulse duration, surge rate, surge decline, and duty cycle. Unfortunately, the markings for these controls are most often linear, usually from 0 to 10, but the actual control of these various parameters may be quite nonlinear.[1] In practical applications, this means that a slight knob movement in the upper portions of the control range may produce disproportionate increases or decreases in comparison to the same control movement in the lower part of the range. Caution should be taken regarding abrupt, extreme changes in the upper part of the control range so as to avoid patient discomfort.

ELECTRODES

The electrode—tissue interface is the site of a conversion between electron flow and ion flow. In addition to the parameters of the stimulating wave form already discussed, several other important factors affect this conversion process.

Electron—Ion Exchange

At any instant in time, the electrode with the greater concentration of electrons, referred to as either the *cathode* or the *negative electrode*, is negatively charged and, therefore, attracts positive ions from the underlying tissues. The electrode with a relative scarcity of electrons, referred to as either the *anode* or the *positive electrode*, attracts negative ions and free electrons from the underlying tissue. Positive ions (mostly sodium and some potassium) flow opposite to negative ions (principally chloride and free electrons). In the vicinity of the cathode, the concentration of negative ions and electrons causes the resting potential difference across the cell membranes to be reduced to the point where spontaneous depolarization occurs. Once the critical threshold has been reached and the depolarization wave begins propagating up and down the cell membrane, further infusion of negative ions and electrons will have no effect until the refractory period has been completed.

Because it is the site of lowest threshold for depolarization, the cathode is also sometimes referred to as the *active electrode*. It is the site where stimulation is first perceived. The anode is sometimes referred to as the *indifferent electrode*. In the vicinity of the anode, the concentration of positive ions tends to hyperpolarize the cell membrane, making it less sensitive to depolarization. With an AC wave form, each electrode is alternately the anode and the cathode. If the wave form is symmetrically biphasic, the perception of stimulation is equal at both electrode sites. In the case of unbalanced wave forms, the charge characteristics of the positive and negative phases of the signal are not equal. As a result, stimulation will be felt more strongly at one of the electrodes.

Tissue Impedance

Different body tissues provide different impedances to current flow (to both ion flow and electron flow). Skin, adipose tissue, and bone tend to be poorer conductors than muscle and nerve tissues. Because the skin and adipose tissues are not pure insulators, DC does flow through these resistive elements. When good conductors, such as a metallic electrode and a bundle of muscle fibers, are separated by more insulating, less conductive, layers of skin and subcutaneous fat, a biologic capacitor exists. As was discussed earlier, capacitors tend to impede DC flow and provide different impedances to different AC wave forms, depending on their frequency. The resulting biologic circuit, therefore, is not a simple resistive one but displays more complex impedance characteristics, which are likely to vary from individual to individual.

The skin provides the greatest opposition element to current flow because it is composed primarily of keratin and contains very little fluid.[2] Skin lesions, such as open wounds and lacerations, and even minor irritation, such as from shaving, can significantly lower skin impedance. Conversely, skin impedance may be abnormally high in certain dermatologic conditions, such as icthyosis. Techniques to reduce skin impedance include mild abrasion, tissue warming, and hydration. In addition to mild physical abrasion to remove the superficial cell layers of the skin, another method has been suggested to avoid skin-heat buildup.[3] The use of high-voltage currents of approximately 100 V can cause sudden, spontaneous breakdown in skin impedance.[2,4] This initial resistance drop is followed by a continued, slower decrease in skin impedance.

The capacitive effects of the skin and adipose layers can be minimized by the use of higher-frequency signals because, in general, the higher the frequency, the lower the impedance to current flow. Carrier frequencies of several kH are sometimes used for the express purpose of increasing current flow across the electrode–skin interface.

Electrode Materials

An electrode must be thought of simply as the contact point between an electrical circuit and the body. The electrode–tissue interface is the site of the electron–ion conversion discussed earlier, and several factors must be taken into consideration when deciding on the proper electrode material to use: (1) Electrodes must be good conductors so that they provide very little resistance to electron current flow. Since metals (such as tin, lead, steel, aluminum, copper, and silver) are all good conductors, they have been used in electrodes for therapeutic stimulation. (2) Attention must be given to the toxicity of the electrode material. For example, zinc/zinc sulfate electrodes have highly desirable electrical properties, but they are highly toxic to exposed tissue (due to the passage into the tissue of free zinc or sulfide ions, or both.[5] (3) The polarizability of electrode materials must be considered. With the conversion from electron to ion flow, there is a tendency in some materials for the electron–ion exchange to occur more readily in one direction than in the other.

The result is the creation of a charge gradient that inhibits current flow. This tendency toward polarization may be particularly important when using DC wave forms.

Carbon-filled silicone electrodes are also used with many electrotherapeutic devices, especially transcutaneous electrical nerve stimulation (TENS) units. Basically, these electrodes consist of silicone rubber impregnated with small carbon particles; they are often referred to as conductive rubber electrodes. Both metallic and rubber electrodes may be coupled to the skin via moistened sponges or pads. More commonly, however, electrolytic gel is used with conductive rubber electrodes. Karaya gum electrodes have also become very popular in recent years. Karaya is a naturally occurring gum that comes from a tree found in India and, when mixed with certain alcohols, it forms a flexible mass that adheres to the skin when moistened. Between 10 and 20 percent of individuals using carbonized silicone electrodes experience some skin irritation, whereas only 1 to 2 percent of those using karaya gum electrodes have shown skin irritation.[6] However, instances of allergic reactions to karaya gum electrode pads have recently been described.[7] Synthetic polymer electrodes and conductive adhesive "tac" gels have also been developed for clinical use.

Size and Placement of Electrodes

Electrodes come in a wide variety of sizes, shapes, and arrangements. Each of these factors can affect a very important stimulation variable—current density. Current density is the amount of current flow per unit area.[7] It is a measure of the quantity of charged ions moving through a specific cross-sectional area of body tissue, and it is expressed in units of milliamperes per square centimeter or per square inch. Current density is an important factor in determining the reaction of biologic tissues to stimulation. In general, the greater the current density, the greater is the "effect" on the tissues. The two obvious determinants of current density are the amount of current applied and the size of the area of its application.

For a given current, larger electrodes tend to disperse the charge better than smaller electrodes, which have more localized effects. The simultaneous use of two different-sized electrodes with an AC wave form will have selective effects in the area of the smaller electrode. When the larger of the two electrodes becomes the "active" cathode, its greater area will result in a lesser current density and a reduced effect compared to when the smaller electrode functions as the cathode.

Electrode placement is another factor that influences current density, and thus tissue response. (The impeding properties of skin, bone, and adipose tissue have already been mentioned.) Placement of electrodes over these tissues will have serious effects on the amount of current flow in the surrounding tissues. Additionally, it is generally true that, the greater the distance between stimulating electrodes, the lesser the current density in the intervening tissues. In other words, with more possible conductive routes, the current will disperse in its travel between electrodes. With large spacings between electrodes, it is difficult to estimate exactly what the current density might be for any particular structure. The greatest current flow will be through the tissues providing the least impedance (usually, muscle and nerve). This tendency for current to disperse when wide electrode spacing is selected can be used to great advantage when the goal is to stimulate deeper tissues. Electrodes have been constructed in a wide variety of shapes and sizes so as to facilitate specific placements for specific applications. Orientation of the electrodes can also have an important effect on the response of the underlying tissues. Muscle tissues are nearly four times more conductive in the longitudinal direction of their fibers than in the transverse direction.[9,10]

Electrode Coupling

In addition to the type of material and the size of the electrode, the current density at the electrode–tissue interface depends on two other factors. The first of these is the pliability of the electrode and its consequent ability to conform to the body part. For instance, rigid metal electrodes may lose some of their contact with the skin when a muscle contracts and changes its shape, whereas more compliant rubber and gum electrodes are more likely to change shape with the muscle and maintain total contact. This pliability is of greater concern with larger electrodes than with smaller ones. If the electrode contact is reduced to half, the current density applied to the skin is doubled. Painful sensations are likely to result.

The use of some conductive liquid or gel medium to facilitate the electron–ion exchange between the electrode and the skin is often highly desirable. Historically, water-soaked gauze or cotton pads have been used for this purpose. Other options include the use of water-soluble electrolyte gels, which are less susceptible to rapid drying and the resultant loss in conductivity. Karaya gum electrodes form a semiliquid, adhesive conductive layer when wet and do not require the use of an additional conductive medium.

Often, additional tape or other adhesive material is used to maintain good contact between the electrode and the skin. Attention should always be given to the prospect of skin irritation which might be caused by the amplitude of electrical stimulation, mechanical shearing produced by electrodes or tape, or reactions to electrode coupling agents or adhesive materials.

SIGNAL MONITORING

There is currently no practical means of monitoring ionic current flow at the cellular level. However, it is feasible and advisable in many situations to monitor parameters of the stimulating wave form being applied to a patient. Basically, three different methods are available for such monitoring.

Analog Meters

An *analog meter* is one that indicates the value of a measured variable using a continuous scale. A household thermometer is an example of an analog indicator. The most popular type of electrical meter incorporates a permanent magnet and moving coil in its movement and has a fixed scale with a moving pointer. Such devices are basically current meters, which deflect when current flows through them. Technically, they are capable of measuring only direct current, but they can be used to measure alternating current if the AC signal is first converted to DC (usually through the use of a rectifying diode network). Because of the mechanical nature of an analog meter, it cannot be expected to accurately indicate abrupt changes in current flow. For example, if a brief DC pulse of only 20 ms were passed through an analog meter, only a very slight deflection of the pointer would be likely to occur. The mechanical inertia of the coil and pointer would not allow an accurate indication of the amplitude of the pulse. The typical analog meter responds to the average value of a current when the current or voltage is a pure sine wave. Since, as we have indicated, the effective (or rms) value of current amplitude is more useful, most meter scales are calibrated to indicate rms. A knowledgeable equipment user should know the units in which each meter is calibrated. Used to measure amperes, typical amp meters found on electrotherapeutic equipment are calibrated in milliamperes. In order to measure current flow within a circuit, the measuring device (meter) must be a part of the circuit; that is, it must be in "series" with all other components in order to measure total current flow.

The basic analog meter movement just described can also be used to measure voltage. Since the meter itself provides some resistance to current flow, Ohm's law can be used to determine the voltage across the meter. Meters used to measure voltage usually have high resistance and therefore do not divert a significant amount of the current being measured from its primary path, although the possible circuit "loading effect" of a voltmeter must be kept in mind. Since potential differences must exist at two different points in any circuit, voltages are always measured across, or "in parallel," with some element of the circuit; for instance, between two electrodes. The same limitations cited for use of analog meters to measure current apply to the use of these meters to measure voltage. Limitations include a very sluggish response to abrupt changes. Alternating current must be internally converted to direct current, and only the average value is accurately displayed (usually on a scale converted to rms). Voltmeters on electrotherapeutic equipment are usually scaled to display units of volts.

The same analog meter movement that we have been discussing can be used to measure the resistance of a particular circuit element; it is then referred to as an *ohmmeter*. Internally, the ohmmeter consists of a battery, a series resistance, and a meter movement. The unknown resistance to be measured is placed in series with the known resistance; the amount of current measured by the meter is an indication of the proportion of the unknown resistance to the known resistance. Depending on the value of the known resistor, the scale of the meter can be marked in ohms, kilohms, or megohms. Such a meter is useful for measuring parameters such as interelectrode skin impedance. A major point to remember is that, in order to accurately measure the impedance of any component in a circuit, the component must be removed from the circuit so that alternate current paths are not possible. Therefore, when measuring interelectrode skin resistance, the stimulator must be detached from the electrodes, or the measurement will include the resistance of the entire stimulator circuit.

Ohmmeters are rarely found as an integral part of electrotherapeutic equipment but usually exist as separate, general-purpose pieces of instrumentation. Most commonly, an ohmmeter is part of a *multimeter* or a volt-ohm-milliammeter (VOM), which combines all three measurement capabilities in one case. A single selector switch controls various inputs to one meter movement.

Digital Meters

Digital meters measure analog quantities and present them in digital form. A typical digital multimeter has three or more digits and a switch (or switches) with which to select an appropriate input range for measuring voltage, current, or resistance. In contrast to the coil movement inside an analog meter, a digital meter contains a signal-processing circuit (to scale the signal) and an analog-to-digital converter circuit. Other components control the display digits. Similar to the analog meter, the analog-to-digital converter of the digital meter can technically measure only a DC input. However, if the signal-processing portion of the meter converts the incoming signal to the average (or rms) value, then the readout can be calibrated properly to measure these parameters of AC signals.

There are several general advantages of digital meters over analog meters. The display of a digital meter is usually much easier to read, including a decimal point and a polarity indicator. Digital meters also usually provide better resolution and accuracy and are faster to read than analog meters. Both types of meters are equally portable although the analog meters tend to be slightly less expensive. Although digital meters may have a faster response than analog meters, they are still grossly inadequate for displaying the quick changes in voltage or current that are important parameters of electrotherapeutic wave forms.

Oscilloscopes

An oscilloscope consists of a cathode ray tube (CRT), with its associated electron gun, deflection plates, phosphor screen, and a variety of electronic components designed to control the deflection of an electron beam in order to produce a trace on the screen. Although the meters described above provide a means of measuring a limited number of parameters about DC and AC wave forms, an oscilloscope makes it possible to display and measure exact details about the amplitude, shape, and timing of nearly any wave form. Because of its very high frequency response, the oscilloscope is the only practical means of monitoring complex, modulated stimuli. Oscilloscope screens sometimes come as an integral part of larger, more stationary stimulator units, but recent advances in electronics miniaturization have made it feasible to use smaller, portable, battery-powered scopes for monitoring stimulating wave forms in most clinical settings.

Figure 2–5 shows a setup for using an oscilloscope to monitor stimulator output characteristics.[11] Normally, an oscilloscope is used to display changes of voltage over time. Attached in parallel with stimulating electrodes (switch position 1 in Figure 2–5), the oscilloscope will display the electrical potential at the electrode sites as influenced by body tissue impedance. In order to assess the stimulating current characteristics, voltage drop across a known resistance can be monitored (switch position 2). The resistor used in this setup (eg, 100 ohm) must have adequate power-dissipating capacity (eg, 1 watt) to prevent overheating and damage when using typical stimulating currents (<100 mA).

SAFETY CONSIDERATIONS

Background
Health care professionals work with patients in hazardous environments, such as hospitals and private clinics. Since the 1960s, a number of sources have

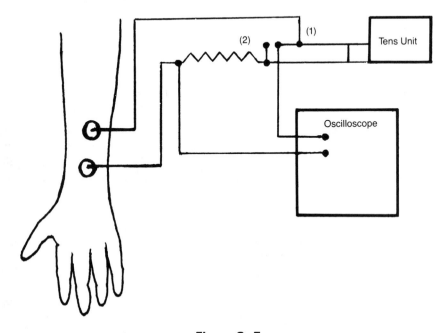

Figure 2–5.

described a variety of electrical hazards and subsequent remedies that can be followed to promote electrical safety.[12-23] The news media has alleged that approximately 12,000 patients per year are electrocuted in hospitals.[20] Electrocution death by common physical therapy equipment has been documented.[21] In 1969, Ben-Zvi reported that approximately 40 percent of all electronic and mechanical equipment inspected at his medical center over a 2-year period was found to be either unsafe or did not meet manufacturer's safety specifications.[22] Electrical hazards are not solely a result of defective equipment. Errors of judgment based on lack of knowledge concerning safety regulations and principles, and facilitated by clinician fatigue or patient medications, contribute significantly to the existence of electrical hazards.

Electrical Shock

Electrical shock is the primary concern of clinicians. Electrical shock involves the flow of current through human tissue, usually with adverse effects. Such effects are related to a number of factors including tissue impedance, current amplitude, size of area contacted, and individual susceptibility (eg, presence of a cardiac pacemaker). For humans, tissue impedance may range from 500,000 ohms for dry skin to 1000 ohms for wet skin, while an intravenous line or a cardiac catheter running directly to the heart may only present a few ohms of impedance.[5,23] *Microshock* (generally imperceptible) is produced by current of less than 1000 μA. Microshock on the order of 20 μA through a ventricular pacing catheter can induce fibrillation. *Macroshock* results from current at or above 1 mA. The physiological effects are detailed in Table 2–1.

Electrical shock commonly results when current passes from a source of high electrical potential, through the body, and to a point of lower potential. Sources of high electrical potential (110 or 220 V) include electrical outlets, equipment power cords and plugs, and internal equipment circuitry. If damaged, these components may allow *fault current* to escape. Electrical shock may also result from *leakage current,* which is a normal characteristic of electrical circuits. Leakage current is produced by circuit capacitance. It also may be induced in circuit wiring by electromagnetic fields from inductors and

TABLE 2–1. PHYSIOLOGICAL EFFECTS OF ELECTRICAL CURRENT*

Current Amplitude	Physiological Effects
1 mA	Threshold for tingling sensation
16 mA	Cannot release grip on electrical conductor due to muscle contraction
50 mA	Pain and possible fainting
100 mA to 3 A	Ventricular fibrillation
6 A	Sustained myocardial contraction, temporary respiratory paralysis, and burns

*Modified from Bruner JMR, 1967, pp 396–425, for 1 second of 60-Hz AC stimulation of intact skin of the hands.23

transformers. Standards have been established that limit leakage current (measured in AC [root = means = square—RMS]) to 100 uA on grounded equipment cases, to 50 uA on ordinary direct patient connections like electrodes, and to 10 uA on isolated patient connections like intra-aortic pressure monitors.[24]

Grounding and Ground Fault Circuit Interrupters

Electrical current enters a wall-mounted electrical outlet by the "hot" wire (coated with black insulation) attached to the narrow prong slot. Current then travels to the equipment power plug and up the "hot" wire of the power cord in order to energize the unit's power supply. The electrical current then exits the unit through the "neutral" wire (coated with white insulation) of the power cord and plug, and it re-enters the wall outlet through its wide prong slot. Contemporary electrical codes and equipment specifications require that wall outlets and equipment plugs and power cables be equipped with a *safety ground* wire (coated with green insulation). At the wall outlet, this wire runs from the circular prong hole to a central ground cable ultimately connected to true *earth ground*. It is the safety ground wire that provides a very low resistance pathway for fault and leakage currents to pass harmlessly to ground. Were this not so, a patient or clinician in contact with a grounded water pipe, metal conduit, or other grounded piece of equipment would be shocked as current passed through them in route to ground.

Maintenance of the safety ground must be ensured. Wall outlets, including metal face-plates and attaching screws, should be tested for ground continuity. One-piece molded three-prong plugs do not allow inspection of the wire to the ground prong. UL-approved hospital grade plugs (coded with a green dot) allow visual and physical inspection. "Cheater adaptors", which allow a three-prong plug to be inserted into a two-prong outlet, should never be used. Although theoretically the adaptor's "pigtail" wire can be attached to a grounded face-plate screw, this wire is easily broken. Three prong extension cords which are repeatedly bent and straightened, suffer from the same continuity problem.

A *ground fault circuit interrupter (GFCI)* is a device that can provide an extra margin of shock protection. The device monitors the difference between the amplitude of the current entering a piece of equipment through its "hot" wire versus that leaving the equipment through its "neutral" wire. A difference in amplitudes indicates the loss of current to ground through an electrical fault. At a present difference limit, usually 5mA, the GFCI interrupts the circuit and shuts off power to the equipment in a fraction of a second. Such a device is beneficial for preventing most levels of macroshock, but it is not activated by current which produce microshock. Also, the GFCI does not protect against shock arising from contact directly between hot and neutral wires. Available in models which can protect single or multiple outlets, this device should be installed wherever electrical equipment is used.[25] Some authorities have cautioned that GFCIs should not be used with life-sustaining equipment, or with other equipment vital to health and safety that rely upon continuous electrical power.[20]

SUGGESTIONS FOR ASSURING ELECTRICAL SAFETY

The following suggestions are intended to stimulate consideration of electrical safety in the clinical environment. This listing is not all inclusive, rather it is meant to prompt development of safety policies and procedures that are in compliance with extant codes and standards for various clinical settings.[25,26]

Some safety recommendations are:

1. An adequate number of three-prong outlets attached to true earth ground should be installed in all clinical areas. Ground continuity and plug-pull tension should be regularly tested.
2. GFCIs should be incorporated in all outlets powering therapeutic and diagnostic equipment, and tested monthly.
3. Bibliographic sources that critically evaluate equipment safety and performance should be consulted prior to placing equipment in a clinic. ECRI (5200 Butler Pike, Plymouth Meeting, PA, 19462) publishes Health Devices, the Hospital Product Comparison System, and the Health Devices Sourcebook.
4. Equipment should be purchased on a trial basis, during which time it can be evaluated by trained biomedical personnel for compliance with safety standards and manufacturer's specifications. Professional staff should also assess the equipment for clinical utility and effectiveness.
5. All equipment should be tested and, where appropriate, calibrated on an annual basis as part of a preventive maintenance and safety program.
6. Three-prong to two-prong "cheater" adaptors and extension cords should never be used.
7. Metal equipment that might easily become grounded should be removed from the vicinity of the patient.
8. External cardiac pacing leads should not contact other electrical devices. Exposed metal lead heads should not be touched without rubber gloves, and the unattached heads should be kept insulated.
9. Power cord plugs should never be removed from an outlet by pulling on the power cord itself.
10. Shoes that provide good insulation should be worn by all personnel, especially in areas likely to have water on the floor.
11. Any equipment that is suspected of being defective should be immediately removed from service, and clearly labeled as to the problem, date, and personnel involved. It may be necessary to file an incident report with the clinical facility. Entry of water into equipment cases, smoke, and unusual equipment odors or sounds should also prompt such action. Equipment should be thoroughly inspected before it is returned to service.
12. Share your experiences concerning equipment problems and hazards with others. Written or phone reports can be filed with the ECRI User Experience Network (5200 Butler Pike, Plymouth Meeting, PA, 19462,

215-825-6000; or TWX at 510-660-8023) and with the Medical Devices and Laboratory Product Problems Reporting Programs (US Pharmacopeia, 12601 Twinbrook Parkway, Rockville, MD, 20852, 800-638-6725, 24 hours a day).

SUMMARY

The informed user of electrotherapeutic equipment must have a fundamental understanding of electrical phenomena, of the wave forms produced and controlled by modern-day instrumentation, and of the factors affecting the choice and placement of electrodes. Additionally, the knowledgeable practitioner must be capable of monitoring the stimuli applied to his or her patients and must be ever-conscious of important safety considerations.

REFERENCES

1. Campbell JA; A critical appraisal of the electrical output characteristics of ten transcutaneous nerve stimulators, *Clin Phys Physiol Meas.* 3:141, 1982
2. Procacci P, Corte D, Zoppi M, et al. Pain threshold measurements in man. In Bonica JJ (ed): *Recent Advances in Pain Therapy*, Springfield, Ill., Thomas, 1974, pp 105–147
3. Newton RA, Karselis TC: Skin pH following high voltage pulsed galvanic stimulation. *Phys Ther.* 63:1593, 1983
4. Mueller EE, et al. Skin impedance in relation to pain threshold testing by electrical means. *J Appl Physiol.* 5:746, 1952
5. Strong P. *Biophysical Measurements.* Beaverton, Ore., Tektronix, 1970.
6. Hymes AC. The use of karaya electrodes with transcutaneous electrical nerve stimulation. A preliminary report. Unpublished paper, 1978
7. Ronnen M, Suster S, Kahana M, et al. Contact dermatitis due to karaya gum and induced by the application of electrodes. *Int J Dermatol.* 25(3):189, 1986
8. Benton LA, Baker LL, Bowman BR, et al. *Functional Electrical Stimulation.* Downey, Calif, Rancho Los Amigos Rehabilitation Engineering Center, 1980
9. Shriber WJ. *A Manual of Electrotherapy*, 4th ed. Philadelphia, Penn., Lea & Febiger, 1975
10. Geddes LA, Baker LE. *Applied Biomedical Instrumentation.* New York, N.Y., Wiley, 1975
11. Barr JO, Nielsen DH, Soderberg GL. Transcutaneous electrical nerve stimulation characteristics for altering pain perception, *Phys Ther.* 66(10):1515, 1986
12. The fatal current (clinic note). *J Am Phys Ther Assoc.* 46:968, 1966
13. Tiny flaws in medical design can kill (clinic note). *Phys Ther.* 48:158, 1968
14. Berger WH. Electrical hazards (letters to the editor). *Phys Ther.* 55:794, 1975
15. Arledge RL. Prevention of electrical shock hazards in physical therapy. *Phys Ther.* 58:1215, 1978
16. Reeter AK, Jensen R. Nursing electrical safety (video tape). Medfilms, Inc, 1983
17. Berger WH. Electrical shock hazards in the physical therapy department. *Clinical Management in Physical Therapy* 5(4):26, 1985

18. *American National Standard for Transcutaneous Electrical Nerve Stimulators.* Arlington, Va. Association for the Advancement of Medical Instrumentation, 1986
19. Mykelbust BM, Robinson AJ. Instrumentation. In Snyder-Mackler L, Robinson AJ (eds): *Clinical Electrophysiology: Electrotherapy and Electrophysiologic Testing.* Baltimore, Md., Williams & Wilkins, 1989, pp 23–58
20. Electrical Safety (Special Issue). *Health Devices,* January 1974
21. Therapist dies in whirlpool. *Progress Report,* September 1984, p 30
22. Ben-Zvi S. The lack of safety standards in medical instrumentation. *Trans New York Acad of Sciences.* 31:737, 1969
23. Bruner JMR. Hazards of electrical apparatus. *Anesthesiology.* 28:396, 1967
24. Standard for medical and dental equipment. UL544 2nd ed. Northbrook, Ill. Underwriters Laboratories Inc, 1985
25. Ritter HTM. Instrumentation considerations: Operating principles, purchase, management and safety. In Michlovitz SL (eds): *Thermal Agents in Rehabilitation.* Philadelphia, Penn., FA Davis Co, 1986, pp 51–72
26. Griffin JE, Karselis TC. *Physical Agents for Physical Therapists,* 2nd ed. Springfield, Ill., Charles C. Thomas Publisher, 1982

CHAPTER 3

Principles of Electrical Stimulation

Gad Alon

The recognition that conduction of electricity through biologic systems alters physiological and pathologic events is as old as the discovery that biologic systems are conductive media. The historical development and evolution of clinical electrical stimulators has been characterized by a cyclic pattern, alternating between popularity and disregard. The latest surge of interest has evolved around the use of electrical stimulation to modulate pain. Over the last 10 to 15 years, this surge of popularity has not only continued but expanded far beyond the application of electrical stimulation used to manage pain.

Many additional physical deficiencies have been reported to respond favorably to electrical energy. Among those are joint swelling and inflammatory reactions,[1-7] tissue healing,[8-15] muscle re-education,[16-27] circulatory impairments,[28-31] joint dysfunction,[7,20,32] postural disorders,[33-35] and pelvic floor disorders.[36-39]

These, as well as many other uses of electrical stimulation, can be found in historical reviews.[40,41] This latest surge of interest in electrical stimulation has attracted the attention of many professionals. Furthermore, numerous commercial stimulators have become available, creating a diversity of parameters, terminology, and many unsubstantiated claims for unique physiological effects and superior clinical results.

Which type of stimulator to be used, a daily decision for many clinicians, may be confusing. Questions such as which physical deficiencies indicate electrical treatment and what treatment protocols can provide predictive results can be problematic to many physical therapists. The present disarray, and the natural tendency to accept nonscientific, subjective, and commercially motivated claims (which are usually promoted outside the profession) may threaten the substantive potential that electrical stimulation can offer as an objective clinical modality.

This chapter will minimize confusion and redirect clinicians and students toward a sound, systemic, objective, and predictive approach to the principles of electrical stimulation. To achieve these goals, a clinical model must be developed. By definition, such a model is subject to parameters whereby electrical, physiological, physical, and procedural concepts are directly applied to clinical practice. The section on therapeutic currents offers functional definitions and is organized so as to provide a framework by which any present or future clinical electrical stimulator can be recognized for its clinical capabilities and limitations. Recently, a committee of the electrophysiological section of the American Physical Therapy Association (APTA) developed a document that attempts to unify and standardize the terms and definitions used by biomedical engineers, researchers, educators, and clinicians. The revision of the section on therapeutic currents incorporates these new terms and definitions as proposed in the document.[42] The section on physiological responses delineates physiological events and processes induced by the stimulation and associates them with the expected clinical results. Surface electrodes are an integral part of the electrical stimulation system, and their size, material, and placement technique dramatically affect physiological responses and clinical results. The section on surface electrodes offers a functional approach to their application and will hopefully resolve many of the present misconceptions. The last section integrates all previous sections by offering those protocols that best predict results for the various clinical problems treated by electrical stimulation.

This chapter is restricted to the transcutaneous (surface) application of electrical stimulation. Invasive electrodes may prove very beneficial in the future, particularly when inserted in denervated muscles, but as present clinical practice does not include them, they are not discussed in this chapter.

THERAPEUTIC CURRENTS

General Considerations

The custom has been to recognize electrical stimulators by the names of their inventors or by the (mostly) inappropriate names promoted by commercial companies. Galvanic, faradic, diadynamic, high voltage, low voltage, low frequency, medium frequency, and TENS are several examples. These names have created tremendous confusion relative to the physiological effects and clinical results. The simple fact is that all are transcutaneous electrical stimulators (TES), and the majority are also TENS (transcutaneous electrical nerve stimulators) because they work transcutaneously and excite the nerves. Thus, as long as surface electrodes are utilized, and as long as the peripheral nerves are excited, the stimulator is a TENS unit.

Discrimination between TENS and transcutaneous muscle stimulators

(TMS) or neuromuscular electrical stimulators (NMES) is also misleading, because the applied stimulation always excites the peripheral motor nerves, which in turn leads to muscle contraction. Direct activation of muscle fibers is possible only if the muscle is denervated. Indeed, only under such conditions may the term TMS be substituted for TENS. (With the exception of Chapter 5, where electrical stimulators of denervated muscles are discussed, all remaining chapters simply recognize TENS devices of different pulse characteristics and different current modulations.) In the field of physical medicine and rehabilitation, electrical stimulators should be classified as either direct current, alternating current (AC) or pulsed current. With the exception of subliminal stimulation, all pulsed and most AC currents are TENS stimulators, regardless of their waveforms or commercial names.

All stimulators must provide sufficient voltage in order to conduct appropriate current against the impedance of the conductive medium. Most clinical stimulators are designed electronically as either constant-current or constant-voltage stimulators. *Constant voltage* means that the voltage output level set by the therapist will remain the same. If the impedance of the tissue or of the tissue–electrode interface (or both) is changed, the current will also change, but the voltage will remain constant. Conversely, any change of impedance during the application of a constant-current stimulator will change the voltage output but will leave the current unaffected, provided that the stimulator is appropriately designed to function in the full range of tissue impedance.

Basic physiological responses and clinical results are most likely to be identical whether constant-voltage or constant-current stimulators are used.[43] The clinical advantage of a constant-voltage stimulator is the automatic reduction of current when electrode size is reduced or if electrode contact with the skin becomes loose. The disadvantage is apparent if the pressure between the tissue and the electrode is suddenly increased. Impedance is reduced, and current amplitude is automatically increased, thus intensifying the stimulation level. The advantage of constant current is the more consistent level of stimulation. The disadvantage is apparent when electrode size or pressure with the skin or both are reduced and lead to a sudden increase of current concentrations. The result is a sudden discomfort of the stimulation and, in extreme cases, electrical burns. This hazard can be eliminated by limiting the maximum voltage output.[44]

Another concept of general concern is the classic term *average current*, which each clinical stimulator provides. This generic term may not be the most appropriate relative to physiological processes. Current flow per unit of time may be better described by the term *total flow*. Mathematically, total current is calculated as coulomb/sec. Clinically, total current can be thought of as the amount of current flow per second. Excessive total current may cause harm, whereas insufficient current will not cause the expected physiological response. The upper limit of safe total current depends largely on current density or current per area of electrode. Application of 10 mA/cm² of surface electrode has been suggested, but more conservative values of 1.5 to 4 mA/cm² are also recommended.[45,46] Because more specific guidelines are yet to be established, the prevailing clinical approach should be to use the lowest total current capable of producing the desired physiological response. Excess, unnecessary current increase patient discomfort and decrease the efficiency of the stimulator.

Direct Current (DC)

Electrical current that flows in one direction for about 1 sec or longer can be defined as *direct current* (DC). (In classic terminology, DC was also called galvanic current.) Direct current that flows unidirectionally for less than 1 sec, especially a few milliseconds or less, is no longer a DC current but rather a pulsed or AC current.

The flow of a DC can be modulated for clinical purposes. The three most common modulations are:

1. Reversed DC
2. Interrupted DC
3. Surged DC

In reversed DC, the direction of current flow is reversed. Since, by definition, DC should flow for about 1 sec or longer, reversal also occurs after about 1 sec or longer. Reversal of the current can be accomplished by using a hand switch or an automatic switch inside the unit. Continuous DC and reversed DC are illustrated in Figure 3–1.

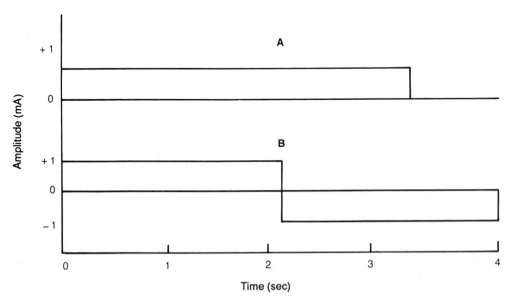

Figure 3–1. Direct current (DC). **A.** Continuous DC. **B.** Reversed DC. Note the time scale.

Interruption of current flow occurs when the current ceases to flow for about 1 sec or longer, usually up to 50 to 60 sec, and then flow again for about 1 sec or longer. Interruption is usually accomplished by a switch on the hand probe or by an automatic switch inside the stimulator. The most common classical purpose of interrupted DC is to cause twitch contraction of denervated muscles during electrodiagnosis or treatment (TMS). When the switch is closed, an ON current flow prevails; switching OFF arrests current flow. Switching ON and OFF occur abruptly. If one wishes to grade the ON and OFF so that current amplitude will increase and decrease gradually, a modulation termed "ramp" can be added. Classically, ramp-up and ramp-down were termed surge-up and surge-down, respectively. Ramping usually occurs over a period of time lasting from 0.5 sec to several seconds. Interruption without ramp, with ramp, and the combination of interruption coupled with reversed DC and ramp are illustrated in Figure 3–2.

Ramping takes place inside the stimulator, but the therapist determines the time of ramping by a switch on the unit panel. With modern clinical methods, there is little use for interrupted DC, with the possible exception of treating denervated muscles. In fact, most applications of electrical stimulation over the last decade have been used to treat intact peripheral nerves and have employed to a limited degree alternating current (AC) and to large extent pulsed currents.

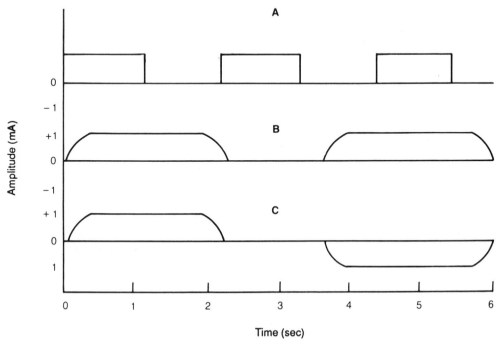

Figure 3–2. Direct-current modulation. **A.** Interrupted DC. **B.** Ramped, interrupted DC. **C.** Ramped, reversed, interrupted DC.

⚡Alternating Current (AC)

As defined, *alternating current* (AC) is a current that changes the direction of flow, with reference to the zero baseline, at least once every second. Continuous AC indicates no modulation, and no intervals between pulses. The typical AC is symmetrical and can be delivered in various shapes including sinusoidal, rectangular, trapezoidal, and triangular. A typical AC can be nonsymmetrical and of various shapes (Fig. 3–3).

Typical to AC are the inverse relations between frequency and pulse and phase durations. Inherent in this relationship is the phenomenon that as the frequency of AC is increased, phase and pulse durations are automatically decreased. The opposite occurs if the pulse frequency decreases (Fig. 3–4). It follows that phase and pulse duration can be calculated as the reciprocal of frequency.

A growing body of knowledge on the physiological and clinical effects of

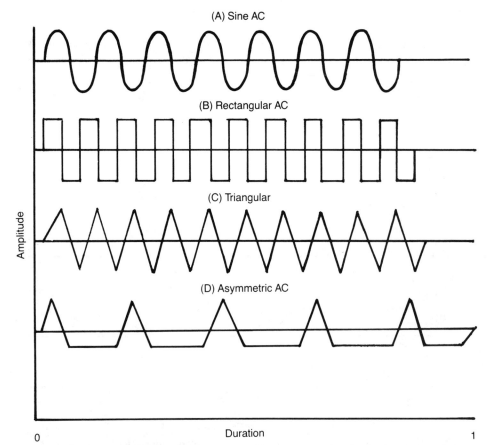

Figure 3–3. Different shapes of continuous (nonmodulated) alternating current (AC).

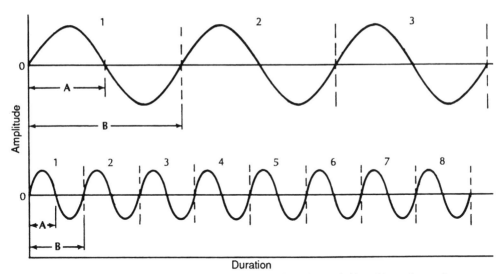

Figure 3—4. Frequency—pulse end-phase duration relationships of continuous sine waves. **A.** Phase duration. **B.** Pulse duration. Note how phase and pulse are shortened as frequency increases.

continuous, unmodulated AC is evident in the medical literature. The most common use to date is of a 60,000-Hz sine wave with a 5 to 10 volts peak-to-peak (P-P) amplitude. Such AC is not designed to excite peripheral nerves and is aimed at promoting soft and osseous tissue regeneration.[47-53] As most of these applications have been predominantly conducted by physicians and bioengineers rather than physical therapists, they are beyond the scope of this chapter.

⚹AC Modulation
AC modulation is recognized by time and amplitude variants. Time-modulated AC can be subgrouped into burst and interrupted modes. Bursting AC is created when the current is permitted to flow for a few milliseconds and then ceases to flow for a few milliseconds, in a repeated cycle (Fig. 3–5). The interval between successive bursts is known as interburst interval and is equivalent to the interpulse interval of pulsed currents. The AC bursts have also been termed polyphasic pulses[54] because physiologically they seem to elicit the same excitation as mono- or biphasic pulses.[55,56] The most common clinical stimulator that is designed to deliver bursts of time-modulated AC is the so-called "Russian" current.

ACcan also be modulated as interrupted AC. This modulation prevails when the current ceases to flow for 1 sec or longer and then flows again for a few seconds in a repeated cycle. Such modulation is different from burst in that the current ceases to flow for a long enough time to permit relaxation from a muscle contraction. The interruption modulation of AC is identical to the interruption of pulsed current.

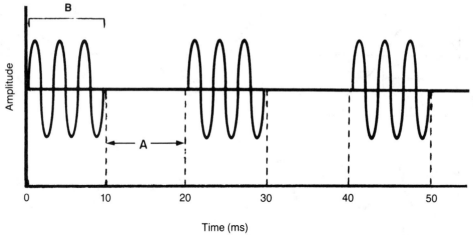

Figure 3–5. Time-modulated AC to form bursts of pulses. **A.** Interburst interval. **B.** Single burst.

Amplitude-modulated AC can be obtained by several electronic approaches. The most common electronic approach is to cause a mix of two AC sources that differ from each other in frequency. This approach has been the electronic basis in the generation of what is clinically known as the *interferential current* (IC). At present there is no known physiological or clinical advantage for amplitude-modulated AC over time-modulated AC or pulsed current.[54,56] Some manufacturers have used this modulation approach to create what they term beat (or "envelop") frequency. Each beat seems to cause excitation of peripheral nerves much like a single pulse of a mono- or biphasic pulse and therefore can be also termed a polyphasic pulse.[54] Amplitude-modulated AC is likely to remain an electronic concept without superior clinical benefit over conventional pulsed stimulators unless new data will prove otherwise in the future.

In continuous, unmodulated AC stimulators, the total current (coulomb/sec) is always between 65 and 70 percent of the peak current. Modulation into bursts (Russian) or beats (interferential) somewhat reduces the total current but typically it remains unnecessarily high (80–100 mA) and may present undesired clinical responses.

Pulsed Currents

A *pulsed current* is defined as an electrical current that is conducted as a signal (or signals) of short duration. Each pulse lasts for only a few milliseconds (msec) or microseconds (μsec) followed by an interpulse interval. Different pulses may exhibit different shapes. Consequently, numerous names (such as pulsating DC, spike, square, faradic, exponential, and triangular) have appeared in the literature over the years and have led to enormous confusion regarding their common and unique correlates with physiological responses.

Discriminating these pulses according to their waveforms eliminates the confusion. Once this is accomplished, the characteristics of each pulse must be recognized. Two pulses of different shape but of the same waveform and similar characteristics are likely to cause similar physiological effects and clinical results.

This approach—namely, discriminating these various devices on the basis of waveform and pulse characteristics, rather than names—is likely to minimize confusion and ambiguity regarding modern stimulators.

WaveForms. Most, if not all, present and future pulsed stimulators can be classified under one of two waveform groups: monophasic or biphasic.

Monophasic. By definition, *monophasic* indicates that there is only one phase to each pulse. This type of stimulator has also been called pulsating DC. Whether the shape of the pulse is square, triangular, twin peak, or halfway rectified sine wave, only one phase occurs in each case. In monophasic pulse, current flow is still unidirectional, indicating negative or positive polarity.

Biphasic. When two opposing phases are contained in a single pulse, the waveform is defined as a *biphasic* pulse. Shapes may include square, triangular, or sinusoidal, but they are all biphasic. Furthermore, biphasic pulses can be symmetrical or asymmetrical. Presently, symmetrical pulses with added interphase interval seem clinically preferred to asymmetrical pulses, particularly if motor nerves are the target of excitation.[43,57–60] In the past, asymmetrical pulses were more common, faradic current one example and compensated monophasic another. A major advantage of a symmetrical biphasic pulse over an asymmetrical pulse is that neither negative nor positive polarity requires any specific physiological or clinical consideration. Illustrations of monophasic and biphasic waveforms are provided in Figure 3–6.

Interpulse Interval. Irrespective of waveforms, all pulsed stimulators are characterized by a space between successive pulses. These spaces have been termed *interpulse intervals,* and each usually lasts from 10 to 999 msec. The

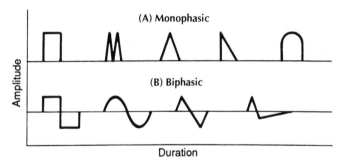

Figure 3–6. Basic pulsed-current wave forms.

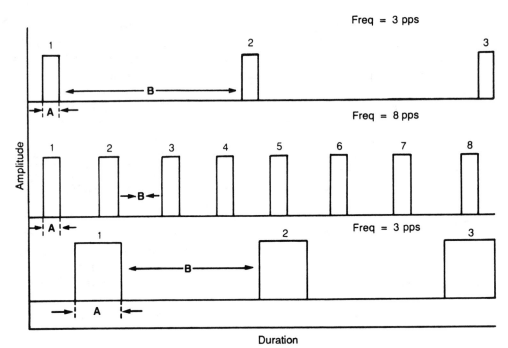

Figure 3–7. Frequency–pulse duration relationships of pulsed current. **A.** Phase duration. **B.** Interpulse interval. Note complete independence of duration and frequency.

exact time depends on the duration of each pulse and on the number of pulses per second (Fig. 3–7).

Pulse Characteristics. Regardless of waveform, pulsed currents exhibit some essential characteristics that must be recognized. To account for all waveform classes, the phase should be considered the basic, fundamental unit of description. The problem in choosing the phase is the traditional clinical selection of the term *pulse*, rather than the term *phase*, as the basic descriptive unit. To avoid misunderstanding, the realization is necessary that, in a monophasic design, phase and pulse are synonymous. In biphasic pulses, each phase should be described. If symmetrical, then the characteristics of both phases are identical, and the description of one phase should suffice. If asymmetrical, the characteristics of both phases should be recognized. An outstanding historical review by Geddes documented Fick as the first scholar to discuss the three important attributes of the phase (stimulus): abruptness of onset (rate of rise of phase amplitude, also known as the leading edge), amplitude, and duration.[41] Other attributes, as well as additional characteristics, must be described. These include phase and pulse duration, phase and pulse amplitude, phase and pulse charge, and pulse rate (frequency).

Phase and Pulse Duration. The elapsed time from the initiation of the phase until its termination is defined as *phase duration.* The phase begins when the current departs from the zero line and ends as the current returns to the zero line. For the biphasic pulse, the pulse duration is determined by adding the two phase durations. Duration of the phases and pulses of monophasic and biphasic waveforms is illustrated in Figure 3–8.

Phase and Pulse Amplitude. The highest point of the phase is defined as *peak phase,* or *peak current amplitude.* When monophasic pulses are used, the terms peak phase current amplitude and peak pulse current amplitude are synonymous. However, when symmetrical or asymmetrical biphasic pulses are considered, two peaks (one for each phase) can be recognized. Electronically, the amplitude refers to the differences between the peaks of the two phases and is measured as peak-to-peak amplitude. Physiologically, investigators usually measure the peak amplitude from zero to one phase peak amplitude (Fig. 3–9). Peak current amplitude must be distinguished from total current amplitude.

One advantage of the pulsed current stimulators is the ability to keep the total current (coulomb/sec) relatively low compared to the peak current amplitude. This low total current is because pulsed currents contain relatively long interpulse intervals at which current amplitude is zero. Thus the average amount of flow per second is much lower (Fig 3–10). The significance of relatively low total current is in the safety of stimulation. Most pulsed current clinical stimulators do not exceed 20 mA of total current and many are limited to only 2 to 5 mA. This limited total current can be contrasted with the total current of time- and amplitude-modulated AC stimulators where the total currents usually reach 80 to 100 mA (see Russian and interferential stimulators, respectively).

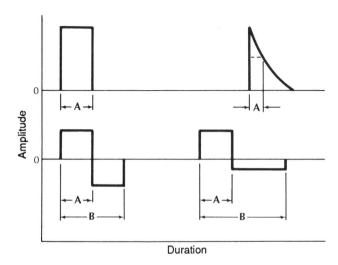

Figure 3–8. Phase and pulse duration. **A.** Phase duration. **B.** Pulse duration.

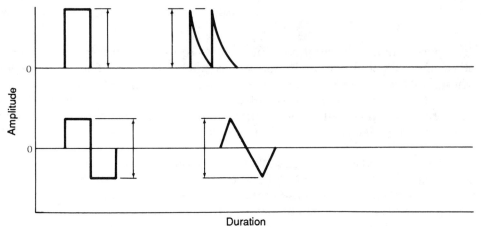

Duration

Figure 3–9. Peak current amplitude.

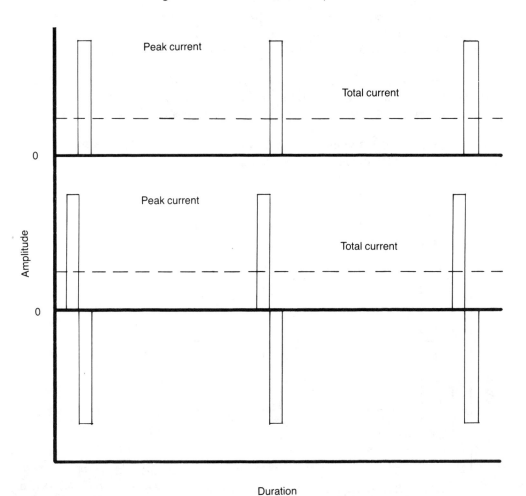

Duration

Figure 3–10. Peak and total current associated with monophasic and biphasic pulses.

Phase and Pulse Charge. Phase charge can be defined as the quantity of electricity delivered to the tissue with each phase of each pulse. Charge quantities of clinical stimulators are measured in microcoulombs (µC). In a monophasic pulse, phase and pulse charge are synonymous, and the total and net amounts of charge are identical and are always greater than zero. In contrast, the charge contained in a biphasic pulse is the sum of charges of the two phases and thus contains a total amount of charge greater than the charge of each phase. The net amount of charge may or may not equal zero. Symmetrical biphasic pulses deliver twice the amount of charge contained in each phase to the tissues, while the net charge delivered remains zero. (Fig.3–11).

When the net charge is different from zero, a DC component is recognized by electronic definition. Such a DC component provides a residue of electrical charge in the tissues. Only monophasic, and a few asymmetrical biphasic pulses exhibit such residue, which may be of physiological and clinical value.[61] Absence of a DC component refers to zero net charge (ZNC) and is characteristic of the symmetrical, biphasic pulses.

Pulse Rate (Frequency). The excitatory responses to the number of pulses of pulsed current seem to be identical regardless of the number of pulses contained in each pulse. For example, 50 monophasic, 50 biphasic, or 50 bursts all provide very similar tetanic contraction.[56] Thus, when the rate of pulsed current is considered, only the term *pulse* is used. The correct terminology should be *pulse frequency*, measured in pulses per second (pps). Alternating current frequency is expressed in Hertz (Hz) or the number of cycles per second (cps), an old term.

In the past, and based on the strict electronic definition, frequency has always been considered inversely proportional to pulse duration.[62] Stated another way, pulse frequency and phase or pulse duration always depend on

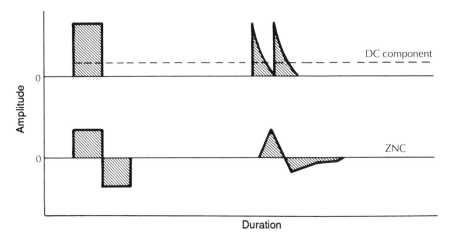

Figure 3–11. Phase and pulse charge.

each other when continuous sine wave is used (see Fig. 3–4). Modern stimulators, however, are designed to produce short pulses with relatively long interpulse intervals (see next section). Such a design leads to complete independence of frequency and duration, at least from a physiological perspective. Indeed, having an interpulse interval allows the therapist to change phase and pulse durations without affecting the frequency, and vice versa (see Fig. 3–7).

At present, a great deal of confusion seems to exist with regard to the recognition of "low"-frequency, "medium"-frequency, and "high"-frequency stimulators. By electronic standards, all clinical electrical stimulators are low frequency. The aforementioned adjectives in the clinic are, therefore, relative to each other. Some clinicians refer to 2 to 5 pps as low frequency and 70 to 100 pps as high frequency. Others refer to 40 to 100 pps as low and 2500 to 4000 pps as medium frequency. Two groups of stimulators have been commercially promoted as medium frequency, and a most unfortunate (and misleading) concept has further added to the clinical confusion. These so-called medium-frequency stimulators use an AC sine wave of frequencies varying between 2000 and 10,000 Hz. Not only do such AC sine waves offer no physiological or clinical advantages over monophasic or biphasic pulses,[43,54,58,59,63] but the real physiological reason for such a frequency level is simply to obtain short phase duration by using the inverse relationship between frequency and duration of a continuous sine wave. These short pulses are then time or amplitude modulated as bursts containing from 1 to 200 pps. These modulated groups represent a physiologically effective frequency—a low frequency identical to the range of the monophasic and biphasic pulse frequencies.[64,65] Claiming that such "medium frequency" provides less skin impedance in comparison to short-duration monophasic or biphasic pulses is incorrect and misleading (see section on calculation).[61,62,66,58,66–69] In summary, all clinical stimulators, whether monophasic, biphasic, or "medium frequency," effectively provide low-frequency operation that range from 1 pps to several hundred pulses per second.

Pulse and Current Modulation. When a pulsed current is flowing continuously at a preset phase duration, amplitude, and rate, there is no pulse or current modulation, and the setting is called *continuous* mode. Modulation of each current can be subdivided into two groups: phase/pulse modulation and current modulation. These two groups are not mutually exclusive and can occur simultaneously.

Phase/Pulse Modulation. Phase/pulse modulation refers to an automatic increase and decrease of the phase/pulse parameters. Usually, phase duration, phase amplitude, or pulse rate are programmed to increase and decrease (automatically) in preset ranges. This concept is illustrated in Figure 3–12.

Phase duration, or amplitude, or rate modulation, or all of these are available in many clinical stimulators; they have, however, failed as yet to provide

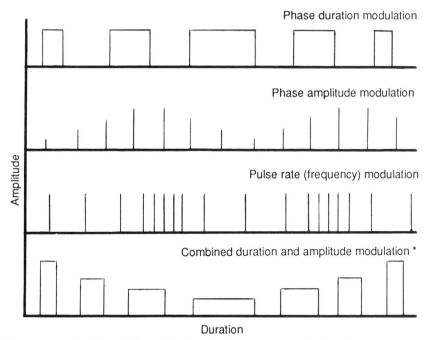

Figure 3–12. Modulation of phase/pulse characteristics. Note the so-called S-D modulation where, as amplitude decreases, duration increases.

either physiological or clinical advantages. The intention of phase-modulation-based stimulations has been to delay perceptual accommodation to current flow. Such a delay may prevail for several minutes, but in a 30- to 60-min treatment, a few minutes are insignificant. No greater pain suppression has yet been noted for automatically modulated pulse rates or durations than for non-modulated pulses, thus contradicting promotional claims.[70–76]

Current Modulation. Current modulation refers to the alteration of the pulsed current as a whole rather than to the parameters of each pulse. One form of such modulation is bursts. Others are interruption (ON–OFF) and ramping of pulsed current flow.

1. *Bursts.* Bursts are created when a pulsed current is permitted to flow for a few milliseconds and then ceases to flow for a few milliseconds in a repeated cycle. Much like the modulation of AC into bursts, such bursts can also occur with monophasic and biphasic pulses (Fig. 3–13). Physiologically, individual pulses, or bursts cause similar excitation thresholds.[55,56] Five bursts or five pulses both cause twitch contractions, although the perception of the bursts is somewhat different from that of individual pulses. The number of bursts per second, much like the number of pulses per second, is predetermined by the therapist.

   Bursts have so far failed to add any advantage to clinical practice

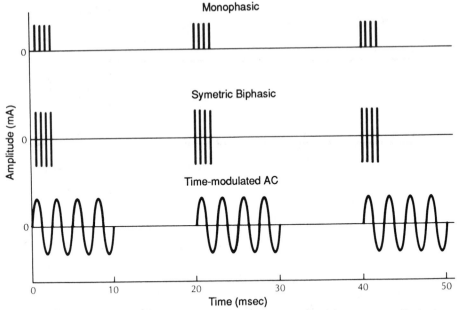

Figure 3–13. Bursts. Monophasic and biphasic pulsed bursts usually last only 1 msec, while AC bursts last about 10 msec. (The limited space of the figure does not allow actual illustration of correct values.)

except confusion.[70,72,74,76,77] The therapist must recognize the fact that bursts and interburst intervals do not cause true interruption of muscle contractions. Thus, intervals should not be referred to as interruptions. Indeed, true interruption of pulsed current flow is a different category of current modulation. Both bursts and interburst intervals are measured in milliseconds, intervals too short to permit relaxation during tetanic contraction.

2. *Interruption.* True interruption modulation occurs when monophasic or biphasic pulses continue to flow for about 1 sec or longer and then cease to flow for 1 sec or longer. Clinically, many stimulators provide an interruption mode where the ON time can usually be varied between 1 and 60 sec and the OFF time between 1 and 120 sec. The interruption mode is of major clinical importance.[19,20,64,78] Many clinical techniques associated with muscle re-education, improving joint range of motion, and enhancing venous blood flow require such current modulation.[54,57]

3. *Ramps.* The last form of modulation that we shall consider is a ramp mode, also recognized by many clinicians as a surge mode. This modulation is associated with the ON portion of the interrupted mode. With a ramp, current amplitude will increase gradually over a predetermined period, usually lasting from 1 to 5 sec. Such modulation is called ramp-up. Many stimulators also provide ramp-down, resulting in a gradual decrease of amplitude toward the end of the ON time (Fig. 3–14). Ramp-

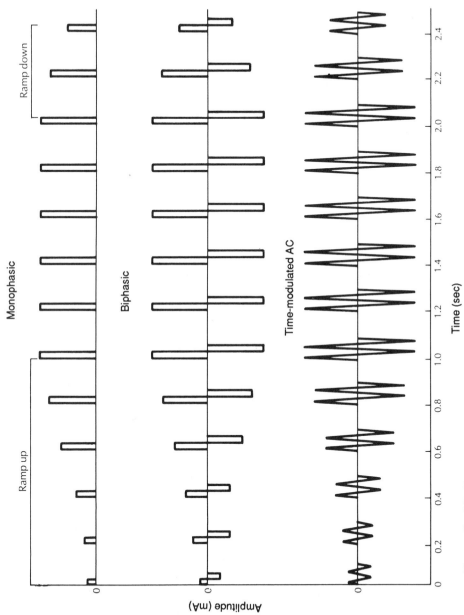

Figure 3–14. Ramp modulation. Note that ramping can be used equally with pulsed and AC-modulated bursts.

down is usually less effective in graduating muscle relaxation. After a strong contraction, a reduction of 10 to 15 percent of amplitude usually causes an abrupt relaxation of the muscle. However, ramp-down is perceived by the subject as offering more comfortable stimulation than would be provided with the ramp-up mode only.

Ramp modulation is either preset as a percentage of the ON time or is manually determined by the therapist. In the former, usually one third of the ON time is a ramp, so that if ON time is 6 sec, then ramp time is 2 sec. The ramp is therefore dependent on the ON time and thus presents an appreciable limitation of clinical flexibility. Manual selection of the ramp, where the therapist determines ramp time independently of the ON time, is clinically far superior to other options.

Summary of Current Modulation. The therapist must recognize that modulation of electrical currents can include both modulation of the individual phase/pulse parameters and modulation of the pulsed current as a whole. At present, automatic variation of individual pulse parameters does not seem to have an added clinical value, whereas interrupted and ramping modulation of the pulsed current as a whole is of major importance for appropriate selection of different clinical protocols.

Finally, there seems to be considerable confusion regarding the differences between phase duration, interpulse interval, burst duration, interburst interval, ON duration, and OFF duration. These terms are differentiated in Table 3–1.

Figure 3–14 shows clearly that interburst intervals are not a physiological interruption. Rather, they are an interval between successive bursts that parallels the interpulse interval of monophasic or biphasic pulses. It then follows that a nonmodulated pulsed current having monophasic or biphasic pulses and a frequency of 50 pps should have an excitatory response very similar to that of an amplitude- or time-modulated AC with 50 bps. Interrupted mode can be added to monophasic and biphasic pulses, as well as to AC bursting current.

If interrupted, a ramp modulation should be added to both pulsed cur-

⚡TABLE 3–1. CURRENT PULSE AND PHASE TERMINOLOGY

Parameter	Synonyms	Measured Time
Phase duration	Pulse width, pulse time	Microseconds[a]
Interpulse interval	Interpulse spacing, rest period	Milliseconds
Burst duration	Packets, beat, envelop	Milliseconds
Interburst interval	Interburst spacing, rest period	Milliseconds
Interrupted current	ON–OFF	Seconds
Ramp	Surge	Seconds

[a]Can also be milliseconds.

Interrupted Current

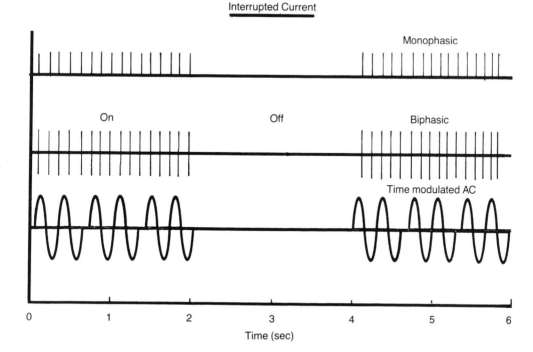

Figure 3–15. Interrupted modulation.

rents as well as to the interrupted time- or amplitude-modulated AC, as illustrated in Figure 3–15.

Identification of Clinical Stimulators

As previously discussed, all noninvasive clinical stimulators are classified as transcutaneous electrical stimulators (TES). The majority of these are also TENS since they all conduct pulsed current through surface electrodes and cause excitation of peripheral nerves. Few of those TENS deliver burst of time-modulated AC, the so-called Russian, or amplitude-modulated AC, the so-called "interferential." Both modulated AC currents can also be recognized as polyphasic pulsed currents.[54] The different names for stimulators, such as low voltage, high voltage, interferential current (IC), Russian, American, medium frequency, TENS, NMES, or EMS, help sales representatives and sales-oriented clinicians, but have little bearing on physiological and objective clinical benefits or on the limitations of these various devices.

In the last few years a new group of TES has been promoted in the clinic that may require a separate classification. Whereas these stimulators conduct their current through surface electrodes, they do not, in most instances, excite the peripheral nerves.[57] Thus, in generic terminology, they are not TENS, but are classified as subliminal or nonperceived TES. The promoters of these devices seem to prefer meaningless names such as Microcurrent, MENS Therapy, Electro-Acuscope, Myopulse, Myomatic, MENS-O-MATIC, "Alfastim," Pain Suppressor Biopulse, and more. The list of names seem to keep growing and with it the confusion, misapplication, and false information to patient and clinician alike.[54]

Evaluation of the various stimulators must not be based on *names*. The astute clinician should examine the pulse characteristics and parameters and identify whether or not these parameters are in agreement with the appropriate stimulation protocols. An appropriate protocol is defined as that which is based on *objective* clinical results or presently valid physiological rationale, or both. The purpose of this section is to examine briefly the most common groups of stimulators and evaluate them according to their pulse characteristics and current modulation, rather than according to their names and promotional misconcepts. Indeed, the more important characteristics and parameters that should be recognized by the astute clinician in each TES are waveform, phase duration, phase charge, pulse rate, total current, and current modulations.

This section should allow the therapist to recognize that clinical stimulators irrespective of name are not unique and simply represent different electronic designs that will achieve the same physiological effects and clinical results. Some stimulators are clinically more versatile than others because they can be set to comply appropriately with more clinical protocols. No single stimulator is optimally designed to provide all clinical treatments.

Low-Voltage Stimulators. The term "low voltage" is a useless and misleading descriptor for a group of classic stimulators. Previous electrotherapy texts nevertheless identify low-voltage devices as a group of three different stimulators including DC, the so-called galvanic, and two pulsed stimulators: faradic and diadynamic. A short description of each follows.

Direct Current (Galvanic) Stimulators. The basic design of a galvanic stimulator incorporates a continuous direct current (DC). Such a current flows unidirectionally for at least 1 sec, but can be reversed, interrupted, or ramped. By definition, the DC stimulator does not have pulses, and thus no waveform or pulse parameters. In the simple galvanic stimulator, there is neither reversal of polarity nor surge capability. Interruption is accomplished manually with a switch on the stimulating electrode. In more sophisticated units, the therapist can set the time intervals of interruption, surging, and reversal of polarity prior to operation, and they are then automatically instituted during treatment.

The major direct physiological responses to galvanic stimulation are the electrochemical changes that occur at the cellular and tissue levels. The change of skin pH under the electrodes causes a reflex vasodilation, thus indirectly increasing arterial blood flow to the skin.[46,79] Because of the prolonged flow of DC, current amplitude must be extremely low, and therefore the direct effect of such current is primarily limited to superficial tissues (such as skin).

Excitatory responses can only be elicited if such DC is interrupted. The excitation only affects very superficial nerve fibers and is usually painful, as discrimination among large sensory fibers, motor fibers, and pain-conducting fibers is difficult to obtain when current flow is of a duration greater than 500 μsec.

When a state of denervation prevails, the therapist can transcutaneously use interrupted DC to directly stimulate the denervated muscle fibers. The superficial effect of such stimulation, the inevitable elicitation of only twitch contractions, and the painful perception of the stimulation render a very limited clinical effectiveness to such DC (see Chapter 5).

The effectiveness of DC in alleviating pain, with or without iontophoresis, has been clinically reported[3,4,80,81] but may not be the treatment of first choice because of the unpleasant and potentially harmful stimulation.[82] Pulsed currents having a short phase duration are likely to be more effective and are much more comfortable to the patient. As a last resort, and particularly when the pain is caused by superficial structures, DC should be considered. The therapist must be aware of the hazard of skin burns with DC, as total current, current density, and treatment time may all contribute to excessive stimulation.

Faradic Current. Faradic current, whether implemented as general or localized faradism, has been used clinically since the late 19th century. The faradic pulse is an asymmetric biphasic pulse. In the early 1940s and until the late 1960s, faradic current was considered more comfortable than galvanic DC. Most physical therapists mistakenly believed that the relative comfort of the faradic pulse derived from its being a form of AC. Present knowledge strongly indicates that the real reason for relative comfort was that the faradic pulse was simply of a shorter duration than the galvanic current. The duration of the main phase of the faradic pulse is typically 1 msec (Fig. 3–16). By today's

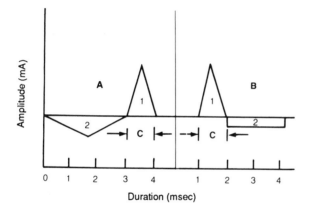

Figure 3–16. Faradic current. **A.** Original wave shape. **B.** Modified wave shape. Note that both waves are asymmetrical biphasic. Phase 1 is the main phase for excitation, usually lasting 1 msec **(C)**. The amplitude of the second phase is too low to cause excitation.

standards, this pulse duration is much too long for maintaining comfort. Indeed, the phase duration of most modern pulses, whether monophasic or biphasic, is only between 20 and 200 μsec. Duration of the phase is responsible for patient comfort rather than the type of current.[54]

Faradic pulse's asymmetric biphasic waveform may render such current obsolete, even with a design of shorter pulses. Today's knowledge suggests that future stimulators will provide either monophasic or symmetric biphasic pulses in order to maintain comfort. Having an asymmetric pulse (such as the faradic pulse) is unlikely to offer any physiological, clinical, or engineering advantage over either monophasic or symmetric biphasic waveforms. Most clinical faradic stimulators have variable pulse rates, usually 1 to 60 pps, but not variable phase duration. Many stimulators also have a ramp-up and ramp-down (surge) mode but no true interrupted mode (Table 3–2). Lack of comfort and limited current modulation reduce the clinical versatility and number of treatment protocols that the classic faradic stimulator can provide.

Diadynamic Current. Diadynamic current is actually a monophasic pulsed current developed in the early 1950s. It is usually a sine wave at a carrier

TABLE 3–2. TRAITS OF ELECTRICAL STIMULATORS

	Stimulator Classes				
Trait	Low-Voltage Faradic	High Voltage	Russian Current	Interferential Current	Optimal Design[e]
Channels	1	1–2	2	1	2–4
Modes	Continuous ramp[a]	Continuous/ interrupted[b]	Interrupted	Continuous	Continuous/ interrupted
Waveform	Asymmetric biphasic	Monophasic	Burst or pulses	Multiphasic	Symmetric biphasic[c]
Phase duration	1000 μsec (fixed)	5–20 μsec (fixed)	200 μsec (adjustable)	125μsec (fixed)	20–200 μsec (adjustable)
Phase charge	60 μC	12–14 μC	30μC	20–25 μC	40 μC
Pulse rate	1–60 pps (adjustable)	1–25 pps (adjustable)	1–100 pps (adjustable)	1–200 pps (adjustable)	1–150 pps (adjustable)
Total current	5–6 mA	1.5 mA	100 mA	80–90 mA	10 mA
Polarity	No[d]	Yes	No	No	No

[a] No true interruption, ramp up/down.
[b] Uncommon.
[c] With 50 to 100 μsec interphase interval.
[d] May have polarity-dependent traits because of waveform
[e] Optimal design should also include option for monophasic waveform. The maximal phase charge of the monophasic waveform should not exceed 15 microcouloumbs.

(Modified from Alon G: Electro-orthopedics: A review of present electrophysiologic responses and clinical efficacy of transcutaneous stimulation. Adv Sports Med Fitness 2:295, 1989)

frequency of 100 Hz, which is either half-wave or full-wave rectified. The result is a monophasic pulse of 10 msec phase duration. Half-wave rectification yields a pulse rate of 50 pps. Full-wave rectification yields 100 pps (Table 3–2). The former has a 10-msec interpulse interval, whereas the latter has no such interval (Fig. 3–17).

Diadynamic current, like other TENS devices, provides direct excitatory responses but, because of its long phase/pulse duration, it is very uncomfortable. The unidirectional current flow, long pulse duration, and relatively short (or absent) interpulse interval render cellular and tissue chemical changes similar to those of continuous DC. Early reports from Europe suggested many different excitatory responses and clinical procedures,[83] but all can be achieved with far greater comfort and ease using the microsecond pulses of modern TENS units. Diadynamic currents are likely to remain obsolete unless comparative data can be presented to demonstrate their superiority over modern TENS.

★ **TENS.** Early in this chapter, the statement was made that most clinical stimulators are TENS (except true "galvanic" DC or subliminal stimulators). TENS includes faradic, diadynamic, interferential, Russian, and high voltage, or any other pulsed stimulator. Unfortunately, too many therapists differentiate TENS units from these other stimulators because they are small and battery powered. Others consider TENS units only when applied to modulate pain.[84] But high-voltage or interferential electrical stimulators can also be battery operated and can be equally effective in reducing pain.[66,85] Hopefully, this chapter has settled this issue by recognizing all pulsed stimulators that are

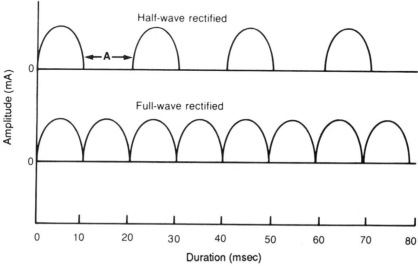

Figure 3–17. Diadynamic current. Full-wave rectification yields 100 pps, while half-wave rectification yields 50 pps. **A.** Interpulse interval.

applied transcutaneously as TENS. They may differ only in their waveform, pulse parameters, and the current modulations that they may or may not offer. Because high-voltage, interferential, and Russian currents are discussed separately in this textbook, only the battery-powered stimulators are summarized here.

Some of these battery-powered TENS units offer monophasic pulses, while others offer symmetrical or asymmetrical biphasic pulses; few offer burst or amplitude-modulated AC pulses. Phase duration usually ranges between 40 and 400 μsec. Maximal peak amplitude reaches between 50 and 100 mA. In some units pulse rate is variable, whereas in others it is fixed. Stimulators that are used for pain management provide phase charge limited to about 20 to 25 μC. They may or may not have automatic modulation of pulse parameters and usually have no current modulation, so that pulses are delivered continuously.

On the other hand, those TENS units that are used for neuromuscular re-education are commonly but unnecessarily called NMES and usually have a fixed phase duration of between 200 and 300 μsec and peak current amplitude of 100 to 150 mA. Their phase charge can reach 25 to 30μC; thus, they are more powerful than the "pain" units. These stimulators are usually modulated to provide interrupted current. Continuous pulses are available only by manually holding a switch.

The major and direct effect of all TENS units takes place at the cellular level. Indirectly, they also affect the biologic system at the tissue, segmental, and systemic levels. The cellular level includes excitation of sensory, motor, and pain-conducting nerve fibers. Many of the pain-management stimulators provide fairly comfortable sensory excitation but limited motor excitation. The neuromuscular re-education TENS units provide stronger motor excitation but many of them may not be sufficiently powerful for vigorous contraction of large muscle groups.

Usually, the battery-powered TENS units are limited to either pain or limited neuromuscular clinical procedures, and thus are not versatile. This limitation is intentional because many units are designed to be used and controlled by the patient. Simplicity of operation, safety, suitability for home use, and low cost are the main reasons for such limited versatility.

Interferential Current. Interferential current has been available in Europe since the early 1950s. Its popularity in the United States has become evident in the last 6 to 7 years following a vigorous advertising campaign. The interferential devices utilize two sinusoidal AC output circuits that differ somewhat in frequency. When these two outputs intersect, the frequency difference causes the sine waves' amplitudes to summate, resulting in the so-called "beat" or "envelope" (Fig. 3–18). From an electrophysiological perspective, each beat represents a polyphasic pulse.[54,57] From a strict electronic perspective, the interferential current can also be recognized as amplitude-modulated AC.[42,56] Detailed explanation of interferential current's electronic concepts are offered in Chapter 9. The significance of such electronic explanation to the physiologi-

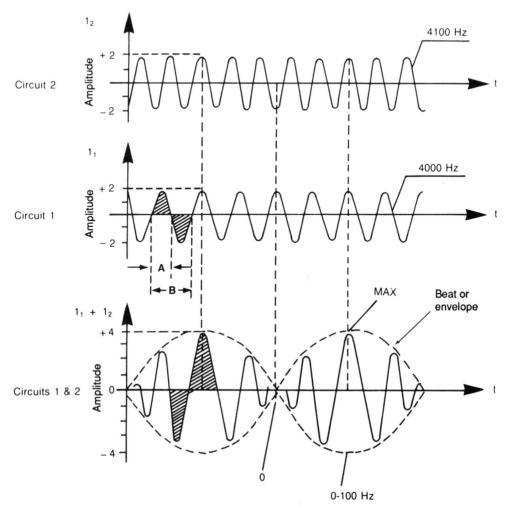

Figure 3–18. Generation of interference current. **A.** Phase duration. **B.** Pulse duration. Note that, when two circuits are in phase, the amplitude of the envelope is twice as high, providing intensity adequate for excitation.

cal responses and clinical results is most likely negligible. The parameters that seem most relevant and meaningful to the researchers and clinicians are often not acknowledged by the manufacturers and users (Table 3–2). Present knowledge strongly suggests that interferential current simply represents a different, and not the most effective, electronic approach to achieve the same basic physiological and clinical responses achieved by other TENS devices.

Objective testing of the many commercial claims used to promote the interferential stimulation proved them false. Interferential stimulators do not offer less skin impedance,[58] cannot penetrate deeper, and are not more effective in pain or edema management compared with other TENS devices. In fact, one clinical study failed to show any advantage of true interferential over placebo interferential current in reducing jaw pain.[86] Objective data showed that interferential current is inferior to symmetric biphasic waveform when comfort of stimulation was the test objective during neuromotor excitation. Recently, the conventional four-electrode arrangement of the interferential stimulator was shown to be less effective in controlling urinary incontinence than the two-electrode system where the interference occurs inside the stimulator (premodulation).[64] These data further discredit the promotional claims for uniqueness of the true interferential concept.[69]

By adding a "vector" system, or claiming a three-dimensional current flow by adding a third output, a mathematical argument occurs.[87] To date, no in-vitro experimental or clinical data have been found to support these concepts. In all likelihood, the therapist will still need to move the electrodes until the patient indicates that the excitatory perception is indeed in the target area that requires the stimulation.[64]

Interferential current, then, is simply a different electronic approach to achieve the same basic excitatory responses that monophasic and biphasic TENS units can achieve. Indeed, such an electronic approach is much less efficient or effective than conventional TENS. Among the reasons for diminished efficiency are excessive (unnecessary) total current as well as the need for four electrodes to establish only one channel.

The maximum total current of most interferential stimulators can reach 70 to 90 mA. In comparison, most other biphasic TENS units reach about 3 to 10 mA. Yet biphasic pulses of appropriate phase parameters can provide all of the basic excitatory responses, much like interferential current but with much less energy.[56]

The claim that automatic modulation of pulse rate can facilitate superior clinical results has not been supported by the literature.[70] Since clinical testing has so far failed to support such a claim for conventional TENS, it is unlikely that such support will be found when interferential current is used.

From an electrophysiological perspective, the main effect of interferential current occurs at the cellular level, much like other biphasic TENS units. Indirect effects of interferential current may involve the tissue, segmental, and systemic levels (see the previous section on TENS).

As a clinical stimulator, interferential units in their present design are not versatile and are quite expensive. They can provide only one or two procedures for pain management, reduction of joint effusion, and inhibition of protective muscle spasm. They are not suitable for muscle re-education because most units lack an interruption mode with independent ON, OFF, and ramp modulation.

They offer only a single channel, an additional drawback for clinical efficiency. Without available clinical data to support their superiority over conventional TENS, the interferential stimulators must be regarded as redundant because any electrophysiological response or clinical results they provide can be achieved more efficiently and at lower cost by other conventional stimulators.

Russian Current. The term *Russian current* applies to stimulators in which a continuous sine wave output of about 2500 Hz is modulated to yield 50 bursts per sec (bps). Each burst is actually a polyphasic pulse waveform.[54] From a strict electronic perspective, Russian current can be defined as time-modulated AC.[42,56] The important characteristics of the Russian current are summarized in Table 3–2. The generation of such current is illustrated in Figure 3–19. Contrary to promotional claims regarding the uniqueness and superiority of such a waveform for muscle activation, electrophysiological evaluation offers sound refutation of these claims. The reason for a carrier frequency of 2500 Hz is unlikely to be a unique medium-frequency effect on comfort of stimulation. Rather, and much as in the case of interferential current, it was selected by Dr. Kots[65] because the reciprocal of 2500-Hz frequency yields single pulse and phase durations of 400 and 200 μsec, respectively. Thus, the phase duration is narrowed to a range that correlates with relatively comfortable stimulation. Yet in accordance with the strength–duration curve, one must compensate for the shorter duration by increasing the pulse amplitude. The amount that the continuous sine wave amplitude under such conditions can be increased is limited, however, because under such conditions, total current is always between 65 and 70 percent of the peak. To limit total current output, the manufacturer of the Russian approach elected to time-modulate the sine wave into 50 bps by creating an interburst interval of 10 msec (Fig. 3–19). Such bursts reduce the total current somewhat and allow peak current amplitude and thus phase charge to increase so that a very powerful motor stimulation can be achieved.

The inefficiency of such an approach is again related to an excessively high total current (90 to 100 mA). Induced muscle contraction at 50 to 65 percent of MVC has been obtained with such current but also with a symmetric biphasic pulse.[21,22,59,63,78,88–91] The latter required only about one tenth of the total current of the former.[56] Other limitations of Russian current include less comfortable perception, fixed pulse rate in earlier units (that severely limited the number of clinical procedures that it could offer), and a fixed phase duration (so that adjustments for individual patient's comfort are not possible).[92,93]

✗The main physiological effect of Russian current is at the cellular level, but (indirectly) the tissue, segmental, and systemic levels may also be affected, as with other TENS stimulators.[21,59,63,65,89]✗Because of its present design, clinical uses are mainly restricted to muscle re-education treatments. Russian current is, therefore, one of the least versatile clinical stimulators presently available and is not cost effective.

High-Voltage Stimulation. As in the case of popular stimulators, many promotional claims regarding high voltage have caused tremendous confusion, misconception, and inappropriate use of these stimulators. A book by Alon and DeDomenico attempted to clarify many of these false claims.[54] This section reiterates the appropriate electrophysiological and clinical attributes of the high-voltage units.

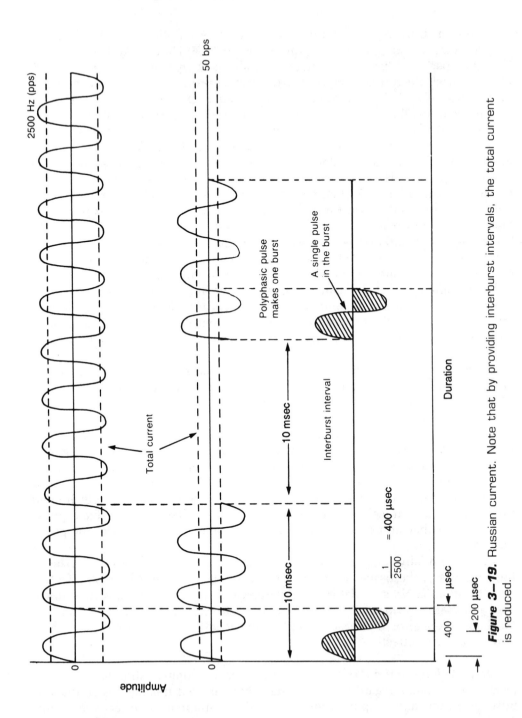

Figure 3–19. Russian current. Note that by providing interburst intervals, the total current is reduced.

is monophasic wave form

A high-voltage stimulator is *not* a galvanic stimulator. Its typical twin-peak pulse has no known significant physiological or clinical uniqueness, and a single peak is probably as effective for excitation as is the twin peak.[61] Thus, high-voltage units should simply be considered a monophasic pulsed TENS, with very short phase duration (5 to 20 μsec) and very high peak current amplitude (2000 to 2500 mA). It is obvious that when phase duration is so short, peak current must be very high (S–D curve), and that to generate such peak current, the voltage must also be high. This is the electrophysiological reason for high voltage. The interpulse intervals are very long and constitute at least 99 percent of each second (Fig. 3–20). Thus, total current is extremely low, reaching a maximum of only 1.2 to 1.5 mA. These and other characteristics are summarized in Table 3–2. Consequently, high-voltage stimulation can be used with both large and small electrodes.

The combination of very short pulse duration and high-peak current allows relatively comfortable stimulation. Furthermore, this combination provides an efficient means of exciting sensory, motor, and pain-conducting nerve fibers. Perceptual discrimination of the responses is relatively easy to achieve.

High-voltage stimulators are TENS units. As such, they directly affect the cellular level.[7,43] Indirect effects are at the tissue, segmental, and systemic levels, much as with other TENS units. Any attempt to attribute unique or different physiological responses to the application of high-voltage stimulation has yet to be demonstrated and is unlikely to succeed. The usefulness of the

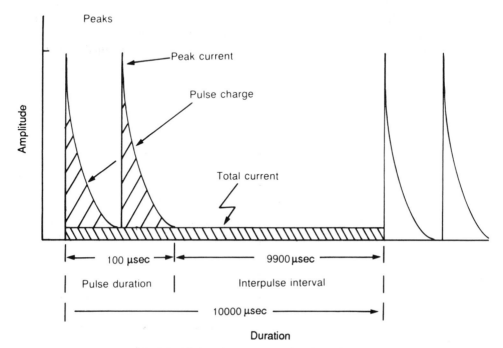

Figure 3–20. High-voltage monophasic pulsed current.

high voltage is therefore in its clinical versatility and not in its physiological superiority.

As clinical stimulators, high-voltage units offer many clinical uses.[54] All clinical methods for pain management,[36-39,85] reduction of joint effusion,[1,2,94] reduction of protective muscle spasm, acceleration of dermal and subdermal tissue regeneration,[8,11,95,96] muscle re-education,[97,98] and increasing venous blood flow are claimed to be achieved by those stimulators. Clinical versatility does not mean that high-voltage stimulators are the best units available and are without limitations. Indeed, they are not optimally designed. They are less than adequate for stimulation of large muscle groups; nor are they suitable for stimulation of denervated muscles or in iontophoresis.[8,58,99]

★ *Symmetrical Biphasic Pulsed Current.* In an effort to optimize stimulation parameters, researchers recently reported that symmetric biphasic waveform with interphase (also termed intrapulse) interval should be favored when excitation of peripheral nerves is the objective.[43,58-60,63,100] Other waveforms including monophasic, asymmetric biphasic, and AC modulated bursts (Russian and interferential) were all compared for perceived comfort of stimulation, but were consistently judged inferior to the symmetric biphasic by the majority of subjects.

The latter waveform was also shown to require less amount of phase charge during sensory and motor excitation compared to the Russian and interferential stimulators.[43,56,60] The interphase interval of 50 to 100 μsec between the two phases (Fig. 3–21) further optimizes peripheral nerve excitation as research have shown that less charge per phase is required compared with no interphase interval.[100] If in addition to the symmetric biphasic waveform

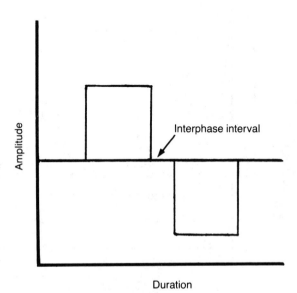

Figure 3–21. Symmetric biphasic waveform.

other parameters and modulation are incorporated in the design (Table 3–2), the relative comfort of stimulation can be ascertained and the most appropriate parameters can be enabled according to available stimulation protocols.

The major deficiency of the symmetric biphasic current could be the absence of polarity. A number of in-vitro and animal studies have indicated that either negative or positive polarity was detrimental to the achievement of non-excitatory effect associated with connective tissue regeneration and osteogenesis.[100–103] In contrast, clinical data may challenge the polarity concept as nonpolarized current consistently showed collagen formation and osteogenesis.[14,15,47,104,105] At present, the significance of polarity to clinical practice remains, therefore, an open question, and the use of symmetric biphasic waveform to effect non-excitatory processes such as tissue regeneration seems warranted.

✳**Subliminal Stimulation.** *for superfic stim* Subliminal or subthreshold TES devices are the ✳newest class of transcutaneous stimulators to be marketed. Although specifications on these stimulators are not readily available through the manufacturers, Table 3–3 provides a general description.

✳The uniqueness of this class of stimulators is their delivery of low total current that is unlikely to cause peripheral nerve excitation; thus the term "subliminal stimulation." The exception of this class of stimulators may occur when a device is set at maximum output and electrodes of 25 mm² or smaller are used. This situation may result from excitation of peripheral nerves if applied over very sensitive body areas (such as the ear or temporal region of the head). The patient may perceive the stimulation as stinging and unpleasant.

Several hypotheses have been offered for the physiological responses to subliminal stimulation. Manufacturers have claimed that such a device can

TABLE 3–3. CHARACTERISTICS OF THE SUBLIMINAL STIMULATORS

Source	Characteristics
Waveform	From reversing DC to monophasic
Mode	Continuous
Phase duration[a]	Inverse of frequency (1.5–500 msec)
Phase charge (maximum)	0.9–300 μC
Pulse frequency[b]	0.3–320 pps (adjustable)
Polarity	Yes
Total current	25–600 μA (adjustable)
Channels	One or two

[a] Shorter duration, higher frequency.

[b] Depends on frequency: lower frequency, higher charge.

(Modified from Alon G: Electro-orthopedics: A review of present electrophysiologic responses and clinical efficacy of transcutaneous stimulation. Adv Sports Med Fitness 2:295, 1989)

detect abnormal distribution of the body's bioelectrical conductivity, and that stimulation can reestablish normal conductive properties. The stimulation serves as a corrective measure to promote healing of various cells and tissues with dysfunction. This correction arrests the progression of pathological processes. Another hypothesis offered is that the servo mechanisms built into the devices augment athletic performance by supplementing the electrical energy required for optimal muscle contraction.[106,107] Subliminal stimulation has been reported to provide the bioelectrical balance needed to achieve alcohol detoxification and control of some psychological states.[108–110]

Supportive data of claims and hypotheses for subliminal stimulation are scarce and unconvincing. Manufacturers of subliminal stimulators frequently refer to studies using conventional TES devices that alter electrical energy in cell metabolism, ATP synthesis, calcium ion concentration, and serotonergic response.[101,111] Because subliminal stimulation is below tactile perception, controlled testing against a placebo is warranted. In one study subjects were asked the weight that they could lift after receiving six 30-minute subliminal stimulation treatments. This study, however, was an uncontrolled and non-parametrial approach to measure effects of subliminal stimulation, and published in an unrefereed journal and distributed by the manufacturer.[106] In a double-blind study in which subliminal stimulation was compared with a placebo during one exercise session, the results did not reveal significant differences between the placebo and stimulation groups for muscle strength, endurance, or postexercise soreness.[112]

Solomon and Guglielmo compared amplitudes of stimulation with control and placebo groups for effects on headaches. They found significant reduction of headaches only in the group that perceived the electrical stimulation, and concluded that subliminal stimulation was no better than placebo.[113] The chiropractic literature is limited to a single report of objective testing of subliminal stimulation on acute and chronic pain, protective muscle spasm, inflammatory reaction, and musculoskeletal/neurological dysfunction.[114] This identical study was published by different authors.[115]

One study used a questionnaire that asked the locations of undefined pain, severity of pain, and the number of treatments for relief to compare "conventional therapy" to "microneural stimulation." Questions on adverse responses, cost, and treatment effectiveness were also compared. The investigators stated that pain was resolved using subliminal stimulation, regardless of diagnosis. The treatment was cost effective because only two to six treatments were required before discharging 66 percent of the subliminal group compared with 21 percent for the conventional therapy group.[116] Numerous flaws limit this study to a pilot approach because different therapists were assigned to treatment groups; lack of homogeneity because of diagnoses not given; subjective, retrospective questionnaire; undisclosed treatment procedures; and commercialism.[116] Competence of the practitioner must be questioned since 36 percent of the patients following conventional therapy were reported to have "severe" yet undefined adverse reactions.

⋆Case studies in which subliminal stimulation is claimed to have relieved alcohol and drug addiction, musculoskeletal, audiological, and even nerve regeneration pathologies have been used in advertisements.[117–121] These same case studies have not been reported in peer reviewed professional journals, and in the absence of objective data they cannot be considered more effective than a placebo.

FUNDAMENTAL PHYSIOLOGICAL RESPONSES

One of the most difficult tasks facing the clinician has been to organize, comprehend, and interpret electrophysiological information into a functional, clinically practical, and integrated data base. Having no such system, much of the physiological data cannot be systematically related to the pathological processes that electrical stimulation may be capable of modifying. The purpose of this section is to offer a new framework that organizes the fundamental physiological responses elicited by transcutaneous stimulation. Such clinically oriented organization can then be used to examine the physiological correlates of either pulsed or nonpulsed currents and will enable the clinician to better integrate such knowledge with the clinical signs and symptoms that electrical stimulation attempts to resolve. (Physiological correlates of electrical stimulators are presented in detail in other chapters.)

Biological Effects

The flow of electrical current through a biological conductive medium results in three basic effects. These direct effects may be recognized as electrothermal, electrochemical, and electrophysical. Theoretically, every time electrical current flows, all three effects occur. They can be identified and measured with appropriate equipment at the cellular level. Recognizing which of the three effects dominates during the stimulation is a prerequisite for the understanding of the physiological responses to electric stimulation.

Electrothermal Effect. The mobility of charged particles in a conductive medium causes microvibration of these particles. This vibration and the associated frictional forces leads to the production of heat.[67,79] The amount of electrical-to-heat conversion is described by Joule's law: The amount of heat production (H) is proportional to the square of the total current (I^2), the resistance (R), and the time (t) for which the current flows, (ie, treatment time). The formula is expressed by the equation:

$$H = 0.24 \ I^2Rt.$$

The heat production is given in gram-calories. From a clinical perspective, high total current, high skin impedance, and prolonged treatment time may all lead to a measurable thermal effect. If DC stimulation is used, skin impedance is usually high, so both the amplitude and treatment time must be minimized to avoid excessive thermal effect. If a continuous AC is used, skin impedance decreases as frequency increases. As long as the total current amplitude is low (up to a few milliamps), the thermal effect will decrease as frequency increases. However, usually there is a need to increase current amplitude with these stimulators; consequently an increase in thermal effect can be calculated. A pulsed current having a very short phase duration (5–200 μsec) and a pulse rate of up to 100 to 200 pps usually results in a much smaller total current compared to AC as well as significant reduction of skin impedance. As a result the thermal effect of pulsed current is usually dramatically lower than that provided by an AC stimulator.[54] Finally, it must be emphasized that the aforementioned differences in thermal effects between DC, AC, and pulsed stimulators are more theoretical than practical as all three stimulator categories cause heat production that is so minimal that it cannot be measured at the tissue level[54] and may not have a known physiological effect even at the cellular level.

Electrochemical Effects. Electrochemical effects are recognized when the conducted current causes formation of new chemical compounds. The steady state of existing chemical compounds is being altered by the current flow, an electrolytic phenomenon most recognized with the application of DC stimulation. The unidirectional flow of DC redistributes sodium and chlorine to form a new chemical compound in the tissue under the electrodes. These changes at the tissue level (see next section) can be summarized as:

$$2Na + 2H_2O \longrightarrow 2NaOH + H_2 \text{ (alkalin)}.$$
$$2Cl_2 + 2H_2O \longrightarrow 4\ HCl + O_2 \text{ (acid)}.$$

The alkalin and acid formation occur under the negative and positive electrode, respectively.[46,79] The release of hydrogen and oxygen may be involved in further chemical reactions, particularly at the cellular level.

As long as these DC-induced chemical reactions are not excessive, the normal response of the intact body is to increase local blood flow in order to restore the normal pH of the tissue. Chemical changes that exceed the body's ability to reverse them and reestablish the steady state will result in blistering or even chemical burns of the stimulated tissue. Decreasing current amplitude, shortening treatment time, or reversing polarity every few seconds or minutes minimizes such hazards.

Practical elimination of chemical change at the tissue level can be obtained if a pulsed rather than DC current is used. Absence of measurable chemical changes at tissue level does not indicate that electrochemical changes do not take place at the cellular level. Indeed, the origin of the electrolytic process is in each cell. But the changes are so minute and transient that the clinical significance of such changes has only recently appeared in the literature. Specifically, it has been proposed that the electrochemical reaction occurs between the mitochondrial membrane-bound H⁶ adenosine triphosphatase (ATPase) and adenosine diphosphate (ADP), which leads to the formation of

ATP. Synthesis of DNA by electrical current has also been demonstrated at the cellular level but the associated chemical reaction has not been elucidated.[93] Enzymatic activity facilitation of succinate dehydrogenase (SDH) and ATPase has likewise been reported.[27,111,122,123] Whether or not such enzymatic facilitation is electrochemically mediated is not clear at the present time. It must be emphasized that these electrochemical cellular changes have been demonstrated to occur through the use of either DC or monophasic pulsed currents.[101,111]

Two of Faraday's laws can be used to quantify the amount of chemical changes during an electrolytic reaction. One law indicates that the amount of chemical reaction is directly proportional to the quantity of electricity passing through the electrolytic solution. Quantification of the electrical current is obtained by calculating the phase charge, total current, or both. The charge delivered by a clinical DC stimulator may reach 5000 to 60,000 μC. "Since current equals coulomb/sec,'" this charge is equivalent to 5 to 60 mA of total current. On the other hand, clinical monophasic stimulators usually reach only 12 to 20 μC and 1.5 to 2 mA of total current. This can explain why burns of the tissue can result from careless application of DC current while the chemical effects of a pulsed current do not present any known significantly harmful effects.

Faraday's second law states that the amount of various electrolytic substances liberated by a given amount of phase charge is directly proportional to their chemical equivalent weights. Thus, at the cellular level the electrolysis is likely to affect the calcium ions more than it affects the potassium or sodium ions. Calcium is highly associated with the cellular process of muscle contraction and relaxation as well as with the formation and remodeling of connective and osseous tissues. In contrast to calcium, potassium, chlorine, and sodium are associated with the process of nerve excitation. The fact that one can observe nerve excitation long before the electrolytic effects on bone, connective tissue, or muscle may be related to the electrolytic quantities and concentration that are required to cause these different physiological changes. To achieve the calcium-dependent electrophysiological effects, a longer treatment time of several hours daily is probably indicated. In fact, the electrical effect on calcium, potassium, sodium, and other ions' concentration and dynamics may not be electrochemical but rather electrophysical.

Electrophysical Effects. Unlike the electrochemical, the electrophysical effects do not cause change in the molecular configuration of ions. Rather, the electrical charge causes movement of the ions whether they are electrolytes or non-dissociated molecules such as proteins or lipoproteins. The electrophysical effect has also been termed electrokinetic effect. The best known physiological consequences of such ionic movement include the excitation of peripheral nerves, where in the presence of adequate phase charge the sodium and potassium ions move across the cell membrane. Such direct cellular effects may lead to many different indirect responses, including the contractions of skeletal or smooth muscles, activation of endogenous analgesic mechanisms, and various vascular responses, all of which are discussed in other chapters of this text and other sources.[54]

Other direct cellular effects are associated with the electrophysical influence on ions that are not part of nerve excitation. Electrolytes such as calcium and magnesium and other ions such as free amino acids and proteins are also forced to move in the presence of current flow through the tissue. Such movement may lead to increases or decreases in their concentration and trigger a host of subsequent indirect physiological responses.[124,125] In a broad sense, many of the direct effects that occur at the cellular level can be classified as excitatory and non-excitatory responses.

Physiological Model

As electrical current is conducted through a conductive biologic medium, alteration in physiological processes can occur at various levels of the total system. Functionally, four levels can be recognized: cellular, tissue, segmental, and systemic.

At each level, many different processes can be affected by the stimulation, which in turn may enhance or suppress the respective physiological activities. Furthermore, the effect of the stimulation can be direct, indirect, or both.

The main effects of the stimulation at each of the four levels are listed in the following outline (D = direct; ID = indirect; * = unknown):

1. Cellular level
   a. Excitation of peripheral nerves (D).
   b. Changes of membrane permeability of non- or less excitatory cells (calcium channels) (D or ID).
   c. Modification of fibroblasts and fibroblastic formation (D or ID).
   d. Modification of osteoblasts and osteoclastic formation (D or ID).
   e. Modification of microcirculation—arterial, venous, and lymphatic (capillary flow) (*).
   f. Alteration of protein and blood-cell concentration (*).
   g. Alteration of enzymatic activity, such as SDH and ATPase (D or ID).
   h. Alteration of protein synthesis (D).
   i. Modification of mitochondrial size and concentration (D or ID).
2. Tissue level
   a. Skeletal muscle contraction and its effects on muscle strength, contraction speed, reaction time, and fatigability (ID).
   b. Smooth muscle contraction or relaxation and its effects on arterial and venous blood flow (ID).
   c. Tissue regeneration, including bone, ligament, connective, and dermal tissues (D or ID).
   d. Tissue remodeling, including softening, stretching, decreasing viscosity, and fluid absorption from joint cavities, and interstitial spaces (D or ID).
   e. Changes in tissue thermal and chemical balance (D).

3. Segmental level
   a. Muscle group contraction and its effect on joint mobility and synergistic muscle activity (ID).
   b. Muscle pumping action effects on the lymphatic drainage, venous, and arterial blood flow of large circulatory and lymphatic vessels (macrocirculation) (ID).
   c. Alteration of lymphatic drainage and arterial blood flow not associated with skeletal muscle contraction (ID).
4. Systemic level
   a. Analgesic effects associated with endogenous polypeptides, such as beta-endorphins, enkephalins, dopamines, and dymorphins (ID).
   b. Analgesic effects associated with neurotransmitters, such as serotonin and substance P (ID).
   c. Circulatory effects associated with polypeptides, such as vasoactive intestinal polypeptides (VIP) (ID).
   d. Modulation of internal organ activity, such as kidney and heart functions (ID).

Regardless of the form of electrical current used, there is always a direct effect, usually electrochemical and electrophysical, at the cellular level under the stimulating electrodes. This direct effect can also prevail at the tissue level if a DC or a very-long-phase-duration (50 to 300 msec) monophasic waveform is used. Provided that pulse rate is extremely high (several hundred to several thousand pulses), even pulses of very short duration can induce direct tissue response, but such clinical stimulators are not presently available. Direct effects at tissue level (mostly electrophysical and possibly electrothermal) may also occur with a symmetric biphasic or polyphasic pulse, if the total current per unit area (current density, phase charge density, or both) is excessively high.

Indirect effects of current flow are expected at all four levels. Indirect alterations of cellular, tissue, segmental, and systemic functions are defined as those physiological reactions or responses that are triggered by the direct effects. They may occur at or remote from the area where the current flows.

The combination of direct and indirect effects results in physiological response to the application of surface stimulation. Depending on the electrical stimulation procedure, the relevant responses must be recognized and must be specified as the physiological targets of the stimulation. Within the limits of present knowledge, the achievement of clinical results seems to be highly dependent on the establishment of appropriate physiological responses.

The use of such a model can be demonstrated in the following example: When electrical stimulation is used to suppress pain, the direct effect occurs at the cellular level, where pulsed or AC modulated currents cause excitation of peripheral nerve cells. The indirect physiological effects predominate at the systemic level, as indicated by the release of endogenous analgesic substances, such as endorphins, enkephalins, and serotonin.

Another example is related to the use of stimulation to retard muscle atrophy because of disuse and to enhance a muscle's capacity to develop contractile force. Direct effect is obtained at the cellular level by the excitation of peripheral nerves. Unlike the previous example, however, where predominantly sensory fibers were excited, the motor fibers are excited as well. The indirect physiological effect occur at both tissue and segmental levels. The contraction of skeletal muscle fibers represents the tissue level. If a sufficient number of motor units is activated, the whole muscle or muscle group will contract. This activity may be coupled with movement at the joint. If few muscle groups are stimulated, few segments are affected simultaneously. Additional, indirect physiologic responses resulting from muscle contraction include cellular-level modification of capillary blood flow and enhancement of SDH and ATPase activity. Indirect segmental response includes large-vessel blood flow associated with the pumping action of the muscles.

A direct physiological effect that simultaneously involves both cellular and tissue levels is usually associated with a DC stimulation. The unidirectional, continuous current flow alters the pH of the cells and tissue under the electrodes. The indirect physiological response is vasodilation of arterial capillaries (cellular) and small arteries (tissue) in an attempt to restore the steady-state pH and temperature of the affected tissue.

The foregoing discussion and examples may suffice to draw a conclusion. Knowledge of the electrical current and its waveform, recognition of its direct and indirect effects, and understanding of the physiological levels at which these effects take place, can provide a systematic, clinically oriented framework. This model can then be used to select the treatment method needed to obtain the best clinical results. Furthermore, the model may serve to improve communication among the various professionals and eliminate the use of undefined, ambiguous terminology; for example, that TENS is used to "improve circulation," "heal tissue," or "balance the body's energy."

Physiological Correlates of Electrical Stimulation

Generally stated, transcutaneous stimulation can induce *direct* physiological responses in both the excitatory and the non-excitatory systems. A short summary of those responses follows.

Non-excitatory Responses. All living cells depend, in part, on various magnitudes of internally generated electrical potentials. The source of these potentials seems to be associated with the concentration gradient of ions across the cell membrane.[126,127] Changes in the concentration gradient may be linked with the opening of ion channels and lead to enhancement of DNA and protein synthesis.[101,122,128,129] One may hypothesize that such protein synthesis and the resultant enhanced formation of collagen fiber is clinically significant. But clinical evidence that resuscitation of dermal and subdermal connective tissues can be accelerated by externally applied electric current is inconclusive.[8,11,13,95] Similarly, bone tissue (and possibly, ligaments and cartilage) can also be remodeled in the presence of appropriate quantities of voltage and current.[48-51]

The exact mechanism by which such stimulation influences the non-excitatory cells is very complex and, at present, has not been elucidated. First, whether the process is electrochemical, electrophysical, or both is not clear and is rarely identified in the literature. Second, different cells at different states (ie, pathological or normal) seem to respond differently to electrical energy. Proteins are an example of charged ions that, when abnormally present in the interstitial spaces or joint cavities, may be displaced into the lymphatic capillaries.[52,53,124,130] On the other hand, the proteins that are the building blocks of collagenous fibrous tissues seem to be synthesized rather than displaced with the stimulation.[13,101,102,104] Other ions (such as sodium, calcium, potassium, and magnesium) play a major role in the function of non-excitatory cells. The mobility and concentration of these ions may also be affected in part by externally induced electrical energy. Consequently, tissue metabolism and nutrition may be enhanced.[131]

Hypothetically, any current flow through a conductive medium should have some *direct* influence on non-excitatory cells. If the current source is DC, then a direct effect on the *tissue* level should also be realized, as pH and temperature changes can occur.[79] Modern pulsed currents *directly* affect only the cells. The *indirect* effect of both current sources is hypothesized to be associated with circulatory response. Pulsed current's effect on cell metabolism may lead to increased microcirculation, including arterial, venous, and lymphatic capillary exchange. Experimental evidence supporting these effects on human subjects is limited,[132] and the most appropriate pulse parameters to achieve effective non-excitatory cell response have not been determined. But the reader must realize that, whether electrical stimulation is used for pain management, muscle re-education, edema reduction, or protective muscle spasm, non-excitatory and excitatory cells are both affected by the current flow.

Excitatory Responses. Excitation of peripheral nerves by transcutaneous stimulation is a well-established phenomenon. Stimulation directly affects the nerve cells. Larger-diameter nerve fibers are known to become excited before smaller-diameter nerve fibers do. Strength–duration (S–D) curves have been established for each of the three main groups of fibers, including those that transmit tactile and pressure stimuli, motor impulses, and painful or noxious stimuli.[133,134] A typical response of these three nerve categories is illustrated in Figure 3–22.

A clinical, functional, interpretation of these excitatory responses (and related literature) may warrant the following observations:

1. The three basic excitatory responses to transcutaneous stimulation are perceived as **sensory, motor, and painful** stimulation.
2. The excitation proceeds in the order of sensory stimulation, motor stim-

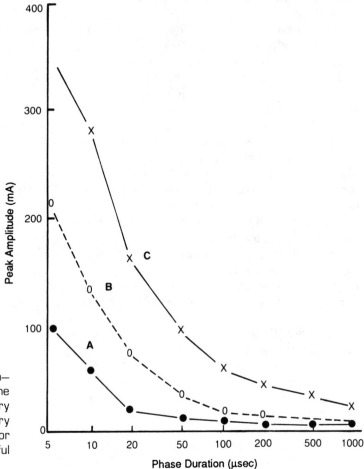

Figure 3—22. Strength–duration curves of the three major excitory responses. **A.** Sensory stimulation. **B.** Motor stimulation. **C.** Painful stimulation.

ulation, and painful stimulation. This order prevails regardless of pulse duration, waveform, or pulse rate, as long as all three nerve groups are at approximately the same distance from the stimulating electrode.

3. Perceptual discrimination among the three responses is more easily achieved if pulse duration is set in the range of 20 to 200 μsec.[133,135] Electrode size also affects this perceptual discrimination.[136]

4. From a physiological perspective that ignores discriminatory perception or electronic efficiency, it should make no difference what combination of pulse duration (in microseconds or milliseconds) and amplitude (in milliamps) is used to achieve the excitation. Once excited, the nerve impulses will propagate and will provide the indirect physiological responses. In contrast, variations of pulse rate alter the frequency of firing of the excited nerves. Different firing rates affect some of the

indirect physiological responses; most notably the types of muscle contraction and (possibly) the endogenous analgesic mechanism.[111,137]

Whereas the direct effect of transcutaneously exciting the peripheral nerves is well understood and the limits well drawn, the indirect effects are numerous, less well defined, and only partially established. The scope of indirect physiological responses may be realized by recognizing that all biologic systems can be influenced by the afferent and efferent neurological pathways. Thus, neuromusculoskeletal, vascular, endocrine, digestive, respiratory, and limbic functions can all be indirectly affected by TENS. Many of these indirect effects are discussed in the remaining chapters of this text, although at present many others have not been established.

The complexity of indirect physiological responses is increased by their simultaneous interaction. For example, motor excitation causes muscle contraction, which leads to waste products. Lactic acid formation requires increased blood flow to remove it.[26] Yet under normal conditions, electrical stimulation may not reduce,[138,139] or even affect, peripheral blood flow.[140] These seemingly contradictory responses are likely to be resolved physiologically by a poststimulation increase in muscle blood flow. Clinically, the resolution of the complex responses may greatly depend on the use of proper stimulation procedures and clinical monitoring of the physiological responses to the stimulation. The question is, how can this be done practically in the clinic?

Establishing specific values of current amplitude, in milliamperes or volts, for each clinical problem is unlikely to yield appropriate physiological responses. Differences in body parts and pathologies, continuous changes in tissue conductivity, intersubject variation, and differences in stimulators and electrode size are just some of the uncontrolled variables that all but prevent the clinician from selecting standard machine settings based on measured current amplitude. A much better approach to providing standardized and systematic treatment techniques is offered on the basis of the direct excitatory responses perceived by the patient.

As discussed earlier, the three categories of perceived excitation are sensory, motor, and painful stimulation. Each of the three can be established despite the aforementioned uncontrolled variables. Once the prescribed excitatory level is achieved, the clinician can estimate (or measure, if possible) some of the indirect physiological responses. For example, when motor excitation is indicated, the therapist can estimate both the strength of a muscle contraction and muscle fatigue. Such estimation should help to promote faster strength development while eliminating muscle soreness. Similarly, neurovascular vasoconstriction usually requires only minimal sensory excitation. By setting current amplitude to such an excitatory level, the therapist can then evaluate skin temperature and color and can ascertain the changes of the indirect physiological responses. Having established the resultant physiological targets of the stimulation, clinical results can be predicted with much greater certainty.

The presented physiological model is sufficiently functional to include most of the clinical situations but nevertheless bears some limitations. It does not include one additional dimension — subliminal, non-perceived stimulation. This is because most clinical problems seem to respond better to perceived excitation. Another difficulty may arise when stimulation is provided to patients with sensory loss, as sensory excitation may not be perceived by the subject. The astute therapist, however, can find several procedures that will overcome such difficulties.

In summary, physiological responses to TENS occur at four levels of the biologic system (cellular, tissue, segmental, and systemic). The effects can be direct and indirect, and they may involve simple, well-established physiological responses as well as a very complex, largely unknown chain of interactive physiological correlates of such stimulation. In daily practice, the therapist must recognize the currently known responses, establish the appropriate treatment method, and set the stimulation parameters to achieve the sensory, motor, or painful perception indicated by treatment goals. Adequate excitatory responses, and evaluation of clinically measurable indirect responses, are likely to provide the therapist with systematic, reproducible, and clinically successful utilization of transcutaneous stimulation.

Relevant Laws and Calculation. There are many laws and equations associated with both the electrical and physiological aspects of electrotherapy. Knowledge of some of them may help the clinician to better understand the interrelationships among the various stimulation parameters and their influence on the clinical application of electrotherapy.

The law of excitation expresses the interaction of voltage, current, charge, and energy required to excite peripheral nerves.[45] Two of these parameters, phase charge and total current, may have immediate clinical relevance. Skin impedance is an additional factor of clinical concern. Phase charge is a term with which most clinicians are not familiar, yet it is the phase charge that determines whether or not a nerve will be excited. Phase charge is a term that defines the quantity of electricity delivered with each phase of each pulse to the tissue. Insufficient charge will fail to excite the nerve, while excessive charge may harm the tissue.

Phase Charge. For a constant-current stimulator having a monophasic square-wave pulse (Fig. 3–23), phase charge (q) is represented by the area under the curve and is expressed as the product of phase duration (t) and peak current amplitude (*I*).

$$q = I \times t. \tag{1}$$

A symmetric biphasic square-wave pulse having two equal phases can be expressed as

$$q = I \cdot t \times 2. \tag{2}$$

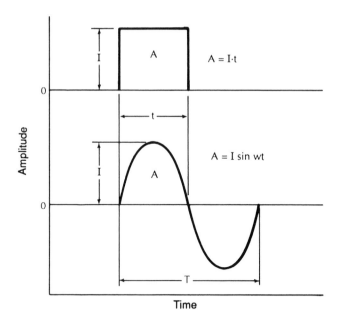

Figure 3–23. Monophasic square wave and symmetrical biphasic sine wave.

A symmetric sine wave pulse (Fig. 3–23) is expressed as

$$I(t) = I \sin \omega T. \tag{3}$$

where

- $I(t)$ = current amplitude in amperes as a function of time (t) in seconds,
- I = peak current amplitude (amperes),
- ω = angular velocity (radians/sec), and
- T = period of one cycle (sec).

Angular velocity (ω) is related to the frequency (f) and the period (T) by

$$f = \omega/2\pi \text{ and } T = 2\pi/\omega. \tag{4}$$

One phase duration is defined by the interval between $t = 0$ and $t = T/2 = \pi/\omega$. Therefore, each phase charge (q) is given by the integral over this time interval, yielding

$$q = I \omega (\cos 0 - \cos \pi/\omega) = 2I/\omega. \tag{5}$$

Since $\omega = 2\pi f$, the phase charge equation can be written as

$$q = I/\pi f. \tag{6}$$

Equations 1 and 6 are used to calculate the phase charge of a monophasic pulse and a burst modulated AC sine wave, respectively. Assuming that peak current amplitude $I = 200$ mA and that phase duration $t = 200 \times 10^{-3}$ msec (200 μsec), then

1. Monophasic square pulse:

$$q = I \times t = 200 \times 10^{-3} \times 200 = 40 \ \mu C.$$

2. One phase of a 2500-Hz burst modulated AC sine wave (e.g., of the Russian current):

$$q = \frac{I}{\pi f} = \frac{200 \times 10^{-3}}{3.14 \times 2500} = \frac{200 \times 10^{-3}}{7.850 \times 10^3} = 25.4 \times 10^{-6} = 25.4 \ \mu C.$$

The following conclusions can be drawn:

- The charge delivered by a square wave is significantly greater than that of the sine wave.
- Comparison of a symmetric biphasic square-wave pulse with a symmetric biphasic sine wave is accomplished by doubling the charge delivered by one phase. In our example, the results are 80 versus 50.8 μC for the square and sine waves, respectively.
- The calculations demonstrate that for equal phase durations one needs significantly less amplitude to excite the nerve with square waves than with sine waves. Thus, sine wave is a less efficient wave form for excitation.
- Any change in phase duration must require a concomitant adjustment of pulse amplitude in order to provide the same charge.

Stimulators known as high-voltage stimulators are designed as constant-voltage, rather than constant-current, stimulators. To calculate phase charge for this monophasic, twin-peak pulse, the following equation is used:

$$q = CV. \tag{7}$$

where

- C = capacitance of output capacitors (μF), and
- V = voltage intensity (volts).

Typically, there are two output capacitors, one (q_1) of 0.010 μF and a second (q_2) of 0.015 μF, representing the first and second peaks of the pulse, respectively. Assuming the maximal voltage output V = 500 volts, the phase charge of the first spike is

$$q = 0.010 \times 10^{-6} \times 500 = 5 \times 10^{-6} = 5 \ \mu C.$$

The phase charge of the second spike is

$$q_2 = 0.015 \times 10^{-6} \times 500 = 7.5 \times 10^{-6} = 7.5 \ \mu C.$$

Summing the two peaks of the pulse:

$$q_p = q_1 + q_2 = 5 \ \mu C + 7.5 \ \mu C = 12.5 \ \mu C.$$

Additional observations can now be made regarding the clinical aspects of phase charge:

- Compared with other TENS units, which can deliver 25 to 40 μC of charge per phase, the presently available high-voltage stimulators may only reach 12.5 μC. Yet the high-voltage stimulators are very effective in causing excitation of sensory, motor, and pain-conducting fibers. The reason for this effectiveness is explained by the law of excitation, which states that at shorter phase durations less charge is needed to cause threshold excitation.[41,133]
- Despite being called high voltage, these stimulators are not powerful. Indeed, one of their deficiencies is phase charge insufficient to strongly activate large muscle groups, such as the quadriceps femoris muscle.[109,112]
- Whether one uses high voltage or low voltage, or whether the pulse is monophasic, biphasic, or polyphasic, makes no difference. As long as there is sufficient phase charge for a given phase duration, excitation of the nerve will occur. This statement holds true whether the charge is negative or positive.[56,138,141]

Total (Averaged) Current Determination. Total current can be defined as the coulomb/sec or the amount of current flow per second. Because most modern clinical stimulators deliver pulsed currents, peak current amplitude is always significantly higher than total current. Determination of the total current of a pulsed current stimulator can be obtained using the following equation:

$$I_{tot} = q/T. \tag{8}$$

where

- q = phase charge (C), and
- T = pulse (period) duration (sec).

using the relationships $f = 1/T$, equation (8) can be written as

$$I_{tot} = q \times f. \tag{9}$$

where

- f = frequency of applied current (Hz).

Knowing the waveform and the number of pulses per second, one can calculate the total current. For example, having a phase charge $q = 20$ μC, the following calculations are made for monophasic and biphasic pulses and burst-modulated AC:

1. Monophasic pulses at 50 pps will yield

$$I_{tot} = 20 \times 10^{-6} \times 50 = 1 \times 10^{-3} = 1 \text{ mA}.$$

2. Symmetric biphasic pulses at 50 pps contain 100 phases. The total current is

$$I_{tot} = 20 \times 10^{-6} \times 100 = 2 \times 10^{-3} = 2 \text{ mA}.$$

3. A burst-modulated AC such as the one used by the Russian current occurs in bursts, each containing 25 sine wave pulses, or 50 phases. Using 50 bursts per second means that 2500 phases are delivered each second. Thus,

$$I_{tot} = 20 \times 10^{-6} \times 2500 = 50 \times 10^{-3} = 50 \text{ mA}.$$

Knowing the total current is of major importance to the clinician because excessive total current (called average current by many clinicians) may be harmful to the tissue. If electrode size is known, total current density is determined through division of the total current by electrode area. The preceding calculations lead to the following observations:

- In pulsed stimulators, the number of pulses per second directly affects the total (averaged) current. Even if peak current amplitude reaches 1000 to 2000 mA, the total current may be only 1 mA if phase duration is short and pulse rate is low.
- Monophasic and biphasic waveforms dramatically deliver less total current than burst-modulated AC such as Russian current if the number of pulses is equivalent.
- Because the objective is to induce the desired physiological responses with the minimum necessary total current, a monophasic or biphasic pulse is far more efficient than the Russian or interferential stimulators. The efficiency reflects both physiological and electronic design criteria. If total current is low, then small electrodes can be used, because density will remain within tolerable and safe limits. The pulsed current stimulators are a good example because of their very low total current. Consequently, both large and small electrodes are used clinically without causing harm. Russian or interferential currents must not be used with small electrodes, because their total current may reach 80 to 100 mA and may cause skin irritation or burn.

Total current is proportionate to the amount of heat production in the tissue. The equation to express electrical-to-thermal energy conversion is:

$$H = 0.24 \ I^2 Rt. \tag{10}$$

where

- H = heat generation (gram-calories, or g-cal),
- I = total current (A),
- R = tissue resistance (ohms, or Ω),
- t = treatment time (sec), and
- 0.24 is a constant.

Let us use the current values of 1, 2, and 50 mA, calculated previously for monophasic, biphasic, and bursts (polyphasic) pulses, respectively. Let us assume electrode–skin impedance of 500 Ω and treatment time of 30 min. The thermal effects are summarized in Table 3–4. Let us assume the following changes:

TABLE 3-4. THERMAL EFFECT OF ELECTRICAL STIMULATION

Waveform	Calculation	Results (g-cal)
Monophasic	$0.24 \times (1.0 \times 10^{-3})^2 \times 500 \times 1800$	0.18
Biphasic	$0.24 \times (2.0 \times 10^{-3})^2 \times 500 \times 1800$	0.81
Polyphasic	$0.24 \times (50 \times 10^{-3})^2 \times 500 \times 1800$	540.00

- Smaller electrode size so that skin impedance is increased to 800 Ω.
- Pulse rate is 100 pps instead of 50 pps. Thus total current is now 2, 4, and 100 mA for monophasic waveforms, biphasic waveforms, and burst-modulated AC, respectively.

The new calculation yields the following results: monophasic, 1.29 g-cal; biphasic, 5.47 g-cal; and burst-modulated AC, 3456.00 g-cal.

The preceding calculations clearly indicate the potentially harmful thermal effect of bursts on the skin.

Skin Impedance. Skin impedance is one major obstacle to current penetration into the deeper tissues, and it should be minimized by proper stimulator design and good treatment technique. The equation denoting impedance (Z) is:

$$Z = \sqrt{R^2 + (X_L - X_c)^2}. \tag{11}$$

where

- R = static resistance (Ω),
- X_L = inductive reactance (Ω), and
- X_c = capacitative reactance (Ω).

Inductive reactance (X_L) is negligible in a biologic medium, and resistance (R) is not altered by pulsed current. Thus, only capacitative reactance (X_c) can be reduced by proper stimulation parameters. The equation denoting XC is:

$$X_C = \frac{1}{2\pi f C}. \tag{12}$$

where

- π = constant (3.14),
- f = frequency of applied voltage (Hz), and
- C = capacitance of tissue (farads).

Equation (12) indicates that, the higher the frequency, the lower the capacitative resistance. This outcome is the basis for the claims that interferential current at frequencies of 4000 to 5000 Hz reduces skin impedance and therefore penetrates better than other TENS units. Frequency, however, is related to phase duration (*t*) by the equations:

$$f = 1/I. \tag{13a}$$

$$t = T/2. \tag{13b}$$

$$t = 1/2f. \tag{13c}$$

where

- f = frequency of applied voltage (Hz),
- I = current amplitude (A),
- T = pulse duration (sec), and
- t = phase duration (sec).

Remembering that phase duration $t = T/2$, it is obvious that the higher the frequency the shorter the phase duration. Thus, phase duration is proportional to skin impedance. Stated differently, the shorter the phase duration, the lower the skin impedance. This statement is true even if the number of pulses is low. The clinical implications are as follows:

- Interferential current does not reduce skin impedance and does not penetrate deeper than other TENS.[58] The phase duration of present interferential units (4000 Hz) is 125 µsec. Any monophasic or biphasic wave form having a 125 µsec phase duration will have the same skin impedance as an interferential current.[50]
- Electrode size and voltage also affect skin impedance. Therefore, claiming that "medium" frequency is the major factor in reducing skin impedance is misleading and is ignored by the astute therapist.

SURFACE ELECTRODES

Surface electrodes serve as the interface between the stimulator and human conductive tissues. They are an integral part of the total stimulation system and play a critical role in whether the desired physiologic response is achieved in the patient. Of great importance in understanding surface electrodes is recognizing lead arrangements, selecting adequate electrode size, and appropriately placing electrodes. The absence of consistent and appropriate terminology has resulted in the misuse of electrodes in clinical practice and has caused clinical efforts to fail. The purpose of this section is to provide functionally appropriate definitions and explanations of the aforementioned concepts.

The Leads

Regardless of the stimulator name, manufacturer, or waveform, there is always a pair of leads emerging from its panel. Contrary to widespread belief, neither lead is a ground. The two leads simply represent the two segments of a circuit that, when connected to the body part, will provide a conductive path for electric-current flow. If not connected to the body, a potential difference (generated by the stimulator) will exist between them, but current will not flow because the circuit is not closed.

If either a direct-current or a monophasic-pulsed current stimulator is considered, then one lead, and the electrode(s) connected to it, will be positive with respect to the second lead: this is equivalent to saying that the second lead is negative relative to the first lead. This factor does not mean, however, that one of the leads is a ground. It is correct to say that there is a polarity difference between the two leads. The recognition of lead polarity is important in those few cases where a treatment method requires specific polarity.

The application of DC stimulation includes a well-established polarity selection, particularly when iontophoresis is used.[82] If a monophasic pulsed current (such as high voltage) is used, stimulation polarity may be important only when applied for skin ulcers and wound healing.[8,61] When treating pain, joint effusion, muscle-disuse atrophy, protective muscle spasm, or joint range-of-motion, there do not seem to be any data in support of polarity consideration.

If either a symmetric biphasic or polyphasic stimulator is used, the polarity of the leads alternates so rapidly that, practically speaking, there is no polarity to consider. Thus, all of the aforementioned clinical problems that do not depend on polarity can be treated with such waveforms, as well as by the monophasic pulses.

The major problem that many clinicians seem to face is recognizing which are the two essential leads that complete the circuit. This outcome is due to the fact that in some stimulators the two leads emerge from the same socket, whereas in others (mostly high-voltage units) one essential lead emerges from the center of the panel and the other extends from the side (Fig. 3–24). In many high-voltage units, the side lead actually appears as two leads. This dual

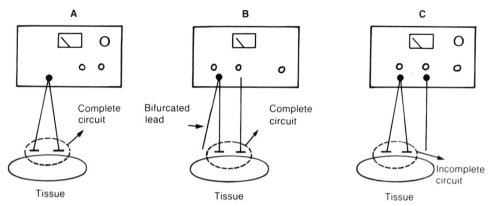

Figure 3–24. Electrode lead connections. In **B**, the bifurcated lead and the center lead can make a complete circuit. In **C**, the circuit is not complete because the "two" leads are actually one lead that has been bifurcated.

lead results because the lead is bifurcated inside the stimulator. The therapist must recognize that this is only one (bifurcated) lead and not the two essential leads that complete the circuit. In fact, bifurcations of either of the two essential leads can take many configurations (Fig. 3-25); but regardless of how many bifurcations are present, they only represent branching of the two essential leads.

The major advantage of a bifurcation is to stimulate more than two areas concurrently. The disadvantage results from the fact that different areas may have different skin impedance. Although the current that passes through the bifurcated leads is identical, the physiological responses may vary significantly, with subliminal stimulation perceived under one electrode and sensory stimulation perceived under the other.

Another disadvantage results from the fact that the total surface area of the electrode connected to one essential lead is the sum of the areas of all of the electrodes connected at the end of the bifurcation (Fig. 3-25). If the total area is larger than the areas of the electrode(s) connected to the other essential lead, then the stimulation is likely to be stronger under the latter electrode due to greater current density. The therapist must recognize these potential problems and must correct them in order to provide the desired physiological responses in the appropriate areas of the body.

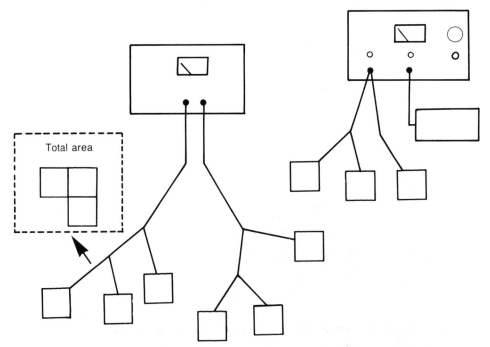

Figure 3–25. Multiple bifurcation of both essential electrode leads.

Electrode Size

The size of surface electrodes is associated with skin impedance, total current density, perceptual discrimination of the excitatory responses, and specificity of stimulation. In general, the larger the electrode size, the smaller the skin impedance. A 100-cm² electrode may offer only 100 to 1000 Ω of resistance, whereas a 1-mm (tip) electrode may reach 50,000 to 100,000 Ω of resistance. The relation of size to impedance may not be linear and in fact has not been adequately described in clinical publications.[136] Clinically, the therapist must first decide how large or small the skin area is that should be stimulated. Only then can the electrode size be selected. Using an electrode that is smaller than the target skin area creates unnecessarily high skin impedance, a practice that frequently occurs when large joints (such as the knee or hip) are stimulated with 5 x 5 cm (2 x 2 in) electrodes. Similar statements can be extended to large muscles such as the quadriceps femoris. The higher the skin impedance, the less the penetration of the current. Using large electrodes may help to resolve this problem.

The effect of electrode size on total current density is obvious; there are several clinical implications. First, current density should not exceed safety limits; therefore, small electrodes should not be used if total current is high (as may be the case with Russian or interferential currents). Second, the electrodes connected to the two essential leads may be identical in size and yet the patient will report more stimulation under one electrode: this is because factors other than size can also affect skin impedance. Increasing the size of this one electrode will decrease current density and should resolve the problem. Third, if the stimulator output is limited, then the use of large electrodes may not provide sufficient current density for the physiologic response to be achieved. Bifurcation of leads may cause the same problem. Reduction of electrode size may restore sufficient current density but may provide less-than-optimal stimulation. Stronger stimulators, which have a higher phase charge, may offer a better solution.

The effect of electrode size on perceptual discrimination between sensory, motor, and pain-fiber excitation was reported by Alon.[136] In essence, larger electrodes produce stronger motor response without pain, whereas smaller electrodes elicit painful stimulation soon after the motor excitation. Sometimes the effective electrode size is smaller than the overall electrode size. This difference in electrode sizes may result in less comfortable stimulation.[142] The clinical implications relate to various stimulation techniques. If vigorous muscle contraction is the objective, electrode size should be large. Size, however, is relative to the muscle mass; therefore, the size appropriate for wrist or elbow extensor groups is much too small when the quadriceps femoris or abdominal muscles are the targets of stimulation. Likewise, patients of different sizes may require different-sized electrodes.

If treatment methods involve brief, intense, painful stimulation of trigger or acupuncture points, very small electrodes are likely to minimize motor stimulation, because motor fibers are usually deeper than sensory and pain-conducting fibers.[85,143,144] The very small electrode thus becomes effectively distant from the motor-nerve fibers. Coupled with very high skin impedance and current density, sensory and pain-conducting fibers are excited before motors fibers. If, however, trigger-point stimulation is accompanied by motor activation without pain, electrode size should be increased.[133,145]

Although large electrodes minimize painful stimulation, they disperse current flow through the tissue, thereby making the stimulation less specific. The clinical consequence is that muscles that are not the target of stimulation may also contract. If this is undesirable, then using smaller electrodes, a bipolar electrode technique, or both (see following section), should eliminate the problem. Smaller electrodes may isolate the individual muscle from the rest of the group (as with nerve conduction testing), but the stimulation may prove painful before sufficient contraction can be achieved. The clinician must therefore change electrode size in accordance with treatment objectives and patient response.

Electrode Placement Techniques

One of the most confusing aspects of clinical electrical stimulation has been the selection and administration of appropriate electrode placement. Again, misleading and inconsistent terminology seems to be a major source of confusion. In fact, there are only two basic techniques of electrode placement: monopolar and bipolar. These two techniques prevail regardless of whether a DC or a pulsed current is used.

Monopolar and bipolar techniques have nothing to do with the polarity of the current, and either technique can be used with any stimulator on the market. The terms monopolar and bipolar simply indicate whether only one essential lead and its electrode(s) are placed over the areas to be stimulated, or both essential leads and their electrodes are placed over the same area(s).

Monopolar Technique. In the monopolar technique, only one of the two essential leads, and the electrode connected to it, are placed over the target area to be affected by the stimulation. This electrode has been called the *treatment*, or *stimulating*, *electrode*. The other lead and its electrode are placed over an area that is not to be affected by the stimulation and can be called the *non-treatment*, or *dispersive*, *electrode*. The target area is where the basic excitatory response should be perceived. Contrary to what is reported in most electrotherapy texts, this area is not only a muscle. Joints, bursae, hematomas, dermal ulcers, and trigger and acupuncture points are also included in the list of target areas, depending on the clinical problem and its appropriate treatment procedure.

The non-treatment electrode is commonly known as the dispersive electrode because it is usually, though not always, a large electrode. Its large size minimizes current density, preventing current from being perceived under it. Thus, any size will suffice, and this electrode can be placed over various body parts, as long as no excitatory response is perceived under it. If the treatment electrode is very small, then the non-treatment electrode need be only somewhat larger. The exact size is therefore relative and is determined by the therapist, based on the response of the patient. A perception of sensory stimulation under the non-treatment electrode is not contraindicated but is unnecessary and should be avoided.

The treatment electrode can be a single electrode or several. The latter arrangement is obtained by bifurcation of the lead. Multiple electrodes are usually justified if the stimulator provides only one channel and if there is more than one target area requiring stimulation (an example would be pain at both sides of the knee joint). Clinicians typically use the high-voltage stimulator for such bifurcated arrangements, but any TENS can be used in the same way. A schematic illustration of a monopolar technique with and without bifurcation is provided in Figure 3-25. It is important that the sum of the areas of the electrodes in a bifurcated lead be less than the area of the non-treatment, dispersive electrode, in order to avoid perception of current under the latter. In those cases where such perception persists, the dispersive lead can also be bifurcated so as to allow an arrangement of two dispersive electrodes.

At present, the only clinical problem that may require use of the monopo-

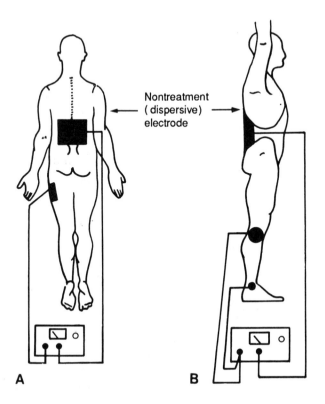

Nontreatment (dispersive) electrode

Figure 3–26. Monopolar technique. **A.** Simple method. **B.** With bifurcated lead so that both knee and ankle can be treated simultaneously.

A   B

lar technique is the treatment of dermal ulcers and wounds. There is some inconclusive evidence that connective-tissue regeneration and bactericidal effects are polarity dependent.[8,62,146,147] Using a monophasic pulse, or DC stimulation and a monopolar technique, allows the therapist to treat the ulcer with positive or negative electrical charges. Which polarity the treatment electrode should be in most cases has yet to be determined. The clinical problems of muscle-disuse atrophy, neuromuscular facilitation, range-of-motion limitation, protective muscle spasm, or circulatory impairment can be treated more efficiently by using the bipolar technique.

None of these problems has any known electrophysiological rationale that requires use of the monopolar technique. The selection of a monopolar or bipolar technique is solely based on clinical convenience and on efficiency of obtaining the appropriate physiological responses. Once the physiological responses (whether sensory, motor, or painful stimulation) have been achieved, the clinical results are most likely to be the same regardless of the electrode-placement technique used.

Trigger- and acupuncture-point stimulation are much more conveniently obtained with the monopolar technique. Other protocols of pain management—joint effusion, interstitial edema, and hematomas—can be conveniently treated using either monopolar or bipolar techniques.

Bipolar Technique. As defined, the bipolar technique requires that both the essential leads and the electrodes connected to them be placed over the target area in order for the area to be affected by the stimulation. It follows that both the complete conductive circuit and the current flow through the tissue should be confined to the area where the clinical problem is present. Unlike the monopolar technique, the excitatory responses are now perceived under both electrodes of the circuit. Obviously, the two electrodes are usually, but not necessarily, of the same size, and the non-treatment, dispersive electrode is not used.

Bipolar placement of the electrodes can be used with any TENS, including high-voltage stimulation. The majority of clinicians have been misled to believe that a dispersive electrode must be used with high-voltage stimulation. This is totally false. It is true that one of the essential leads of high-voltage stimulator is customarily connected to a large dispersive electrode, but this electrode can be easily replaced with a smaller electrode if a bipolar technique is indicated.

As in the monopolar placement, bifurcation of the leads may be accomplished with a bipolar technique. Indications for bifurcation of electrode leads include a situation where the target area is large but the available electrodes are too small. (An example could be a radiating pain that covers a large part of dermatomal distribution, or a protective muscle spasm across the whole lower back.) Figure 3-27 illustrates bipolar and bifurcated bipolar techniques.

Like the monopolar technique, the bipolar technique is used regardless of whether the pulsed current is monophasic, biphasic, or in bursts (polyphasic).

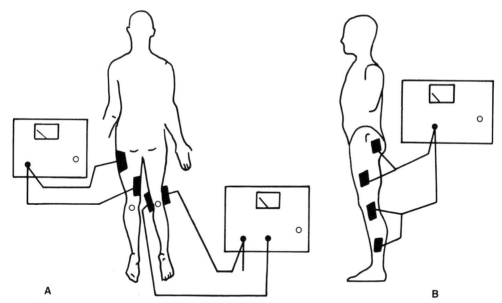

Figure 3–27. Bipolar techniques. **A.** Simple method over a joint or muscle. **B.** Bifurcated along dermatomal distribution.

The symmetrical biphasic and burst waveforms do not present a polarity factor; thus, it makes no difference which of the two electrodes is placed proximally and distally on the skin over the target muscle. If monophasic pulses or some of the asymmetrical biphasic pulses are used, polarity may affect the excitatory response. Classically, the assumption has been made that excitation occurs only under the negative electrode.[44,145] This assumption must be seriously questioned, as it is very easy to demonstrate excitation under the positive electrode. Thus, when the two electrodes are placed on the skin over the target muscle, the selection of which should be negative and which positive is simply based on ease and comfort of excitation.

Many of today's stimulators offer two or more channels. When two channels are used simultaneously over the same target area, each channel is still arranged as a bipolar placement technique. The dual-channel arrangement, however, can take several configurations, as illustrated in Figure 3-28. Using different configurations to improve pain relief has been advocated.[146] However, no objective clinical data have been found to support such a contention. Therefore, any of these dual bipolar techniques can be used. Changing the arrangement may only provide anecdotal, unpredictable improvement.

Bipolar should be selected over monopolar placement if the presented clinical problems are muscle-disuse atrophy, neuromuscular facilitation, range-of-motion limitation, protective muscle spasm, or circulatory disorders. Particularly when the clinical problem requires motor stimulation, the bipolar technique should be less time consuming and should provide more specific

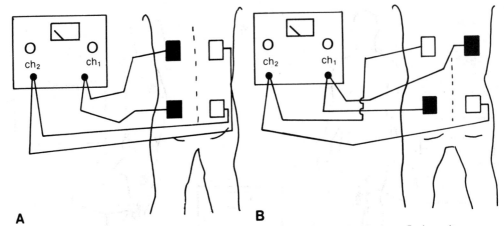

A   **B**

Figure 3—28. Bipolar placement using two-channel stimulation. **A.** Longitudinal paravertebral configuration. **B.** Crossed pattern arrangement.

excitation of the target muscles. If only sensory excitation is indicated, then either bipolar or monopolar placement techniques can be equally efficient.

CLINICAL PROCEDURES

Ever since the discovery of electricity, attempts have been made to use this energy for the alleviation of medical problems. The increased interest of the last 15 years is no exception, and many clinicians have been using the modality in an attempt to improve numerous physical and symptomatic problems. Many objective and subjective results have been reported. Unfortunately, it has been extremely difficult to develop appropriate treatment procedures because of confusing or absent terminology and because of conflicting reports. Furthermore, many claims for success have been promoted that lack supporting clinical data. Indeed, many of the procedures associated with clinical problems that may be helped by TENS have not yet been established. Many techniques can be established, however, using present knowledge.

The purpose of establishing systematic procedures is to enhance prediction of success and failure and to serve as a baseline from which improvement of existing procedures can evolve. Any suggested method represents present knowledge as it applies to a group of patients suffering from similar clinical signs and symptoms; individual adjustments must be considered. Yet using the same baseline should help in selecting the appropriate stimulator, preferred electrode placement, and treatment time. The application of modality should then become more efficient, and the trial and error that prevail in the clinic today are likely to be minimized.

The procedures outlined below are categorized on the basis of general clinical problems. Each technique provides ranges of pulse parameters and

East
Pasco
Medical
Center

7050 Gall Boulevard • Zephyrhills, FL 33541 • (813) 788-0411
An Adventist Health System/Sunbelt Facility

treatment times. Parameter ranges simply indicate that any stimulator that provides characteristics within, or close to, that range can be used (regardless of the manufacturer) with similar results. Ranges of treatment time are based on the achievement of clinical results. The decision whether to add, reduce, or terminate treatment must rest with the individual therapist and should be based on the desire to avoid adverse responses while promoting desired treatment objectives.

For some clinical problems, more than one procedure is offered, in suggested order of selection. Should the first method fail to yield the results, the second should be used. Many other modifications are available but, with a few anecdotal exceptions, continued manipulation is unlikely to improve the results.

I. Pain Management
   A. Procedure A (acute musculoskeletal pain; acute or chronic neurogenic pain)
      1. Parameter setting
         a. Waveform: monophasic, biphasic, time/amplitude-modulated AC
         b. Phase duration: 20 to 200 μsec
         c. Pulse rate: 40 to 100 pps
         d. Polarity: makes no difference
         e. Amplitude: sensory stimulation
      2. Current modulation mode: continuous pulses
      3. Electrode placement: monopolar or bipolar over painful area
      4. Treatment time: 20 to 30 min or longer, based on the degree of pain suppression and lasting effect
   B. Procedure B (chronic musculoskeletal pain)
      1. Parameter setting
         a. Waveform: monophasic or biphasic
         b. Phase duration: 20 to 100 μsec
         c. Pulse rate: 15 to 200 pps
         d. Polarity: makes no difference
         e. Amplitude: motor stimulation
      2. Current modulation mode: continuous pulses
      3. Electrode placement: monopolar over trigger points
      4. Treatment time: 1 to 5 min per point, based on pain suppression and lasting effects
   C. Procedure C (general systemic pain)
      1. Parameter setting
         a. Waveform: monophasic or biphasic
         b. Phase duration: 20 to 200 μsec
         c. Pulse rate: 2 to 5 pps
         d. Polarity: makes no difference
         e. Amplitude: motor stimulation (twitch contraction)
      2. Current modulation mode: continuous pulses or bursts

    3. Electrode placement: monopolar or bipolar over painful area, or remote area

    4. Treatment time: 30 to 45 min, based on pain suppression and lasting effects

Comments

    1. Procedure A, followed by B or C, is the order for acute musculoskeletal pain. Procedure B followed by A or C is the order for chronic musculoskeletal pain.

    2. If two to three treatments have failed to reduce pain, switch to next procedure.

    3. Terminate any procedure if pain increases or if no further pain reduction is observed.

II. Joint Effusion/Interstitial Edema

  A. Procedure A (acute swelling)

    1. Parameter setting

      a. Waveform: monophasic, biphasic, burst

      b. Phase duration: 20 to 200 μsec

      c. Pulse rate: 80 to 100 pps

      d. Polarity: makes no difference

      e. Amplitude: sensory stimulation

    2. Current modulation mode: continuous pulses

    3. Electrode placement: monopolar or bipolar, over the target joint or inflamed area

    4. Treatment time: 2 to 4 hr daily

  B. Procedure B (chronic edema)

    1. Parameter setting

      a. Waveform: symmetrical biphasic preferred, but monophasic or polyphasic (burst) can also be used.

      b. Phase duration: 20 to 200 μsec

      c. Pulse rate: 40 to 50 pps

      d. Polarity: makes no difference

      e. Amplitude: motor stimulation

    2. Current modulation mode: interrupted pulses

      a. ON time: 5 to 10 sec

      b. OFF time: 15 to 120 sec

      c. Ramp time: 2 to 5 sec

    3. Electrode placement: bipolar over target muscles in the swollen area

    4. Treatment time: No clinical data to suggest

Comments

    1. Procedure A may only prove effective in acute cases and should be initiated as soon as possible.

    2. Procedure A can be used in combination with cold baths or ice packs.

    3. Procedure B has very well-documented physiological rationale but no clinical data to support it.

III. Protective Muscle Spasm
  A. Procedure A (motor nerve inhibition)
    1. Parameter setting
      a. Waveform: symmetrical biphasic preferred, but monophasic or polyphasic can also be used
      b. Phase duration: 20 to 200 μsec
      c. Pulse rate: 100 to 150 pps
      d. Polarity: makes no difference
      e. Amplitude: motor stimulation
    2. Current modulation mode: continuous pulses
    3. Electrode placement: bipolar, over target muscles
    4. Treatment time: No clinical data to suggest treatment time
  B. Procedure B (contract-relax)
    1. Parameter setting
      a. Waveform: symmetrical biphasic preferred, but monophasic or polyphasic (burst) can also be used.
      b. Phase duration: 20 to 200 μsec
      c. Pulse rate: 40 to 50 pps
      d. Polarity: makes no difference
      e. Amplitude: motor stimulation
    2. Current modulation mode: interrupted pulses
      a. ON time: 5 to 10 sec
      b. OFF time: 60 to 120 sec
      c. Ramp time: 2 to 5 sec
    3. Electrode placement: bipolar over target muscles in spasm
    4. Treatment time: no clinical data to suggest treatment time
  Comments
    1. In procedure A the objective is to induce vigorous, nonpainful, continuous contraction in order to inhibit the motor nerves and thus the muscles. Since patients may be sensitive, current amplitude must be increased gradually and must be adjusted every few minutes once the patient accommodates to the stimulation.
    2. Procedure B should provide strong contraction followed by long relaxation.
    3. Either procedure is indicated for trunk and cervical musculature.
    4. Reduction of protective spasm should be evaluated by increased range of motion.
IV. Muscle-Disuse Atrophy
  A. Procedure A (induce muscle strength)
    1. Parameter setting
      a. Waveform: biphasic preferred, but monophasic or bursts can also be used
      b. Phase duration: 20 to 200 μsec
      c. Pulse rate: 40 to 60 pps
      d. Polarity: makes no difference

    e. Amplitude: high amplitude motor stimulation

  2. Current modulation mode: interrupted pulses

    a. ON time: 5 to 15 sec

    b. OFF time: 15 to 120 sec

    c. Ramp time: 1 to 5 sec

  3. Electrode placement: bipolar, over target muscles

  4. Treatment time: from few repetitions (muscle contractions) to many

Comments

  1. Patient should contract muscle(s) volitionally, in combination with the electrically induced contraction.

  2. Muscle cramps must be avoided.

  3. The ON/OFF ratio is based on prevention of muscle fatigue. The greater the tendency to fatigue, the shorter the ON and the longer the OFF selected.

  4. Ramp time is determined by patient comfort.

  5. Pronounced muscle soreness 24 to 48 hours after stimulation may indicate overstimulation.

  6. The therapist must move the electrodes until the most vigorous, yet most comfortable, stimulation is achieved.

V. Dermal Ulcers and Wounds

  A. Procedure A (electrical theories)

    1. Parameter setting

      a. Waveform: monophasic

      b. Phase duration: 20 to 100 μsec

      c. Pulse rate: 80 to 100 pps

      d. Polarity: positive for healing effects, negative for bactericidal effect

      e. Amplitude: sensory stimulation

    2. Current modulation mode: continuous phase

    3. Electrode placement: Monopolar, treatment electrode inside ulcer, nontreatment electrode over convenient place (low back)

    4. Treatment time: 30 to 60 min daily

  B. Procedure B (activation of VIP)

    1. Parameter setting

      a. Waveform: monophasic, biphasic

      b. Phase duration: 20 to 200 μsec

      c. Pulse rate: 2 to 5 pps

      d. Polarity: makes no difference

      e. Amplitude: motor stimulation (twitch contraction)

    2. Current modulation mode: continuous pulses or bursts

    3. Electrode placement: bipolar over web space of left hand and hypothenar muscle group of the same hand or along peripheral nerves proximal to the ulcer

    4. Treatment time: 30 to 45 min daily (or bid)

Comments
1. Selection of polarity in procedure A has been an unsettled issue.
2. Bleeding from the ulcer should be avoided.
3. Treatment electrode in procedure A is a sterile gauze wet with sterile 0.9-percent saline solution.
4. A preference between procedures A and B has not been established.
5. Necrotic tissue debridement is accomplished as indicated.

VI. Circulatory Disorders

A. Procedure A (venous insufficiency)
1. Parameter setting
   a. Waveform: biphasic, monophasic
   b. Phase duration: 20 to 200 μsec
   c. Pulse rate: 40 to 60 pps
   d. Polarity: makes no difference
   e. Amplitude: motor stimulation
2. Current modulation mode: interrupted pulses
   a. ON time: 5 to 10 sec
   b. OFF time: 10 to 20 sec
   c. Ramp time: 1 to 5 sec
3. Electrode placement: Bipolar, over target muscles
4. Treatment time: 10 to 20 min

B. Procedure B (neurovascular disorders)
1. Parameter setting
   a. Waveform: biphasic, monophasic
   b. Phase duration: 20 to 200 μsec
   c. Pulse rate: 40 to 100 pps
   d. Polarity: makes no difference
   e. Amplitude: minimal sensory stimulation
2. Current modulation mode: continuous pulses
3. Electrode placement: bipolar or monopolar, over painful segment
4. Treatment time: 20 to 30 min

Comments
1. Mild muscle contraction during procedure is sufficient. Avoid muscle cramps.
2. Acute venous disorders are contraindicated for stimulation.
3. Only minimal sensory stimulation is indicated in procedure B. Overstimulation may cause vasoconstriction instead of vasodilation.
4. In neurovascular disorders, procedure B (under V., dermal ulcers and wounds) can also be used.

In summary, it must be stressed that these procedures only represent those that are most commonly used. They are an attempt to integrate the clinical data available to date. Although some have been objectively reproduced, others lack sufficient clinical support. None can be considered optimal, and any part of each of them may be challenged by further clinical studies. The reader must also realize that electrical stimulation is only one modality that, when effective, can be combined with other modalities and treatment techniques. If used systematically, based on present and future improvements in our knowledge, electrical stimulation should prove to be a very powerful modality in regard to many aspects of the therapist's daily practice.

REFERENCES

1. Crisler GR. Sprains and strains treated with the ultra faradic M-impulse generator. *J Fl Med Assoc.* 11:32, 1953
2. Quillen S. Data presented at a seminar on high voltage stimulation. Annual Conference of the American Physical Therapy Association, Anaheim, CA, 1982
3. Harris P. Iontophoresis: Clinical research in musculoskeletal inflammatory conditions. *J Orthop Sports Phys Ther.* 4:109, 1982
4. Delacerda FG. A comparative study of three methods of treatment for shoulder girdle myofascial syndrome. *J Orthop Sports Phys Ther.* 4:109, 1982
5. Bettany JA, Fish DR, Mendel FC. Influence of high voltage pulsed galvanic stimulation on edema formation following impact injury. *Phys Ther.* 69:395, 1989 (abstract)
6. Bettany JA, Fish DR, Mendel FC. Influence of high voltage pulsed galvanic stimulation on edema formation following hyperflexion injury. *Phys Ther.* 69:389, 1989 (abstract)
7. Michlovitz S, Smith W, Satkins M. Ice and high voltage pulsed stimulation in treatment of acute lateral ankle sprains. *J Orthop Sports Phys Ther.* 9:301, 1988
8. Alon G, Azaria M, Stein H. Diabetic ulcer healing using high voltage TENS. *Phys Ther.* 66:775, 1986 (abstract)
9. Gault WR, Gatens PF. Use of low intensity direct current in management of ischemic skin ulcers. *Phys Ther.* 56:265, 1976
10. Kaada B. Promoted healing of chronic ulceration by transcutaneous nerve stimulation (TMS). *VASA.* 12:262, 1983
11. Feedar JA, Kloth LC. Acceleration of wound helping with high voltage pulsating direct current. *Phys Ther.* 65:741, 1985 (abstract)
12. Carley PJ, Wainapel SF. Electrotherapy for acceleration of wound healing: Low intensity direct current. *Arch Phys Med Rehabil.* 66:443, 1985
13. Kloth LC, Feedar JA. Acceleration of wound healing with high voltage, monophasic, pulsed current. *Phys Ther.* 68:503, 1988
14. Karba R, Uvdovnik L, Presern-Strukelj M, et al. Experience with the use of electrical stimulation in healing of wounds of different etiologies. *Proceedings Bioelectrical Repair Growth Society.* 9:45, 1989
15. Likar B, Rencel S, Presern-Strukelj M, et al. Analysis of changes of thermal conditions in wounds due to electrical stimulation. *Proceedings Bioelectrical Repair Growth Society.* 9:45, 1989
16. Eriksson E, Haggmark T. Comparison of isometric muscle training and electrical stimulation supplementing isometric muscle training in the recovery after major knee ligament surgery: A preliminary report. *Am J Sports Med.* 7:169, 1979

17. Johnston DH, Thruston P, Ashcroft PJ. The Russian technique of faradism in the treatment of chondromalcia patellae. *Physiother Can.* 29:266, 1977
18. Gould M, Donnermeyer D, Gammon GG, et al. Transcutaneous muscle stimulation to retard disuse atrophy after open meniscectomy. *Clin Orth Rel Res.* 178:190, 1983
19. Bowman BR, Baker LL, Waters RL. Positional feedback and electrical stimulation: An automated treatment for the hemiplegic wrist. *Arch Phys Med Rehabil.* 60:497, 1979
20. Baker LL, Yeh C, Wilson D, et al. Electrical stimulation of wrist and fingers for hemiplegic patients. *Phys Ther.* 59:1495, 1979
21. Delitto A, McKowen JM, McCarthy JA, et al. Electrically elicited co-contraction of thigh musculature after anterior cruciate ligament surgery. *Phys Ther.* 68:45, 1988
22. Delitto A, Rose SJ, McKowen JM, et al. Electrical stimulation versus voluntary exercise in strengthening thigh musculature after anterior cruciate ligament surgery. *Phys Ther.* 68:660, 1988
23. Arvidsson I, Arvidsson H, Eriksson E, et al. Prevention of quadriceps wasting after immobilization—An evaluation of the effect of electrical stimulation. *Orthopaedics.* 9:1519, 1986
24. Arvidsson I, Eriksson E. Postoperative TNS pain relief after knee surgery—An attempt to objective evaluation. *Orthopaedics.* 9:1346, 1986
25. Morrissey MC, Brewster CE, Shields CL, et al. The effect of electrical stimulation on the quadriceps during postoperative immobilization. *Am J Sports Med.* 13:40, 1985
26. Phillips CA. Functional electrical stimulation and lower extremity bracing for ambulation exercises of the spinal cord injured individual: A medically prescribed system. *Phys Ther.* 69:842, 1989
27. Wigersstad-Lossing I, Grimby G, Jonsson T, et al. Effects of electrical muscle stimulation combined with voluntary contraction after knee ligament surgery. *Med Sci Sports Exerc.* 20:93, 1988
28. Tichy VL, Zanket HT. Prevention of venous thrombosis and embolism by electrical stimulation of calf muscles. *Arch Phys Med Rehabil.* 30:711, 1949
29. Doran FSA, White M, Frury M. A clinical trial designed to test the relative value of two simple methods of reducing the risk of venous stasis in the lower limbs during surgical operations, the danger of thrombosis, and a subsequent pulmonary embolus, with a survey of the problem. *Br J Surg.* 57:20, 1970
30. Kaada B. Vasodilation induced by transcutaneous nerve stimulation in peripheral ischemia (Raynaud's phenomenon and diabetic polyneuropathy). *Eur Heart J.* 3:303, 1982
31. Bodenheim R, Bennett H. Reversal of Sudeck's atrophy by the adjunctive use of transcutaneous electrical nerve stimulation. *Phys Ther.* 63:1287, 1983
32. Munsat TL, McNeal DR, Waters RL. Preliminary observations on prolonged stimulation of peripheral nerve in man. *Arch Neurol.* 33:608, 1976
33. Axelgaard J, Brown JC. Lateral electrical surface stimulation for the treament of progressive idiopathic scoliosis. *Spine.* 8:242, 1983
34. Axelgaard J, Nordwell A, Brown JC. Correction of spinal curvature by transcutaneous electrical muscle stimulation. *Spine.* 8:453, 1983
35. Eckerson LF, Axelgaard J. Lateral electrical stimulation as an alternative to bracing in the treatment of idiopathic scoliosis. *Phys Ther.* 64:483, 1984

36. Morris L, Newton RA. Use of high voltage pulsed galvanic stimulation for patient with levator ani syndrome. *Phys Ther.* 67:1522, 1987

37. Sohn N, Weinstein MA, Robbins RD. The levator syndrome and its treatment with high voltage electrogalvanic stimulation. *Am J Surg.* 144:580, 1982

38. Nicosia JF, Abcarian H. Levator syndrome: A treatment that works. *Dis Colon Rectum.* 28:406, 1985

39. Oliver GC, Rubin RJ, Salvati EP, et al. Electrogalvanic stimulation in the treatment of levator syndrome. *Dis Colon Rectum.* 28:662, 1985

40. McNeal DR. 2000 years of electrical stimulation. In: Hambrecht FT, Reswick JB, eds. *Functional Electrical Stimulation: Applications in Neural Prosthesis.* New York, Marcel Dekker, 1977: 3–35

41. Geddes LA. A short history of the electrical stimulation of excitable tissue. *Physiologist.* 27 (suppl):1, 1984

42. Kloth L, Cummings JP, et al. *Standards of Electrotherapeutic Terminology. Report of the Electrotherapy Standards Committee of the Section on Clinical Electrophysiology of the Americal Physical Therapy Association,* Alexandria, VA, 1990 (in press)

43. Bowman BR, Baker LL. Effects of wave form parameters on comfort during transcutaneous neuromuscular electrical stimulation. *Ann Biomed Eng.* 13:58, 1985

44. Baker LL. Neuromuscular electrical stimulation in the restoration of purposeful limb movements. In: Wolfe SL, ed. *Electrotherapy.* New York, Churchill Livingstone, 1982: 38–39

45. Ray CD, Maurer DD. A review of neural stimulation system components useful in pain alleviation. *Med Prog Technol.* 2:121, 1974

46. Kovacs R. *Electrotherapy and Light Therapy,* 5th ed. Philadelphia, Lea & Febiger, 1947: 88

47. Brodsky AE, Khalil MA. Update of experience with electrical stimulation for enhancement of lumbar spine fusion. *Trans Biol Repair Growth Soc.* 8:25, 1988

48. Brighton CT, Pfeffer GB, Pollack SR. In vivo growth plate stimulation in various capacitatively coupled electrical fields. *J Orthop Res* 1:42, 1983

49. Nogami H, Aoki H, Okagawa T, et al. Effects of electrical current on chrondrogenesis in vitra. *Clin Orthop Relat Res.* 163:243, 1982

50. Frank C, Schachar N, Dittrich D, et al. Electromagnetic stimulation of ligament healing in rabbits. *Clin Orthop Relat Res.* 175:263, 1983

51. Ricci J, Zimmerman M, Parsons JR, et al. Preliminary studies of tendon cell colony formation on carbon fiber electrodes with direct current stimulation. *Trans Biol Repair Growth Soc.* 3:35, 1983

52. Murray JC, Lacy M. Pulsing electromagnetic field can modulate the production of degradative enzymes by synovial cells. *Trans Biol Repair Growth Soc.* 3:7, 1983

53. Zecca L, Ferrario P, Furia G, et al. Effects of pulsed electromagnetic field on acute and chronic inflammation. *Trans Biol Repair Growth Soc.* 3:72, 1983

54. Alon G, DeDomenico G. *High Voltage Stimulation: An Integrated Approach to Clinical Electrotherapy.* Chattanooga, Chattanooga Corp, 1987: 129–146

55. Johnston RM, Kasper S. Compound nerve action potentials produced by signals from clinical stimulators. *Phys Ther.* 66:85, 1986 (abstract)

56. Kantor G, Alon G, Ho HS. Charges Associated with threshold excitation of peripheral nerves using various wave forms. IEEE Trans Biomed Eng 11th Annual International Conference Proceedings, 1660–1661, Nov. 1989

57. Alon G. Electro-orthopedics: A review of present electrophysiologic responses and

clinical efficacy of transcutaneous stimulation. *Adv Sports Med Fitness.* 2:295, 1989

58. Plevney BL, Nutter PB. *Comparison of Subject Comfort Using Three Electrical Stimulation Systems.* Research project submitted to the department of physical therapy in partial fulfillment of the requirements for the master of science degree, University of Southern California, 1981

59. Baker LL, Borup C, Mann M. Comparison of three wave forms for comfort during electrical stimulation. *Phys Ther.* 67:799, 1987 (abstract)

60. Baker LL, Cornell S, Flannery A, et al. Wave form and comfort of electrical stimulation in the upper extremity. *Phys Ther.* 69:372, 1989 (abstract)

61. Alon G. *High Voltage Stimulation: A Monograph,* Chattanooga, Chattanooga Corp, 1984

62. Alon G. *Electrical Stimulators—Video Presentation.* Chattanooga, Chattanooga Corp, 1985

63. Baker LL, McNeal DR, Dewart KP, et al. Effects of carrier frequency on comfort with medium frequency electrical stimulation. *Phys Ther.* 69:373, 1989 (abstract)

64. Laycock J, Green RJ. Interferential therapy in the treatment of incontinence. *Physiotherpy.* 74:161, 1988

65. Lai HS, DeDomenico G, Strauss GR. The effect of different electro-motor stimulation training intensities on strength improvement. *Aust J Physiother.* 34:151, 1988

66. DeDomenico G. *Basic Guidelines for Interferential Therapy.* Sydney, Australia, Theramed, 1981

67. Ward AR. *Electricity Fields and Waves in Therapy.* Marickville, Australia Science Press, 1980: 17

68. Goodgold J, Eberstein A. *Electrodiagnosis of Neuromuscular Disease,* 2nd ed. Baltimore, Williams & Wilkins, 1977, p 150

69. Alon G. Letter to the editor: Interferential current news. *Phys Ther.* 67:280, 1987

70. Leo K: Perceived comfort levels of modulated versus conventional TENS current. *Phys Ther.* 64:745, 1984

71. Barr JO, Weissenbuehler SA, Bandstra EJ, et al. Effectiveness and comfort level of transcutaneous electrical nerve stimulation (TENS) for elderly with chronic pain. *Phys Ther.* 67:775, 1987 (abstract)

72. Barr JO, Nielsen DH, Soderberg GL. Transcutaneous electrical nerve stimulation characteristics for altering pain perception. *Phys Ther.* 66:1515, 1986

73. Leo KC, Dostal WF, Bossen DG, et al. Effect of transcutaneous electrical nerve stimulation characteristics on clinical pain. *Phys Ther.* 66:200, 1986

74. Jette DU. Effect of different forms of transcutaneous electrical nerve stimulation on experimental pain. *Phys Ther.* 66:187, 1986

75. Jette DU. Effect of TENS frequency and intensity on exercise induced muscle soreness. *Phys Ther.* 67:765, 1987 (abstract)

76. Mannheimer C, Carlsson CA. The analgesic effect of transcutaneous electrical nerve stimulation (TENS) in patients with rheumatoid arthritis: A comparative study of different pulse patterns. Pain. 6:329, 1979

77. Barr JO Forrest SE, Potratz PE, et al. Effectiveness of transcutaneous electrical nerve stimulation (TENS) in the elderly with chronic pain. *Phys Ther.* 69:396, 1989 (abstract)

78. Packman-Braun R. Relationship between functional electrical stimulation duty cycle and fatigue in wrist extensor muscles of patients with hemiparesis. *Phys Ther.* 68:51, 1988

79. Shriber WJ. *A Manual of Electrotherapy*, 4th ed. Philadelphia, Lea & Febiger, 1974: 128–129

80. Bertolucci LE. Introduction of anti-inflammatory drugs by iontophoresis double blind study. *J Orthop Sports Phys Ther.* 4:103, 1982

81. Garzione JE. Salicylate iontophoresis as an alternative treatment for persistent thigh pain following hip surgery. *Phys Ther.* 58:570, 1978

82. Boone DC. Application of iontophoresis. In Wolf SL (ed). *Electrotherapy*. New York, Churchill Livingstone 1982, pp 111–114

83. Pabst, HW. Treatment of peripheral circulatory disorders with frequency modulated impulse currents. *Arch Phys Ther, Balneologie.* 12:230, 1960

84. Manheimer JS, Lampe GN. *Clinical Transcutaneous Electrical Nerve Stimulation.* Philadelphia, FA Davis, 1984: 199–218

85. DeGirardi CQ, Seaborne D, Goulet FS, et al. The analgesic effect of high voltage galvanic stimulation combined with ultrasound in the treatment of low back pain: A one-group pre-test/post-test study. *Physiother Can.* 36:327, 1984

86. Taylor K, Newton RA, Personius WJ, et al. Effects of interferential current stimulation for treatment of subjects with recurrent jaw pain. *Phys Ther.* 67:346, 1987

87. Wadsworth H, Chanmugan APP. *Electrophysical Agents in Physiotherapy*, 2nd ed. Marrickville, Australia, Science Press, 1983: 276–280

88. Kramer JF. Effect of electrical stimulation current frequencies on isometric knee extension torque. *Phys Ther.* 67:31, 1987

89. Soo CL, Currier DP, Threlkeld AJ. Augmenting voluntary torque of health muscle by optimization of electrical stimulation. *Phys Ther.* 68:333, 1988

90. Currier DP, Mann R. Muscle strength development by electrical stimulation in healthy individuals. *Phys Ther.* 63:915, 1983

91. Reismann MA. A comparison of electric stimulators eliciting muscle contraction. *Phys Ther.* 64:751, 1984 (abstract)

92. Protas EG, Dupny T, Gardea R. Electrical stimulation for strength training. *Phys Ther.* 64:751, 1984 (abstract)

93. Owens J, Malone T. Treatment parameters of high frequency electrical stimulation as established on the electro-stim 180. *J Orthopaed Sports Phys Ther.* 4:162, 1983

94. Michlovitz S, Smith W, Watkins M. Ice and high voltage pulsed stimulation in treatment of acute lateral ankle sprains. *J Orthop Sports Phys Ther.* 9:301, 1988

95. Akers TK, Gabrielson AL. The effect of high voltage galvanic stimulation on the rate of healing of decubitus ulcers. *Biomed Sci Instrum.* 20:99, 1984

96. Thurman B, Christian E. Responses of a serious circulatory lesion to electrical stimulation. *Phys Ther.* 51:1007, 1971

97. Le Doux J, Quinones MA. An investigation of the use of percutaneous electrical stimulation in muscle reeducation. *Phys Ther.* 61:737, 1981 (abstract)

98. Wong RA. High voltage versus low voltage electrical stimulation: Force in induced muscle contraction and perceived discomfort in healthy subjects. *Phys Ther.* 66:1209, 1986

99. Mohr T, Carlson B, Sulentic C, et al. Comparison of isometric exercise and high volt galvanic stimulation on quadriceps femoris muscle strength. *Phys Ther.* 65:606, 1985

100. Van der Hornet C, Mortimer JT. The response of the myelinated nerve fiber to short duration biphasic stimulating current. *Ann Biomed Eng.* 7:117-125, 1979

101. Bourguignon GJ, Bourguignon LYW. Electric stimulation of protein and DNA synthesis in human fibroblasts. *FASEB J.* 1:398, 1987

102. Owoeye I, Spielholz NI, Fetto J, et al. Low intensity pulsed galvanic current and the healing of tenotomized rat achilles tendons: Preliminary report using load-to-breaking measurements. *Arch Phys Med Rehabil.* 68:415, 1987

103. Kincaid CB, Lavoie KH. Inhibition of bacterial growth in vitro following stimulation with high voltage, monophasic, pulsed current. *Phys Ther.* 69:651, 1989

104. Stefanovska A, Vodovnik L, Benko H, et al. Exogenous electrical current: Influence on wound healing. *Trans Bioelectr Repair Growth Soc.* 7:22, 1987

105. Brighton CT, Pollack SR. Treatment of recalcitrant nonunion with a capacitively coupled electrical field. *J Bone Joint Surg* 67-A:577, 1986

106. Scott J, Picker R. A double-blind study to evaluate muscle strength. Paper presented at the annual meeting of the International Society of Electro-Acutherapy, Los Angeles, 1983

107. Matteson JH. Cybernetic technology and high-performance athletic training. *Nat Strength Condit Assoc J.* 6:32, 1984

108. Schmitt R, Capo T, Frazier H, et al. Cranial electrotherapy stimulation treatment of cognitive brain dysfunction in chemical dependence. *J Clin Psych.* 45:60, 1984

109. Patterson MA, Firth J, Gardiner R. Treatment of drug, alcohol and nicotine addiction by neuroelectric therapy: Analysis of results over 7 years. *J Bioelectricity.* 3:193, 1984

110. Gibson TH, O'Hair DE. Cranial application of low level transcranial electrotherapy vs relaxation instruction in anxious patients. *Am J Electromed,* 1:18, 1987

111. Cheng RSS, Pomeranz B. Electroacupuncture analgesic could be mediated by at least two pain-relieving mechanisms: Endorphin and non-endorphin. *Life Sci.* 25:1957, 1979

112. Alon G, Fink AM, Anderson PA, et al. The effect of subliminal stimulation on elbow flexors strength, fatigue and soreness. *Phys Ther.* 68:789, 1988 (abstract)

113. Solomon S, Guglielmo K. Treatment of headache by transcutaneous electrical stimulation. *Headache.* 25:12, 1985

114. Lerner FN, Kirsch DL. Microstimulation and placebo effect. *J Chiropr.* 15:101, 1981

115. Meyer FP, Nebrensky A. Microstimulation and placebo effect. *Calif Health Rev.* 2 (Aug–Sept):1983

116. Noto K, Grant P. A comparative study of neural stimulation and conventional physical therapy modalities. *Neurol Report.* 10:40, 1986

117. Royal FF. Cybernetics and electro-medicine. *J Ultramol Med.* 2:41, 1984

118. Letko P. This prescription a winner for Joe. *Toronto Times.* August 3, 1985

119. Matteson JH. The advantages of using "intelligent" cerebral electrical stimulation in drug and alcohol rehabilitation. *Prof Nurs Quart.* p 24, Winter, 1986

120. Huey L. Spinal cord rehabilitation using the Electro-Acuscope and Myopulse. *Health Express.* June 1983

121. *The Electromedical Times.* Fall-winter, 1984–1985

122. Stanish WD, Valiant GA, Bonen A, et al. The effects of immobilization and electrical stimulation on muscle glycogen and myofibrillar ATPase. *Can J Appl Sport Sci.* 7:267, 1982

123. Cabric M, Appell JH, Resic A. Effects of electrical stimulation of different frequencies on the myonuclei and fiber size in human muscle. *Int J Sports Med.* 8:323, 1987

124. Cook HA, Morales ML, La Rosa EM, et al. *Effects of Electrical Stimulation on Lymphatic Flow and Limb Volume in the Rat.* Research paper submitted as partial

fulfillment of a bachelor degree, University of Maryland, School of Medicine, Department of Physical Therapy, Baltimore, 1989

125. Reed BV. Effect of high voltage pulsed electrical stimulation on microvascular permeability to plasma proteins. *Phys Ther.* 68:491, 1988

126. Jehle H. Charge fluctuation forces in biological systems. *Ann NY Acad Sci.* 150:240, 1969

127. Pilla AA. Electrochemical information transfer at living cell membrane. *Ann NY Acad Sci.* 240:149, 1976

128. Pilla AA, Gary K. Electromagnetic modulation of enzyme function: Application to Na-K AtPase in human erythrocytes. *Trans Biol Repair Growth Soc.* 2:44, 1982

129. Doty S, Van Ostenbridge J. Differential response of cell membrane-associated and lysosomal enzymes to pulsating electromagnetic fields. *Trans Biol Repair Growth Soc.* 3:66, 1983

130. Martinovitz U, Heim M, Horoszwski H, et al. Transcutaneous electric nerve stimulation (TENS) for relief of symptoms in hemophiliac patients with acute hemarthrosis. Proceedings of the XV World Federation of Hemophilic Congress, Stockholm, Sweden, June, 1983

131. Tepper SH, Alon G, Stickney SC, et al. The effect of neuromuscular stimulation on body metabolism. Presented at Annual Conference of American Physical Therapy Association, Anaheim, CA, 27 June 1990

132. Cabric M, Appell JH, Resic A. Stereological analysis of capillaries in electrostimulated human muscles. *Int J Sports Med.* 8:327, 1987

133. Alon G, Allin J, Inbar GE. Optimization of pulse duration and pulse charge during transcutaneous electrical stimulation. *Aust J Physiother.* 29:195, 1983

134. Li CL, Bak A. Excitability characteristics of the A- and C- fibers in a peripheral nerve. *Exp Neuro.* 50:67, 1976

135. Howson DC. Peripheral nerve excitability. *Phys Ther.* 58:1467, 1978

136. Alon G. High voltage stimulation: Effects of electrode size on basic excitatory responses. *Phys Ther.* 65:890, 1985

137. Szeto AYJ, Nyquist JK. Transcutaneous electrical nerve stimulation for pain control. *IEEE Eng Med Bio.* 2:14, 1983

138. Hecker B, Carron H, Schwartz DP. Pulsed galvanic stimulation: Effects of current frequency and polarity on blood flow in healthy subjects. *Arch Phys Med Rehabil.* 66:369, 1986

139. Walker DC, Currier DP, Threlkeld AJ. Effects of high voltage pulsed electrical stimulation on blood flow. *Phys Ther.* 68:481, 1988

140. Wong RA, Jette DV. Changes in sympathetic tone associated with different forms of transcutaneous electrical nerve stimulation in healthy subjects. *Phys Ther.* 64:478, 1984

141. Forbes MP, Stambaugh JN. The effect of transcutaneous electrical nerve stimulation on the compound action potential of sensory nerves. *Phys Ther.* 68:789, 1988 (abstract)

142. Omata C, Baker LL, Daymon S, et al. Comparison of three commercial electrodes for neuromuscular electrical stimulation. *Phys Ther.* 69:372, 1989 (abstract)

143. Melzack R. Prolonged relief of pain by brief intense transcutaneous somatic stimulation. *Pain.* 1:357, 1975

144. Mao W, Ghia JN, Scott DS, et al. High versus low intensity acupuncture analgesic for treatment of chronic pain: Effects on platelet serotonin. *Pain.* 8:331, 1980

145. Lane JF. Electrical impedances of superficial limb tissue, epidermis, dermis and muscle sheath. *Ann NY Acad Sci.* 238:812, 1974
146. Bolton L, Foleno B, Means B, et al. Direct current bactericidal effect on intact skin. *Antimicrob Agents Chemother.* 18:137, 1980.
147. Wolcott LE, Wheeler PC, Hardwick HM, et al. Accelerated healing of skin ulcers by electrotherapy: Preliminary clinical results. *South Med J.* 62:795, 1967

CHAPTER 4

Electrical Stimulation of Healthy Muscle and Tissue Repair

John Cummings

When an electrical stimulus of sufficient amplitude and duration is applied to the nerve supplying a healthy muscle, a brisk contraction of the muscle results. The electrical stimulation of healthy muscle is used (1) to facilitate strengthening muscles that have atrophied from immobilization or disuse; (2) to treat and correct scoliosis; (3) to treat urinary dysfunction in both the paralyzed patient and in the patient with urinary incontinence; and (4) to aid in numerous programs of "functional" electrical stimulation. This chapter discusses both the specific clinical applications of neuromuscular electrical stimulation (NMES) of healthy muscle and the basic principles of electrical stimulation as they relate to the stimulation of innervated, healthy muscle. Covered are specific techniques employed in stimulating healthy muscle; the influence of NMES on the anatomy, biochemistry, and physiology of skeletal muscle; and general precautions and contraindications relevant to NMES. The chapter concludes with a consideration of the use of electrical stimulation to facilitate tissue repair. The discussion addresses the use of electrical stimulation in the healing of open wounds, tendons, and ligaments.

REVIEW OF PRINCIPLES GOVERNING STIMULATION OF HEALTHY MUSCLE

Electrical Excitability
The expression *electrical excitability of a healthy muscle* refers to the capability of the nerve innervating the muscle to respond to an electrical stimulus. When stimulating innervated, "healthy" muscle with electricity, we are stimu-

lating the neurolemma of the axon, and not the sarcolemma of the muscle, as in the case of electrical stimulation of "unhealthy," denervated muscle.

Electrical excitability is an important concept, because numerous factors may affect the capability of intact motor nerves (efferent axons) to respond to electrical stimuli. Under certain pathologic conditions, nerves may demonstrate increased (hyper) or decreased (hypo) excitability to an electrical stimulus. Hyperexcitability to electrical stimulation may occur (1) when the central nervous system has lost its inhibitory influence over the peripheral motor axons (eg, hemiplegia); (2) during the first stages of peripheral nerve injuries; and (3) in the early stages of systemic peripheral neuropathies. Hypoexcitability of a nerve to an electrical stimulus may be found (1) in lower motor-neuron lesions (eg, amyotrophic lateral sclerosis); (2) following prolonged immobilization; (3) in advanced stages of peripheral neuropathies; and (4) during the later stages of peripheral nerve injuries.[1]

Efferent axons also demonstrate changes in electrical excitability relative to the polarity of the stimulating electrode. When stimulated by the cathode, the excitability of the axon increases, raising the resting potential of the membrane toward threshold, whereas stimulation by the anode will result in the axon becoming less excitable, displacing the resting membrane potential away from threshold. The relation between excitability and polarity is demonstrated by Pfleuger's law.

Pfleuger's Law

In 1858, Pfleuger first observed that a healthy muscle would contract with less current if stimulated by the cathode rather than the anode.[2] He also reported that, when being stimulated with the cathode, the axon was more excitable when the circuit was closed (making the circuit) than when the current was applied by opening (breaking) the circuit. By stimulating healthy, innervated muscle using four variants, and by noting the minimal amount of current (threshold current) required to elicit minimal muscle contraction for each of these variants, he arrived at the following formula:

$$CCC > ACC > AOC > COC.$$

where

- CCC = cathode closing current,
- ACC = anode closing current,
- AOC = anode opening current, and
- COC = cathode opening current.

This formula states that, when stimulating a healthy muscle with current of the *same amplitude*, the contraction of the muscle elicited when closing the cathode (active electrode) is greater than the contraction elicited when closing the anode (active electrode); which in turn is greater than the contraction elicited when opening the anode (active electrode); which in turn is greater than the muscular contraction resulting from opening the cathode (active electrode). Therefore, when stimulating healthy muscle with direct current, the cathode is the electrode of choice for the active electrode, since the amount of current required to elicit a muscular contraction is less than when using the anode as the active electrode.

Accommodation

As excitable tissues, both nerve and muscle are capable of accommodating to an electrical stimulus. *Accommodation* is defined as the automatic rise in the threshold of excitation resulting from a gradually increasing stimulus applied to excitable tissue.[3,4] The process of accommodation occurs much more rapidly in nerve than in muscle. Therefore, nerve fibers will accommodate to a gradually increasing electrical stimulus before muscle will accommodate to the same stimulus. An understanding of this concept is important when stimulating innervated muscle, because the electrical stimulus must be applied to the healthy muscle (motor axons) rapidly enough to avoid accommodation. Therefore, the *rise time* (rate or speed of rise) of the stimulus must be rapid enough to avoid accommodation when stimulating innervated muscle.

The Law of DuBois-Reymond

In 1843, DuBois-Reymond observed that to electrically stimulate a nerve there must be a sudden variation in the current flow.[5] For example, if a current is instantaneously applied to a nerve, the nerve may be stimulated at a threshold of 1 V; however, the same nerve may require a current of 5 V to effectively stimulate the nerve if the current is applied slowly (ie, slow to reach peak amplitude) rather than instantaneously. As the current is slowly applied to the nerve, the nerve will accommodate to the stimulus, raising (in effect) the excitation threshold of the nerve and necessitating a greater voltage to reach threshold. To avoid accommodation when stimulating with interrupted direct current, the rise time of the stimulus should be less than 60 μsec.

The Strength–Duration Curve

To achieve a better understanding of the excitability of nerves and muscles, we must consider the strength (amplitude) and the duration (ON time) of the applied current, since a relation exists between the strength and the duration necessary to elicit a threshold response from nerve and muscle. By varying the strength and duration of the electrical stimulus, it is possible to plot a curve called the strength–duration (S–D) or amplitude–time (A–T) curve that gives a graphic illustration of the excitability of nerve and muscle. The strength–duration curves for nerve and muscle are very characteristic and are readily reproducible (Fig. 4–1).

Although the shape of the S–D curve is similar for both nerve and muscle, the position of the curve on the graph will vary according to the innervation status of the muscle (innervated, partially denervated, or completely denervated). Two important numerical values that can be determined from the S–D curve are the rheobase and the chronaxie. The *rheobase* (threshold) is the

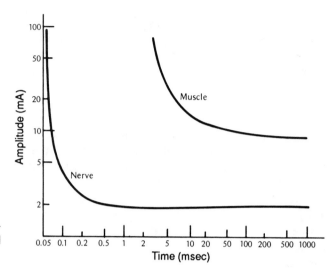

Figure 4–1. Strength–duration curves for nerve and muscle.

minimal strength of an electrical stimulus of infinite duration that is capable of exciting a tissue (nerve or muscle). *Chronaxie* is the duration of an electrical stimulus of twice the rheobase value that will cause a minimal response (ie, muscle twitch). The chronaxie of an intact nerve (healthy, innervated muscle) is much lower (approximately 0.03 msec) than that of a denervated muscle (approximately 10 msec). These values illustrate the fact that healthy, innervated muscle is much more excitable than is unhealthy, denervated muscle. Therefore, healthy, innervated muscle will respond best to a stimulus of sufficient amplitude and of short duration, whereas an impulse of long duration and of greater amplitude is required to effectively stimulate denervated muscle. Therefore, the S–D curve (Fig. 4–1) illustrates the relationship between the time (duration) that an electrical stimulus is applied to a nerve or muscle and the amplitude of the stimulus required to produce a threshold response (muscle twitch).

INFLUENCE OF ELECTRICAL STIMULATION ON HEALTHY MUSCLE

Healthy skeletal muscle undergoes numerous histochemical, physiological, and morphologic changes when subjected to prolonged periods of increased activity. Increased muscular activity may result from either increased exercise or chronic NMES. The changes that occur in healthy muscle in response to increased exercise are the same as those that occur during prolonged NMES. These changes occur so that the muscle may be better-suited to changes in the functional requirements of the muscle. This section discusses the effect of NMES on the histochemistry, metabolism, physiology, and structure of healthy muscle.

Histochemical–Enzyme Changes

Healthy, skeletal muscle is capable of adapting to new patterns of use. For example, if a continuous, low-frequency pattern of activity (such as NMES) is imposed on the fast muscles of the rabbit for several weeks, the fast muscles acquire the biochemical and physiological characteristics of slow muscles.[6] This orderly transformation of fiber types involves changes in myosin, a major contractile protein that exists in polymorphic forms. The involvement of both heavy- and light-chain components of myosin in the transformation has been shown by gel electrophoresis, myosin paracrystal formation, and immunocyto-chemistry.[7–10]

Changes in myofibular proteins following chronic electrical stimulation are not confined to myosin. Roy and associates demonstrated that the ratio of alpha to beta forms of tropomyosin changes to that ratio characteristic of slow muscles after 3 weeks of chronic electrical stimulation.[11]

In another chronic, low-frequency stimulation study of fast muscles, Hudlicka and coworkers concluded that long-term, low-frequency stimulation of fast muscles can cause some contractile properties of fast muscle to resemble those of slow muscles, regardless of the frequency of stimulation, provided that the total number of stimuli is comparable, the duration of the stimuli is long enough (a minimum of 2 weeks), and all of the motor units are activated.[12] These findings indicate that enzymatic plasticity in healthy mammalian muscles is influenced by NMES.

Metabolic Changes

The NMES of healthy muscles also has a direct effect on the metabolic activity of muscles. Long-term NMES of fast muscles at a frequency naturally occurring in nerves leading to slow muscles improves muscle performance and produces changes from predominantly anaerobic to predominantly aerobic metabolism.[13,14] Altman and associates have demonstrated that blood flow and oxygen consumption increase more during contraction in chronically stimulated rabbit muscles than in nonstimulated controls.[15] This increase in both blood flow and oxygen consumption occurred to the same extent in muscles stimulated continuously at frequencies of 10 or 40 pps with three 5-sec trains/min. They also showed that glucose consumption increased in chronically stimulated muscles and that lactate output was lower in chronically stimulated muscles than in nonstimulated controls. The chronically stimulated muscles also fatigued considerably less than did the controls. Altman and associates also concluded that, regardless of its frequency, chronic NMES of healthy muscle for 14 to 28 days accentuates aerobic metabolism and improves muscular performance. They also stated that total activity may be more important for the changes observed in the metabolism of muscle and muscular performance than the specific frequency of NMES. According to Pette and associates, intermittent, long-term (28 days) NMES of fast rabbit muscles with a frequency pattern resembling that of slow muscles (10 pps) leads to a sequential rearrangement of the activity of key metabolic enzymes.[13] Decreases of extramitochondrial enzymes of glycogenolysis (phosphorylase), glycolysis (lactate dehydrogenase), and energy-rich phosphate transfers were found initially, along with increases in enzymes involved in glucose phosphorylation (hexokinase) and fatty acid activation (palmitoyl-CoA synthetase). Later, an increase in key enzymes of the citric acid cycle (citrate synthase) and fatty acid oxidation, as well as ketone body utilization, were evident. From these findings, Pette and co-workers concluded that, assuming that NMES leads to a transformation of the fast fibers into slow fibers, this transformation is accompanied by the formation of an intermediate fiber type that is morphologically equivalent to slow-contracting fibers, and that an increase in the population of these intermediate fibers must be expected in muscles electrically stimulated at 10 pps for long periods of time.

In a clinical study comparing isometric muscle training with NMES supplementation of isometric muscle training following knee surgery, Erickson and Haggmark showed that electrical stimulation could successfully prevent the fall in oxidative enzyme activity that was observed in the quadriceps femoris muscle of individuals receiving only isometric muscle training.[16] They randomly divided eight patients undergoing reconstruction of the anterior cruciate ligament into two groups. The controlled group received a standard plaster cast and isometric muscle training of the quadriceps femoris muscle, whereas the experimental group received a standard plaster cast, isometric muscle training, and transcutaneous electrical stimulation of the quadriceps femoris muscle during the recovery period. NMES of the distal part of the quadriceps femoris muscle was given with one electrode through a window in the cast and with the second electrode over the femoral nerve in the groin. A stimulus of 200 pps was applied for 5 to 6 sec, followed by a 5-sec rest period. The muscles were stimulated for 1 hour each day, 5 days a week, for 4 weeks. The patients were examined clinically, with repeated muscle biopsies before surgery, one week following surgery and 5 weeks after surgery. The electrically stimulated group consistently had better muscle function and significantly higher succinate dehydrogenase activity than the control group. The results of this study suggest that transcutaneous electrical stimulation of healthy muscle may be effective in preventing the muscular atrophy that occurs in the quadriceps femoris muscle following major knee surgery. This study also suggests that one factor contributing to the development of quadriceps femoris muscle atrophy is a fall in succinate dehydrogenase activity, which is (in effect) inhibited by NMES.

In another clinical study of the effects of immobilization and NMES following knee surgery, Stanish and associates found similar effects as did Erickson and Haggmark with NMES on the activity of myofibrillar ATPase.[17] They augmented a conventional rehabilitation program with daily (Monday through Friday) NMES using a 2500-Hz sinusoidal waveform modulated at 50 bursts per sec. Each session consisted of 10 quadriceps femoris muscle contractions of 15-sec duration, followed by a 45-sec rest period. The results of the study showed that the decrease in myofibrillar ATPase resulting from mobilization was prevented. However, the authors did not suggest that NMES may lead to an increase in ATPase activity in subjects who have not been, or are not involved in, a period of immobilization.

Membrane Changes

Muscle impulse activity has also been considered an important factor in maintaining the membrane properties of muscle.[18,19] For example, Jansen and associates have shown that chronic NMES prevents the spread of acetylcholine sensitivity, which follows denervation, and that reinnervation can even be prevented by electrically induced muscular activity.[20] Lomo and associates have demonstrated that chronic electrical stimulation of frequencies greater than 40 pps of denervated muscle can slow the speed of muscle contraction and can actually convert a muscle with predominantly slow-twitch fibers into a muscle with a majority of fast-twitch fibers.[21] Similarly, other investigators have demonstrated that fast-twitch fibers can be transformed into slow-twitch fibers through chronic electrical stimulation at low frequencies.[13,22,23] Although there is a fair amount of controversy concerning whether or not nerve-generated activity is the only factor responsible for the maintenance of healthy muscle, these experiments indicate that impulse activity (impulse frequency) does have a profound effect on the membrane properties of muscle and, therefore, on the contractility of skeletal muscle.

NMES OF HEALTHY MUSCLE IN MANAGEMENT OF SCOLIOSIS

The NMES of healthy muscle is utilized by the physical therapist in the treatment of progressive idiopathic scoliosis. Lateral curvature of the spine of unknown etiology (idiopathic scoliosis) comprises 75 to 80 percent of all cases of scoliosis in the United States.[24] Prior to the mid-1970s, the conservative management of idiopathic scoliosis was limited to a program of bracing and strengthening exercises in an attempt to halt the progressive curvature of the spine.[24-28] Since many physical and psychological problems were associated with bracing, and since the patient had to wear the brace for 23 hours a day, alternate methods of treatment were sought. One alternative investigated was the use of NMES of the paravertebral muscles as a means of strengthening the back muscles, which in turn would result in slowing the progression of the curvature.

Neuromuscular electrical stimulation of the paraspinal musculature using implanted electrodes for the treatment of scoliosis was initially performed in 1974.[29] Although early studies showed that progression of the major curve was halted in 83 percent of cases, the initial technique was not practical, because the patients had to undergo surgical procedures to implant, service, and remove the intermuscular electrodes.[29] Therefore, the possibility of using noninvasive, transcutaneous, NMES techniques was investigated. In 1976, Axelgaard and associates demonstrated that an acute scoliosis of up to 50 percent could be induced in cats following NMES of the lateral trunk muscles.[30] In a subsequent study on humans, Axelgaard and associates reported that progressive idiopathic scoliosis could be reduced by NMES, with the greatest correction of the curvature being achieved when the electrodes were placed at the midaxillary line.[31] In a study of lateral electrical surface stimulation (LESS) in individuals with progressive idiopathic curves of 20 to 45 degrees, Axelgaard and Brown reported that progression of the curve was halted in 84 percent of the patients.[32] The placement of the electrodes is critical in achieving positive results using this procedure.[33]

A specific protocol for electrode placement has been described by Eckerson and Axelgaard.[34] Following a thorough initial assessment and determination of electrode placement site, the physical therapist instructs the patient and parents in the use of a dual-channel, portable electrical muscle stimulator for the home-treatment program. The dual-channel unit delivers trains of rectangular, constant-current pulses with a pulse duration of 220 μsec, a frequency of 25 pps, and a stimulus sequence of 6 sec on and 6 sec off. The amplitude of the stimulus is slowly increased until an acceptable level (50 to 70 mA) is obtained. Circular, carbon-rubber electrodes, with snap connectors and various coupling agents, are used (depending on the tolerance level of the individual patient). The treatment time is increased gradually until the patient can tolerate 8 hours of stimulation nightly while he or she sleeps. The stimulation is continued nightly, without the need for additional treatment or exercises, and with only periodic checkups, until skeletal maturity is reached.

In a study of 57 patients receiving LESS for the treatment of idiopathic scoliosis, Eckerson and Axelgaard reported that many brace-related problems (eg, skin breakdown, negative psychologic changes, and noncompliance) were eliminated and that patient acceptance of the treatment program was high.[34] Therefore, LESS is an effective alternative to the use of braces in the treatment of progressive idiopathic scoliosis in children and adolescents.

NMES FOR URINARY DYSFUNCTION

A hyperreflexic (spastic, inhibited, irritable, hyperactive, or hypertonic) bladder is an unsolved urologic problem that presents itself as urgency, frequency, and incontinence. The medical treatment of a hyperreflexic bladder remains insufficient. Surgical intervention to alleviate the problem, although often effective, frequently results in complications, such as pelvic floor paralysis and impotence.[35] Treating urinary incontinence with NMES of the pelvic floor has been studied.[36] Although Glen has reported positive results with pelvic floor electrical stimulators, these devices have not gained general popularity, primarily because the anal plug electrodes are not well-tolerated by the patients.[37] Another problem with the anal plug approach is the large current loss along the rectal mucosa, which inhibits current flow and impedes effective stimulation of the pelvic floor.[38]

Since there are numerous technical and practical problems associated with direct electrical stimulation of the pelvic floor, McGuire and associates employed NMES of those acupressure points traditionally stimulated (by the practitioners of traditional Chinese medicine) to inhibit bladder activity. In 22 patients with a variety of neural lesions and detrusor instability, surface electrodes were affixed bilaterally to either both posterior tibial nerves or to both common peroneal nerves. Using a commercially available, transcutaneous electrical nerve stimulator, the appropriate points were stimulated at an amplitude of 5 to 8 V, a frequency of 2 to 10 pps, and a pulse duration of 5 to 20 msec. Although constant stimulation was necessary to achieve continence, McGuire and associates reported that detrusor activity had been inhibited in approximately 90 percent of their patients, with 12 patients remaining dry during stimulation.[38] Therefore, it appears that reflex detrusor activity can be inhibited indirectly through the bilateral transcutaneous electrical stimulation of either the posterior tibial nerves or the common peroneal nerves.

A similar potential use for NMES is in the facilitation of bladder emptying in patients with hyoptonic (hyporeflexic, areflexic) bladder dysfunction. Abbate and associates stimulated the thoracic spinal cord in patients with multiple sclerosis using a square-wave pulse with adjustable pulse duration and rate.[39] They found an objective improvement (cystometry and electromyography) in 42.5 percent of the patients. Those showing improvement had an increased bladder capacity and demonstrated an ability to void to completion. In another study, Merrill implanted 155 electrical stimulators into the base of the bladder in patients with either upper or lower motor neuron lesions and neurogenic bladders. He found that the procedure was most effective in patients having vesical hypofunction and in patients with multiple sclerosis. Sixty-two percent of the 24 patients with multiple sclerosis showed marked improvement.[40]

The possibility that NMES of the hypotonic bladder may occur not only through direct, intravesical surface stimulation but also by stimulating peripheral nerves, was suggested by Jones.[35] He further recommended that the following parameters be used in the NMES of the peripheral nerves: frequencies of 15 to 25 pps, pulse durations of 0.5 to 5 msec, and a voltage of 1.5 to 15 V. Flanigan and colleagues presented a case study on the effect of NMES on improving bladder emptying in a 19-year-old female multiple sclerosis patient with a hypotonic bladder. They used a conventional neurostimulator, producing a modified square-wave pulse, with a pulse rate of 2 to 110 pps and a variable pulse duration of 40 to 200 μsec. Following 15 to 30 min of NMES on the inner thighs the patient could initiate voiding and could void to near completion. Clinical follow-up one for 1 year revealed that the patient could consistently empty the bladder to less than 10 cc of residual following NMES of the inner thighs. They concluded that the improvement in bladder emptying in this case was directly dependent on the NMES, because the withdrawal of NMES rapidly reversed the bladder to its prestimulation state.[41]

Although the mechanisms responsible for the effectiveness of NMES on both hypotonic and hypertonic bladder function remain uncertain, numerous investigators are attempting to identify the most appropriate parameters of stimulation for future clinical use. The successful identification of the stimulation parameters could lead to an increase in the use of this approach as an alternative to the correction of urinary problems through medical and surgical intervention alone.

ELECTRICAL STIMULATION IN HEALING OF OPEN WOUNDS

The use of electricity equal to or below sensory threshold amplitude to facilitate the healing of open wounds is well documented.[42–48] Electrically charged gold leaf has been used in the healing of open wounds such as ischemic skin ulcers and decubitis ulcers,[43,44] while continuous, monophasic low-intensity no longer correct term but was in 60s direct current (LIDC) has been used to enhance wound healing in animals[46,50] and in humans.[46,47,50] Recently, the use of monophasic pulsating current has been reported to facilitate the healing of open wounds in human subjects.[48]

A potential mechanism for the role of electrical stimulation in healing open wounds has been proposed by Becker and Murray.[51] They have described a "current of injury" that can be measured on the surface of an open wound following injury. Becker and Murray believe that this current of injury is responsible for triggering the repair process. Theoretically, either amplification or augmentation of the current through electrical stimulation may facilitate the healing process. The current of injury theory proposes that the electrical potentials initially responsible for triggering the healing process are positive potentials, and that placement of the anode of the direct current circuit directly on the wound would facilitate the healing process.

Several studies have used continuous, low-amplitude (less than 1.0 mA) unidirectional current to enhance the healing of superficial wounds.[44,46,50] Using this approach Wolcott and associates[46] reported that the electrically stimulated wounds healed at rates 2 to 3.5 times faster than non-stimulated wounds. Wolcott's group used current amplitude ranging from 200 to 800 μA, with the cathode initially placed over the wound for either 3 days or until the wound was asceptic. Following this period of asepsis the electrodes were reversed with the anode applied to the wound and the cathode placed 25 cm proximal or cephalic to the wound. Stimulation was provided for a total of 6 hr/day in three 2-hr sessions, separated by two 4-hr periods of no stimulation.

More recently, Carley and Wainapel[47] contrasted electrotherapy and conventional therapy for the treatment of open wounds. Using current amplitudes of less than 1 mA, and stimulating several hours a day with the anode directly over the wound, they reported that the electrically stimulated wounds healed 1.5 to 2.5 times faster than the non-stimulated wounds. Carley and Wainapel also stimulated for periods of 2 hr, two to three times a day, until the wounds were closed.

Electrical stimulation using a continuous, low-amplitude, unidirectional current also has an apparent bactericidal effect under the cathode of a direct current circuit.[52,53] Rowley and colleagues[52] reported a 38.8 percent reduction in the growth of *Escherichia coli* in vitro following the application of continuous, low-amplitude, unidirectional current. Although cathodal and anodal stimulation have both been reported to have a bactericidal effect, the cathode has been used in most human studies.

The use of "high voltage" monophasic, pulsating current has recently been reported as effective in facilitating the healing of open wounds in humans.[48] In a well-controlled study in 16 human subjects, Kloth and Feedar[48] reported a 100 percent healing rate of stimulated wounds (mean treatment period 7.3 weeks) while the non-stimulated wounds increased in area an average of 28.9 percent over a mean period of 7.4 weeks. Patients in the treatment group received electrical stimulation to the ulcer site 5 days a week. The stimulator used in the study was a commercially available "high-voltage" unit. Specific stimulation parameters included a pulse frequency of 105 pps, a 50 μsec interpulse interval, and an amplitude just below motor threshold. The investigators initially placed the anode over the wound with the cathode placed 15 cm caudal or distal to the anode. When the proliferation of granulation tissue apparently plateaued, the cathode was placed over the wound, and the anode was moved 15 cm rostral or medial to the cathode. Subjects in the control group had electrodes applied to the wounds but were not attached to the stimulator.

From these studies it is apparent that certain types of electrical stimulation may effectively accelerate the rate of wound healing in humans.

ELECTRICAL STIMULATION IN HEALING OF TENDONS AND LIGAMENTS

Realizing that electrical stimulation had been demonstrated to augment healing of bone and open wounds, Owoeye and associates[54] designed a study to determine whether electrical stimulation could facilitate the healing of another type of soft tissue injury, tendon ruptures. They investigated the effect of low-amplitude (75 μA), pulsed (10 pps), monophasic currents on the healing of tenotomized Achilles tendons. Each pulse in the waveform consisted of a pair of short-duration spikes that decayed exponentially, with approximately 100 μsecs between the onset of the first and second spike. This type of waveform has traditionally been associated with high-voltage "galvanic" stimulators.

Following surgical tenotomy and suturing of the right Achilles tendon in 60 male Sprague-Dawley rats, Owoeye and associates[54] randomly assigned 20 animals to each of three treatment groups. Group one received anodal stimulation to the tenotomy site, group two cathodal stimulation, and group three no stimulation. The "active" Teflon-coated, stainless steel electrode was implanted along the distal stump of the tendon with one end of the wire directly over the tendon defect. A second wire, the "indifferent" electrode, was implanted along the proximal stump of the tendon. Following closure of the wound, a plaster cast was applied to maintain the ankle in plantar flexion and knee extension. The tenotomy sites were treated via the implanted electrodes once daily for 15 min over a 2-week period. After 2 weeks the healing tendon was surgically removed and tested for the load required to rebreak the tendons at the tenotomy site. The investigators demonstrated that the tendons receiving anodal stimulation withstood significantly greater loads ($P<0.001$) than did either the group treated with cathodal current, or the non-treated control groups.

Owoeye and associates[54] emphasized that although their finding indicated that the current delivered by this type of stimulator appears beneficial in facilitating tendon repair, the study represents a preliminary investigation into the use of electric currents in the treatment of ruptured tendons. The study did not address whether one type of current may be better than any other (eg, constant versus interrupted; unidirectional versus bidirectional) in the healing of tendons. The investigators also point out that they chose this type of stimulation since the type of stimulator used in the study is readily available in most rehabilitation departments. They also stress that considerably more research, including histological studies, is needed to answer a host of related questions.

The potential benefit that electrical stimulation may have on tendon healing was further supported in a study by Nessler and Mass[55] on the effect of direct current on tendon healing in vitro. Using the whole-tendon culture method, the investigators studied the effect of continuous 7 μA direct current on the conversion of ^{13}C proline to ^{13}C hydroxyproline (a measure of collagen synthesis) at 7, 14, 21, and 42 days of incubation. The ^{13}C hydroxyproline counts indicated a higher activity in the stimulated tendons at three (7, 21, and 42 days) of the four time intervals. The difference was statistically significant at 7 days ($P = 0.0084$), with the stimulated tendons having 255% greater activity than controls. At 42 days the hydroxyproline activity remained 60% greater in the stimulated tendons, therefore indicating increased collagen synthesis. This study, like the in-vivo study of Owoeye and colleagues,[54] demonstrated a potential role for electrical stimulation in the enhancement of tendon healing.

Enwemeka and Spielholz demonstrated augmented tendon healing following anodal electrical stimulation, although no histological study of the injury site was made. In a series of experiments they confirmed previous findings that high-voltage current (monophasic twin-peaked) accelerates tendon healing when the anode is applied over the injured tendon and retards healing when the cathode is used over the injury site. Use of the so-called "microcurrent" (subliminal) electrical stimulation after eight treatments did not show statistical significance when compared with the high-voltage treatments.[56]

A possible role for electrical stimulation in ligament healing was recently reported by Akai and associates[56] in a study of the effects of electrical stimulation on healing a full-thickness defect of the patellar ligament in rabbits. They demonstrated that although electrical stimulation did not change the collagen content of newly formed tissue, the stimulation did restore the tensile stiffness in a short period of time, and decreased the relative proportion of Type III collagen more rapidly than in non-stimulated controls. According to the investigators the decrease of Type III collagen indicates a progressing separative process of the ligament. Akai and colleagues concluded from the study that electricity enhances the healing of ligaments by changing the ratio of collagen types.

CONCLUSIONS

The electrical stimulation of healthy muscle has been proven effective in facilitating muscle strengthening following disuse atrophy, in the treatment of scoliosis, in the management of urinary dysfunction, and in numerous programs of "functional" electrical stimulation. Future uses for the electrical stimulation of innervated muscle continue to be investigated and developed. The future also looks promising for the use of electrical stimulation to facilitate the healing of open wounds, tendons, and ligaments.

REFERENCES

1. Kovacs R. *Electrotherapy and Light Therapy*, 6th ed. Philadelphia, Lea & Febiger, 1953: 122–123
2. Pfleuger EFW. Ueber die tetanisierende Wirkung des constanten Stromes und das Allgemeingesetz der Reizung. *Virchow's Arch.* 3:13, 1858
3. Erlanger J, Blair EA. The irritability changes in nerve in response to subthreshold constraint currents, and related phenomena. *Am J Physiol.* 99:129, 1931
4. Hill AV. Excitation and accommodation in nerve. *Proc Royal Soc.* B119:305, 1936
5. DuBois-Reymond E. Untersuchungenüber tierische Elektrizität, *Virchow's Arch.* 2:258, 1845
6. Salmons S, Henriksson J. The adaptive response of skeletal muscle to increased use. *Muscle Nerve* 4:94, 1981
7. Pette D, Muller W, Leisner E. Vrbova G. Time dependent effects on contractile properties, fibre population, myosin light chains, and enzymes of energy metabolism in intermittently and continuously stimulated fast twitch muscle of the rabbit. *Pfluegers Arch.* 364:103, 1976
8. Sreter FA, Pinter K, Jolesz F, et al. Fast to slow transformation of fast muscles in response to long-term phasic stimulation. *Exp Neurol.* 75: 95, 1982
9. Sreter FA, Romanul FCA, Salmons S, Gergely J. The effect of a changed pattern of activity on some biochemical characteristics of muscle. In: Milhorat AT, ed. *Exploratory Concepts in Muscular Dystrophy II.* Amsterdam, Excerpta Medica, 1974: 338–343
10. Rubinstein NA, Kelly AM. Myogenic and neurogenic contributions to the development of fast and slow twitch muscles in rat. *Dev Biol.* 62:473, 1978
11. Roy RK, Mabuchi K, Sarkar S, et al. Changes in tropomyosin submit pattern in

chronic electrical stimulated rabbit fast muscles. *Biochem Biophys Res Common.* 89:181, 1979

12. Hudlicka O, Tyler KR, Srihari T, et al. The effect of different patterns of long-term stimulation on contractile properties and myosin light chains in rabbit fast muscles. *Pfluegers Arch.* 393:164, 1982

13. Pette D, Smith ME, Staudte HW, Vrbova G. Effects of long-term electrical stimulation on some contractile and metabolic characteristics of fast rabbit muscles. *Pfluegers Arch.* 338:257, 1973

14. Hudlicka O, Brown M, Cotter M, et al.: The effect on long-term stimulation of fast muscles on their blood flow, metabolism, and ability to withstand fatigue. *Pfluegers Arch.* 369:141, 1977

15. Altman TJ, Hudlicka O, Tyler KR. Long-term effects of tetanic stimulation on blood flow, metabolism, and performance of fast skeletal muscle. *J Physiol (London).* 295:36P, 1979

16. Eriksson E, Haggmark T. Comparison of isometric muscle training and electrical stimulation supplementing isometric muscle training in the recovery after major knee ligament surgery. *Am J Sports Med.* 17:169, 1979

17. Stanish WD, Valiant GA, Bonen A, Beleastro A. The effect of immobilization and electrical stimulation muscle glycogen and myofibrillar ATPase. *Can J Appl Sport Sci.* 7:267, 1982

18. Gutmann E. Considerations on neurotrophic relations in central and peripheral nervous system. *Acta Neurobiol Exp (Warsaw).* 35:841, 1975

19. McComas AJ. Discussion. In: Korr IM, ed. *Neurological Mechanisms in Manipulation Therapy.* New York, Plenum Press, 1977: 369–370

20. Jansen JKS, Lomo T, Micolaysen K, Westgaard RH. Hyperinnervation of skeletal muscle fibers: Dependence on muscle activity. *Science.* 181:559, 1973

21. Lomo T, Westgaard RH, Dahl HA. Contractile properties of muscle: Control of pattern of muscle activity in rat. *Proc R Soc Lond (Biol).* 187:99, 1974

22. Salmons S, Vrbova G. Influence of activity on some contractile characteristics of mammalian fast and slow muscles. *J Physiol (London).* 201:535, 1969

23. Salmons S, Sreter FA. Significance of impulse activity in the transformation of skeletal muscle type. *Nature.* 263:30, 1976

24. Harrington PR. The etiology of idiopathic scoliosis. *Clin Orthop.* 126:17, 1977

25. Mellencamp DD, Bount WPL, Anderson AJ. Milwaukee brace treatment of idiopathic scoliosis: Late results. *Clin Orthop.* 126:171, 1977

26. Moe JH, Winter RB, Bradford DS, et al. *Scoliosis and Other Spinal Deformities.* Philadelphia, WB Saunders, 1978: 359–427

27. Blount WP, Moe JH. *The Milwaukee Brace.* Baltimore, Williams & Wilkins, 1980: 76–82, 107–109

28. Carr WA, Moe JH, Winter RB, et al. Treatment of idiopathic scoliosis in the Milwaukee brace. *J Bone Joint Surg (Am).* 62:599, 1980

29. Bobechko WP, Herbert MA, Friedman HG. Electrospinal instrumentation for scoliosis: Current status. *Orthop Clin North Am.* 10:927, 1979

30. Axelgaard J, Brown JC, Harada Y, et al. Lateral surface stimulation for the correction of scoliosis. *Proceedings of the 30th Annual Conference on Engineering in Medicine and Biology.* Los Angeles, The Alliance for Engineering in Medicine and Biology, 1976:282

31. Axelgaard J, McNeal DR, Brown JC. Lateral electrical surface stimulation for the

treatment of progressive scoliosis. In: Popovic D, ed. *Proceedings of the 6th International Symposium on External Control of Human Extremities.* Dubrovnik, 1978: 63–70

32. Axelgaard J, Brown JC. Lateral electrical surface stimulation for the treatment of progressive idiopathic scoliosis. *Spine.* 8:242, 1983

33. Axelgaard J, Nordwall A, Brown JC. Correction of spinal curvatures by transcutaneous electrical muscle stimulation. *Spine.* 8:463, 1983

34. Eckerson LF, Axelgaard J. Lateral electrical surface stimulation as an alternative to bracing in the treatment of idiopathic scoliosis: Treatment protocol and patient acceptance. *Phys Ther.* 64:483, 1984

35. Jones U. Experimental considerations and clinical application of electrostimulation for bladder evacuation. *Acta Urol Belg.* 47:515, 1979

36. Torrens MJ, Griffith HB. The control of the uninhibited bladder by selective sacral neurectomy. *Brit J Urol.* 46:639, 1974

37. Glen E. Control of incontinence by electrical devices. In: Caldwell KPS, ed. *Urinary Incontinence.* New York, Grune & Stratton, 1975:89

38. McGuire EJ, Zhang SC, Horwinski ER, Lytton B. Treatment of motor and sensory detrusor instability by electrical stimulation. *J Urol.* 129:78, 1983

39. Abbate AD, Cook AW, Atallah M. Effect of electrical stimulation of the thoracic spinal cord on the function of the bladder in multiple sclerosis. *J Urol.* 117:285, 1977

40. Merrill DC: Electrical vesical stimulation. *Acta Urol Belg.* 47:110, 1979

41. Flanigan RC, August Jr HM, Young B, et al. Cutaneous stimulation of the bladder in multiple sclerosis: A case report. *J Urol.* 129:1047, 1983

42. Carey LC, Lepley. Effect of continuous direct electrical current on healing wounds. *Surgical Forum.* 13:33, 1962

43. Kanof N. Gold leaf in the treatment of cutaneous ulcers. *J Invest Dermatol.* 43:441, 1964

44. Wolf M, Wheeler PC, Wolcott LE. Gold leaf treatment of ischemic skin ulcers. *JAMA.* 196:693, 1966

45. Assimacopoulos D. Wound healing promotion by the use of negative electric current. *Am J Surg.* 34:423, 1968

46. Wolcott LE, Wheeler PC, Hardwicke HM, et al. Accelerated healing of skin ulcers by electrotherapy: Preliminary clinical results. *South Med J.* 62:795, 1969

47. Carley P, Wainapel S. Electrotherapy for acceleration of wound healing: Low intensity direct current. *Arch Phys Med Rehabil.* 66:443, 1985

48. Kloth LC, Feedar JA. Acceleration of wound healing with high voltage, monophasic, pulsed current. *Phys Ther.* 68:503, 1988

49. Alvarez OM, Mertz PM, Smerbeck RV, et al. The healing of superficial skin wounds is stimulated by external electrical current. *J Invest Dermatol.* 81:144, 1983

50. Gault WR, Gatens PF. Use of low intensity direct current in management of ischemic skin ulcers. *Phys Ther.* 56:265, 1976

51. Becker RO, Murray DG. Method for producing cellular dedifferentiation by means of very small electrical currents. *Trans NY Acad Sci.* 29:606, 1967

52. Rowley B. Electrical current effects on E. coli growth rates. *Proc Soc Exp Biol Med.* 139:929, 1972

53. Rowley B, McKenna J, Chase G. The influence of electrical current on an infecting microorganism in wounds. *Ann NY Acad Sci.* 238:543, 1974

54. Owoeye I, Spielholz N, Fetto J, Nelson A. Low-intensity pulsed galvanic current and the healing of tenotomized rat Achilles tendons: Preliminary report using load-to-breaking measurements. *Arch Phys Med Rehabil.* 68:415, 1987

55. Nessler JP, Mass DP. Direct-current stimulation of tendon healing in vitro. *Clin Orthop.* 217:303, 1987

56. Enwemeka CS, Spielholz NI. Modulation of tendon growth and regeneration by electrical fields and currents. In: Currier DP, Nelson RM. *Excitable and Connective Tissue: Recent Advances/Clinical Concepts.* (submitted for publication, 1990)

57. Akai M, Oda H, Shirasaki Y, Tateishi T. Electrical stimulation of ligament healing: An experimental study of the patellar ligament of rabbits. *Clin Orthop.* 235:296, 1988

CHAPTER 5

Electrical Stimulation of Denervated Muscle

Neil I. Spielholz

With sincerest apologies to the Bard of Avon, this chapter might well be subtitled "To stimulate or not to stimulate, that is the question." Unfortunately, the answer to this seemingly simple inquiry has been anything but. While the reason for stimulating denervated muscle appears logical enough, contradictory findings concerning the efficacy of such treatment have sprung up incessantly. The purpose of this chapter is to guide the student through the maze of hypotheses, imaginative guesses, experimental findings (and their refutations), and to review some of the more recent considerations, which though adding to the present confusion may ultimately clarify much of our ignorance concerning nerve–muscle interaction. Let us begin then with the basic question: Why stimulate denervated muscle at all? (Other reviews have appeared.[1,2])

RATIONALE FOR STIMULATING DENERVATED MUSCLE

Denervated muscle is stimulated to maintain it in as healthy a state as possible while awaiting re-innervation. Intuitively, this is logical. After all, the function of muscle is to contract, and it is common knowledge that an exercised muscle is stronger, bigger, and more efficient than one that is primarily inactive. Denervated muscle, which cannot be exercised either voluntarily or reflexively, atrophies and weakens. However, since denervated muscle can be made to contract by using appropriate electrical currents, perhaps such artificial activation can substitute for the real thing and prevent the multitude of negative changes associated with denervation. Furthermore, if stimulation is indeed capable of maintaining denervated muscle healthier than it otherwise would be, functional use might return faster when re-innervation finally does occur.

These conjectures are of more than just academic interest. Physical therapy has long played a role in the comprehensive care of patients with peripheral nerve injuries, and this has gained added importance with the advent of microsurgical techniques. But the reattachment of an amputated part, though requiring utmost skill and ingenuity in repairing severed vascular, neurological, and bony components, represents only the beginning of a patient's rehabilitation. How much good is it, for example, if the tissue is revitalized and the bones heal, yet the patient never regains functional use of the part? The muscles of the amputated segment are, after all, denervated. Following surgical reattachment, these muscles remain paralyzed until their nerves regenerate. Since this may take months or years depending upon the distance between the site of nerve section and the muscle, what do we do for the patient in the meantime?

To answer this question, we must first know what happens to denervated muscle before re-innervation occurs (if it ever does).

DENERVATION AND ITS CONSEQUENCES

Denervated muscle is profoundly different from normal muscle. Clinically, the most obvious consequences attending the complete disruption of motor innervation are (1) immediate loss of voluntary and reflex use of the muscle; followed by (2) progressive muscular atrophy over the ensuing weeks and months. These clinical sequelae, however, represent only the tip of the iceberg as denervated muscle fibers are biochemically, mechanically, electrically, as well as morphologically different from normal muscles.

In view of this plethora of both obvious and subtle changes, it is logical to ask which if any is best to measure if one is interested in determining whether a therapeutic intervention, such as electrical stimulation, is effective or not. This section therefore, will discuss in more detail some of the differences between normal and denervated muscle for. the purpose of further exploring this point.

Atrophy, Degeneration, and Fibrosis

Atrophy is a wasting away, or diminution in size, of a cell, organ, or body part. When we speak of "muscle atrophy," the clinical picture that comes to mind is that of a shrunken or wasted muscle. As a result of muscle atrophy, the contour of the affected part flattens and adjacent bony structures become more prominent. Although an experienced practitioner can not only recognize atrophy but can even differentiate changes in it, subjective assessments such as "better or worse" or "more or less" are unacceptable for the purposes of scientific research. Serious investigation of muscle atrophy requires quantitative methodology.

In experimental situations, the two most common methods for quantifying atrophy are (1) weighing a denervated muscle and comparing it to the contralateral control (a macroscopic technique); and (2) measuring diameters or areas of denervated muscle fibers and contrasting these values to contralateral normal muscle fibers (a microscopic technique). Note that these methods are not simply different ways of accomplishing the same thing. The first weighs the entire muscle, and this value may be influenced by factors such as proliferation of connective tissue, edema, and perhaps differences in the amounts of muscle the investigator cut out for weighing (obviously, of course, every effort is taken to remove equal proportions). With the second method, conversely, the investigator looks specifically at the individual muscle fibers themselves, quantifying changes in them and in their connective tissue matrix. Furthermore, by combining microscopy with histochemical techniques, one can determine whether Type I and Type II fibers are affected similarly or differently by denervation (or by any other condition, for that matter). Both techniques (weighing and microscopy) have been used to study the natural history of denervation atrophy and the effects of neuromuscular electrical stimulation (NMES) on it.

With respect to weight, denervated muscles lose mass relatively quickly (Fig. 5–1). Sunderland, reviewing an extensive literature on this topic, summarized his experimental findings and those of others as follows:

> There was a rapid initial loss of weight, the muscle sustaining a 30 percent loss in 29 days which had increased to 50 to 60 percent by 60 days. The process then slowed and a relatively stable state was reached somewhere about 120 days, from which time onwards the weight loss varied between 60 and 80 percent. . . . Thus there is general agreement concerning the marked loss of weight within the first two months of denervation.[3]

How fast denervated muscles lose weight is species-dependent. In a study

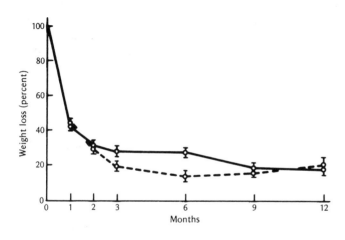

Figure 5–1. Percentage loss of weight in the extensor digitorum longus (solid line) and the soleus (interrupted line) in the rat. Abscissa: months after denervation. *(From Gutmann E, Zelena. J. Morphological changes in the denervated muscle. In: Gutmann E, ed. Denervated Muscle. Prague, Publishing House of the Czechoslovak Academy of Sciences, 1962, with permission.)*

comparing five species of mammals, Knowlton and Hines proposed that the differences found could be related to factors such as the metabolic rate of the species and its average life span.[4] Basically, a high metabolic rate and short life span are associated with fast atrophy. Compared to rats and rabbits therefore, human muscle would atrophy slower.

Figure 5–1 also shows that the curve relating weight loss to time after denervation flattens (in animals) after approximately 3 months. The residual weight after this time represents not only remaining muscle mass but non-muscle elements as well, such as connective tissue, blood vessels, and fat.[3] Indeed,it has been estimated that 10 to 25 percent of the weight of normal muscle is connective tissue.[4,5]

The fact that weight measurements are not the best index of muscle atrophy is more clearly shown by experiments that compared residual weight (as a percentage of normal) to muscle fiber size (also as a percentage of normal). As summarized by Sunderland:

> At all stages of denervation, the percentage decrease of muscle fiber diameters exceeded the percentage weight loss of the entire muscle. From this it is apparent that the fibres suffer more severely than the loss in weight indicates so that the calibre of the fibres provides a more accurate measure of the effects of denervation than does the weight of the muscle. The difference between the weight loss and the reduction in fibre calibre is accounted for by the relative increase in the amount of connective tissue which compensates in some measure for the greater atrophy of the fibre.

Microscopy, then, is obviously indispensable for studying denervation changes. It becomes an even more powerful tool when combined with histochemical techniques. These procedures, which differentially stain one fiber type or the other, are based on the fact that slow (Type I) and fast (Type II) muscle fibers posses different levels of certain enzymes relating to energy metabolism (Figure 5–2). When these techniques were employed in studies of denervation, some investigators reported that Type II fibers atrophy to a greater extent than Type I fibers.[6,10] Not surprisingly, however, these findings of "preferential atrophy" are not universally accepted.[11,12] Jaweed and associates[12] suggest the controversy might reflect (1) differences in the muscles examined (not all muscles react similarly to denervation); (2) the region of the muscle from which the biopsy was taken, and (3) whether muscles were studied early or late in denervation.

Two other questions of importance to understanding denervation atrophy and to determining whether NMES is useful or not are (1) Is denervation atrophy the same as disuse atrophy? and (2) Do denervated fibers ever actually degenerate so that ultimately they are no longer muscle? If this does occur, what time frame are we talking about?

When I was a student, some 30 years ago, we were taught that disuse atrophy, synonomous with "simple" atrophy, was completely different from denervation atrophy. The former occurred in conditions that curtailed volun-

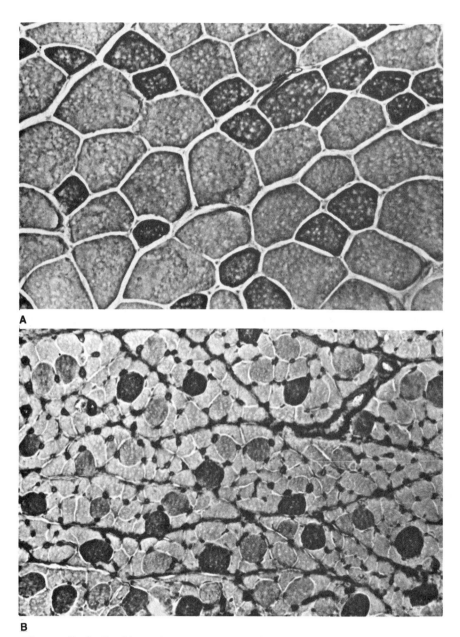

A

B

Figure 5–2. **A.** Normal rat extensor digitorum longus (EDL) muscle, ATPase histochemistry, with preincubation at pH 4.6. With this method, Type I fibers stain more darkly than Type II. Note also that in this muscle, Type II fibers are normally bigger than Type I. **B.** Denervated rat EDL (45 days), same stain as in (**A**). Both fiber types have atrophied considerably but Type I fibers (dark stain) are now bigger than the Type II. Calibration bars in (**A**) and (**B**) equal μ. *(Slides for photomicrographs courtesy of Dr. Bruce Pachter.)*

tary use of the muscle but left its lower motor neuron innervation intact. These clinical situations included immobilization (such as result of splinting, casting, tenotomy, or enforced bed rest), or upper motor neuron lesions (such as in spinal cord injury during the spinal shock stage, or in stroke). In these conditions, the only changes then recognized as occurring in muscles were a relatively mild atrophy associated with relatively mild loss in strength and endurance.

Contrasted to this seemingly benign and uncomplicated picture was the denervated muscle, which was not only paralyzed and wasting to a much greater extent, but was also fibrillating, exhibited marked hypersensitivity to acetylcholine (the agent that normally stimulates it), had totally different chronaxie and strength–duration relationships, and contracted sluggishly (instead of briskly) to long-duration monophasic pulses.

Today it is recognized that disuse atrophy is anything but simple. Though there are still morphological, electrical, mechanical, and biochemical differences between denervation and disuse, it is now apparent that normally innervated muscle reacts to unaccustomed inactivity in more ways than merely becoming smaller.[13,14] These muscles not only change in many of the parameters mentioned (for example, "slow" muscle becomes "fast" when immobilized), but in experimental animals, a muscle's reaction to enforced inactivity also depends upon (1) the length at which it is immobilized (or which it preferentially assumes)[11,15–17]; (2) the muscle itself (eg, soleus versus peroneus longus,[18] or soleus versus plantaris and gastrocnemius)[19]; (3) the species studied; (4) the time period under consideration; and (5) the condition used to effect inactivity (eg, casting, tenotomy, and upper motor neuron lesion). In humans, factor 5 has already been shown to be operative.[20,21] It is apparent, then, that although inactivity and denervation effect muscles differently, the distinction between them is not as great as was once thought. How these inactivity changes relate to the efficacy of stimulating denervated muscles will be brought out later, but let's return now to the question of whether denervated muscle fibers actually degenerate, and if so, within what time frame?

Why is this important to know? People unfamiliar with the problems associated with muscle re-innervation think of the process only in terms of axons regrowing to appropriate muscle fibers. For this to occur, nerve regeneration is obviously a prime requirement, but another is that there must be viable muscle fibers present that are capable of being re-innervated. If denervated muscle fibers ultimately degenerate and are replaced by fibrous tissue before the nerve regenerates to them, the regeneration might just as well not occur. And this brings up a related phenomenon, namely that as intramuscular fibrosis proceeds, it might act as a physical barrier to further retard re-innervation of remaining muscle fibers.[22]

Now we are getting to the heart of the problem: Muscle fiber degeneration and fibrosis are the real enemy, not atrophy itself. An atrophic muscle fiber, as long as it remains a muscle fiber, is capable of undergoing hypertrophy once it is reinervated. The race, then, so to speak, is between nerve regrowth on one hand and muscle fiber degeneration and fibrosis on the other. This is why it is important to know how much time we have before denervated muscle is irreversibly lost.

Not surprisingly, there is no unanimity of opinion concerning ultimate degeneration of denervated muscle fibers. While some investigators have reported considerable degeneration,[23-26] others have reported minimal if any.[27-30] These discrepant findings, however, may reflect the fact that different muscles were studied, different species were studied, different times after denervation were studied; and, of extreme importance to physical therapists, differences existed in the care rendered (or not rendered) the animals after the nerves were cut. (This translates, as will be seen later, into some guidelines for appropriate treatment of patients.) In the studies just cited, the article by Bowden and Gutmann[27] concerns humans and is therefore closest to what we are really interested in. In these cases, which of course were not experimental, degeneration of muscle was not found until at least 3 years following the onset of the lesion.

What causes the degeneration of denervated muscle fibers? Sunderland speculates that this is the result of prolonged intramuscular vascular stasis. He reasons (and gives experimental evidence to support his claims) that denervation leads to both vasoconstrictor paralysis and loss of muscle-pump action. These two factors lead to pooling of blood within the muscle. Prolonged intramuscular stasis, congestion, and possibly thrombosis, so impair the nutrition of the muscle fibers that they ultimately degenerate. According to this hypothesis, denervated distal muscles (hand or foot), because of their dependent position, would be at greater risk than more proximal muscles.

Another factor that might lead to degeneration of denervated muscle fibers is that of associated or superimposed trauma.[31,32] Denervated muscle is apparently more sensitive to trauma (including excessive heat and cold) than normal muscle, possibly related to the impaired nutritional state just described. In other words, normal muscle fibers have all the resources needed to repair even considerable damage to themselves whereas denervated fibers do not. Because of this deficiency, what might otherwise be minor trauma, or the cumulative effects of it, leads to more and more degeneration as time goes by.

The implications of all this for physical therapy (ignoring for now the question of electrical stimulation) is that steps must be taken to (1) limit edema and stasis; (2) maintain flexibility of the part, and (3) avoid further injury to the muscles as much as possible.

Other Changes with Denervation

As mentioned earlier, denervated muscle differs from normal muscle in a number of ways. These include:

1. *Fibrillation*. This involves spontaneous, uncoordinated contractions of individual muscle fibers, manifested as a persistent fine rippling of the surface of an exposed denervated muscle. Fibrillation was first reported

by Schiff in 1851,[33] long before the advent of electromyography. His report was also the first indication that denervated muscle is *not* totally quiescent but actually in fairly constant motion. This fibrillatory activity, however, is too fine to be seen through the overlying skin.

2. *Acetylcholine (ACh) hypersensitivity.* This is an example of the so-called Law of Denervation Supersensitivity.[34] This "law" states that after a period of time, a denervated structure (which could be skeletal muscle, smooth muscle, or gland) becomes hypersensitive to agents that normally activate it. ACh hypersensitivity develops in a denervated muscle because ACh receptors, which are normally present only in the endplate region of the sarcolemma, become incorporated into the entire length of the fiber's membrane.[35]

3. *Other membrane changes.* The resting potential of denervated muscle fibers falls (becomes less negative), and the transmembrane resistance increases.[36–38] Furthermore, the denervated endplate membrane develops pacemaker characteristics, which apparently accounts for the spontaneous fibrillation mentioned earlier.[39,40] The fibrillation is not secondary to the ACh hypersensitivity.

4. *Other electrical and mechanical changes.* Since the late 1800s, it has been known that denervated muscles lose their ability to respond to short-duration electrical pulses. To a long-duration pulse, however, say greater than 10 msec, denervated muscle will contract sluggishly. We are referring, of course, to the well-known changes in chronaxie and strength–duration relationships that help distinguish the innervated from the denervated states. Indeed, it is because denervated muscle retains the ability to respond to long-duration stimuli that we can activate them at all. In addition, because denervated muscle contracts and relaxes slowly, low-frequency stimuli of appropriate duration can fuse these contractions into a tetany. As will be shown, this ability to tetanize denervated muscle is of considerable importance to our topic. But first, a few points concerning re-innervation of denervated muscle should be made.

How Do Muscle Fibers Become Re-innervated?

To regain control of a denervated muscle fiber, a terminal nerve fiber must regrow to the endplate and establish a functional synapse with it. But how this re-innervation comes about depends upon whether all fibers in a muscle were denervated or only some of them. In other words, how muscle fibers become re-innervated depends upon whether the lesion partially or completely denervated the structure in the first place.

Let's first consider what happens when a peripheral nerve lesion disrupts all axons innervating a particular muscle. Although complete loss of voluntary function starts immediately, Wallerian degeneration of axons distal to the lesion proceeds over a period of days to weeks. Concomitant with this progressive distal degeneration, the anterior horn cells that gave rise to the axons change their metabolism, gearing to their new priority of replacing what they have lost. If all goes well, regeneration proceeds from the tip of each axon's proximal stump at a rate of about 1 to 2 mm/day, or about an inch per month. Ultimately, the target muscle, and its appropriate muscle fibers, are reached. Because this regeneration occurs slowly, it may take years before a competely denervated hand or foot muscle is re-innervated following a proximal nerve lesion.

A totally different scenario exists if a muscle is partially denervated, that is, if the lesion spares some of the axons that innervate it. In this case, denervated fibers can be re-innervated by intact axons "adopting" them. This re-innervation occurs via the process of *collateral sprouting*, of which two types, nodal and terminal, are now recognized.[41]

In nodal sprouting, an intramuscular axon lying not too far from a denervated muscle fiber sprouts an extension originating from a node of Ranvier (ie, where the axon is bared of its myelin sheath). This sprout enters a vacated endoneurial connective tissue tube and follows it to a denervated muscle fiber. In terminal sprouting, a terminal nerve fiber that is already innervating a muscle fiber sends out another twig that finds a nearby denervated muscle fiber.

Obviously, re-innervation by sprouting occurs much faster than in the first situation described because sprouts from intact intramuscular nerves need to grow only relatively short distances. It should also be recognized that re-innervation by either type of sprouting increases the size of the remaining motor units.

NMES IN DENERVATION

The literature concerning the effects of neuromuscular electrical stimulation on denervated muscle is enormous. This section is therefore based on articles representative of the various findings and conjectures.

Reid[42] is generally credited for first suggesting (in 1841) that electrical stimulation may be beneficial for denervated muscle.[3] From his time up to about the middle of this century, atrophy was the main if not the only parameter studied, first in terms of muscle weight and later with respect to histology.

During the First World War, Langley and Kato[43] rekindled interest in the topic when they compared a number of physical therapy modalities, namely massage, passive range of motion (ROM), and NMES, on their abilities to either prevent or retard weight loss of denervated muscles in rabbits. In those days, these techniques were used "after the severance of nerves in man . . . based on the view that muscle atrophy is due to inactivity." The authors wanted to determine (1) whether the techniques were indeed useful; and (2) if any insights could be uncovered concerning the cause of the atrophy.

Though theirs was a superficial study by today's standards (only seven animals, all of whom received different combinations of treatments and over different time periods), Langley and Kato concluded that "electrical stimulation with condenser shocks delays the atrophy, that rhythmic extension of the muscles has a similar but less effect, and that gentle massage for a like time has little if any effect."[43] They also noted that electrical stimulation (as they gave it) had no effect on fibrillation (which they looked for in exposed muscles) nor did it prevent the sluggish contractions of denervated muscles.

Why did the electrical stimulation only retard the atrophy, not prevent it? Langley and Kato raised three possibilities: (1) only superficial fibers were activated by the stimulation—more amplitude would have been needed to contract deeper fibers but such higher amplitudes would have damaged the superficial fibers (apparently a common belief in those days); (2) the number of contractions per day was insufficient, and (3) "the change in the muscle following nerve section is not simply an 'inactivity atrophy.' "[43] In view of today's thoughts concerning the possibility of neurotrophic factors and their suggested involvement in the regulation of muscle[1,37,44–47], this last conjecture by Langley and Kato, over 70 years ago, seems visionary.

In a follow-up to the 1915 paper, Langley[48] studied the effects of more prolonged stimulation (daily treatments for 2½ hours instead of for a few minutes). This investigation, however, used only two rabbits, sacrificed 21 and 23 days after neurectomy (a third rabbit was "treated" with passive ROM). Langley reported that "neither electrical stimulation nor passive movement had any definite effect in preventing loss of weight," and "it may fairly be concluded that the atrophy of denervated muscle is not due to the absence of contraction."[48]

Langley then went on to propose a radical but intriguing idea, namely that denervation atrophy was due to muscle fatigue, not disuse![48] The fatigue that Langley hypothesized was secondary to the almost-constant fibrillation. This activity, Langley suggested, might so sorely tax each fiber's energy supply that not enough remained to maintain the fiber's normal size. If this hypothesis was true, he continued, then electrical stimulation of denervated muscle would be contraindicated since the extra activity would only further deplete muscle fibers of their energy.

In this same paper, Langley[48] attempted to test his fatigue hypothesis by dissolving $CaCl_2$ in the milk given to cats. This procedure was done because Ca^{++} applied locally on a denervated muscle or injected into the muscle's bloodstream stops fibrillation. Langley, however, wanted long-term inhibition of this activity, which he tried to achieve by having the cats ingest relatively large amounts of the ion everytime they drank milk. Unfortunately, at the time of sacrifice, fibrillation was still observed and atrophy was still present.

Langley's fatigue hypothesis received a serious setback when Solandt and Magladery[49] reported prolonged inhibition of fibrillation with the drug quinidine but that atrophy still occurred.

Langley's puzzlement concerning whether NMES did (Langley and Kato[43]) or did not (Langley[48]) benefit denervated muscle seemed to set the stage for the contradictory reports that followed. Over the ensuing years, many studies (involving animals or clinical trials in humans) reported that neuromuscular electrical stimulation was either ineffectual or actually deleterious to denervated muscles.[25,50–54] Furthermore, although not directly related to denervated muscle, Cook and Gerard[55] reported that NMES of the distal stumps of severed nerves (ie, nerves that were already in the process of degenerating) hastened their degeneration. Other investigators, however, were equally assertive in claiming that NMES was indeed worthwhile.[22,56–65]

Why these differences? Recalling what was said earlier in this chapter concerning discrepancies regarding just the natural history of denervation atrophy, the reader might start wondering about such factors as species differences and variability between muscles studied. While these possibilities indeed deserve consideration (eg, Pollock and associates[54] did find differences between cats and rats), another variable that we must now consider is the treatment itself. In other words, all electrical stimulation is not equal. Today's informed therapist recognizes that merely knowing whether an investigator did or did not find NMES beneficial is insufficient information. The more important data that one wants concern the specifics of the treatment protocol that gave the results. Different protocols, though all may fall under the aegis of "electrical stimulation," may produce completely different results.[22,57,59,60,63–65] Therefore, when discussing this therapeutic technique, particular attention must be paid to the following:

1. Current or waveform used (eg, monophasic, biphasic, or sinusoidal).
2. Duration of the stimulating pulse (with sinusoidal currents, this is inversely related to the frequency; ie, the lower the frequency, the longer the negative pulse; with monophasic current, the duration of the negative pulse is chosen by the therapist; with classical biphasic current, the negative pulse is 1 msec).
3. Type of contraction used to "treat" the muscle (eg, twitch or tetanus). These, as the student knows (or should know), are related to (1) the muscle's chronaxie; (2) the contraction and relaxation times of the muscle, and (3) the frequency of the stimulus employed.
4. Strength of contraction produced (eg, minimal, weak, strong, or maximum). Related to this, was the contraction isometric or isotonic? Also, was the length of the muscle at the start of the contraction stretched, rest length, or shortened? If the contraction was isotonic, did the muscle shorten against resistance or no resistance?
5. Number of such contractions produced per treatment session.
6. Duration of each such contraction if a tetanus (the duration of a twitch cannot be controlled by the therapist).
7. How much rest was given between contractions.
8. Number of treatment sessions per day.
9. Number of treatment sessions per week.
10. How soon after denervation treatments were started.
11. How long after denervation the study ran (eg, 14 days? 6 months? 2

years?). This last point is particularly important. For example, to a clinician it is only of academic interest to know that 14 days after denervation, muscles treated with a particular stimulation protocol are not quite as atrophic as untreated ones. What we really need to know is how effective the treatment is for muscles that have been denervated 12, 24, or 36 *months*. To my knowledge, no animal study has ever been carried this far.

To this point, we have been talking about the effects of electrical stimulation on just one aspect of denervation, namely atrophy as measured by muscle weight. In a much more ambitious study, Gutmann and Guttmann,[22] studying rabbits, measured not only muscle weight but also circumference of limbs, fiber diameters, connective tissue changes, time to onset of recovery, quality of contractions, and presence of fibrillation, while also systematically varying treatment protocol in terms of treatment duration, number of treatments per day, and when treatment was begun after denervation. Using monophasic pulses strong enough to produce "vigorous contractions" (a typical 20-min treatment would produce 500 to 600 single contractions), they reported:

1. Delayed or diminished atrophy in treated muscles.
2. Best results obtained with daily treatments of 20 to 30 min duration.
3. The earlier the treatments were started, the better the results.
4. Histologically, muscle fibers were larger and connective tissue less in treated muscles (Figure 5–3).
5. Muscle fatigue caused by the treatment did not seem to matter.

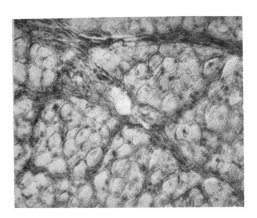 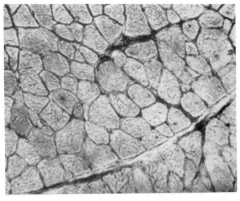

A   **B**

Figure 5–3. Cross sections of untreated (**A**) and treated (**B**) muscles of a rabbit 67 days after denervation. Treatment sessions were for 20 minutes daily, commencing 7 days after neurectomy. Fibers are more atrophic and connective tissue more plentiful in the untreated muscle. *(From Gutmann &* *Guttmann, 1944, with permission.[22])*

6. The rate of re-innervation, as evidenced by return of reflex or voluntary function, was neither hastened nor retarded by the treatment.

So far we have mainly considered atrophy measured either by weighing a muscle or looking at it microscopically. Obviously, neither technique is applicable to serial studies in humans. Osborne[62] developed a volumetric technique that he used to study the effects of NMES. His paper is based on the finding that in 20 healthy subjects, the volumes of both upper extremities, measured by immersion into a cylinder, are quite similar. Therefore, the atrophy of an affected extremity can be estimated by comparing its volume to that of its counterpart. Osborne also pointed out, however, that unlike animal investigations, peripheral nerve injuries in humans are usually associated with other medical problems (such as wound healing and infections) that preclude immediate institution of NMES. Therefore, in the "real" world (and in his study), some amount of denervation atrophy occurs before patients start treatment.

Another problem that Osborne described is that out of fifteen patients, only seven were able or willing to continue with the months or years of treatments (a problem we will address again later). In these seven patients, however, daily stimulation with currents adjusted to produce as strong contractions as the patients could tolerate, resulted in no change in atrophy in three, slight reversal of atrophy in two, and slightly increased atrophy in one. Although Osborne was generally supportive for using NMES as a treatment for denervated muscles, the study contained no control subjects for comparisons. For example, the volumes of the affected limbs may have stayed the same (or even increased) not because atrophy was stopped or reversed but because compensatory hypertrophy occurred in the muscles that remained. Since no control patients were included, we have no way of knowing how much to credit NMES and how much to credit other factors. Furthermore, it must be recognized that a volume measurement is relatively gross and does not tell us specifically what is occurring in muscle. An increase in one area can mask a decrease in another, and a volume measurement will not differentiate between them.

Looking at the problem in a somewhat different way, Wakim and Krusen[64] investigated in rats how NMES effects denervated muscle functionally instead of anatomically. Denervation was accomplished unilaterally by removing segments of both the sciatic and femoral nerves. Treatment consisted of square wave pulses, 1 msec in duration at 16 pps, strong enough to produce maximal contractions of the whole extremity. What was varied between eight groups of animals was the duration of the treatment and how many times a day it was given. After 25 to 30 days (which is, of course, of questionable significance to humans), muscles were tested for their ability to perform mechanical work and their endurance (the interested reader is referred to the article for details to how this was done). Basically, their findings were that 30 min of stimulation once daily was of some benefit (compared to no stimulation); 30 min twice a day was considerably better; 5 min every half hour over an 8-hr day (with 1 hr off for lunch) was as beneficial as longer periods of stimulation also performed every half hour. Should these findings be applicable to humans, patients would be spending so much of their time just waiting around for the next treatment session that gainful employment would be practically impossible. To make matters worse, although stimulated muscles were stronger and had more endurance than non-stimulated controls, treated muscles at best achieved only 50 percent of normal (ie, non-denervated) power and endurance. In other words, stimulation, as done by these investigators, could not substitute totally for the real thing.

In another study comparing the strength of denervated non-stimulated to denervated stimulated muscles, Nix[66] found that after 22 to 49 days, muscles treated daily with submaximal tetanic contractions for 8 hr/day had lower twitch and tetanic tensions in response to supramaximum 0.3-msec pulses. But with longer duration testing pulses, strength was essentially equal in the two groups. Nix also found that when muscles started to become re-innervated, the latency between stimulating the nerve and the onset of the muscle response averaged 13.4 msec in denervated non-stimulated muscles but 14.4 msec in the denervated stimulated ones. In normal controls, this latency averaged 4.8 msec. At best, then, these mechanical and electrical parameters of function were certainly no better in the stimulated denervated muscles than in the non-treated ones. In fact, some people may interpret the findings as showing that the stimulated muscles were worse.

And indeed, reports that NMES may have deleterious effects on denervated muscles have appeared. As far back as 1939, Chor and co-workers[25] reported in monkeys that stimulated muscles had more degenerated fibers than non-stimulated controls (ie, just the opposite of what we're trying to accomplish). And more recently, Nix and Dahm[67] reported in rabbits that 20 minutes of daily strong isometric tetanic contractions (1-msec pulses delivered at 40 pps for 100 msec each second) resulted in mechanical and histological evidence of severe atrophy of fibers with considerable fibrosis and contracture formation at the end of 28 days. However, muscles stimulated at only 1 pps for 20 minutes daily over that same time period showed no contracture formation and statistically significant less atrophy than non-stimulated denervated muscles. But although the differences in atrophy at this lower frequency of stimulation were statistically significant, the stimulated fibers were only about 10 percent less atrophied than the non-stimulated ones. In other words, the treated muscles still atrophied considerably.

Furthermore, in a study on rats up to 7 weeks after denervation, Schimrigk, McLaughlin, and Gruninger[68] reported histological evidence suggesting delayed re-innervation of treated muscles, while Jansen and associates,[69] also using rats, found that NMES inhibited re-innervation by a "foreign nerve," (that is, by a nerve that normally did not innervate that particular muscle. Re-innervation by the usual nerve, however, was not affected. In a somewhat different vein, Girlanda and co-workers,[70] studying rabbits 50 days after denervation, found that NMES *accentuated* the atrophy of Type I fibers in the extensor digitorum longus and soleus muscles and increased the weight loss of the latter. These authors concluded, that "the results obtained raise further doubts about the clinical utility of electrotherapy."[70] In this paper, however, electromyographic evidence of re-innervation appeared at the same time in treated and non-treated animals.

WHY MIGHT NMES BE DELETERIOUS?

From what has been said so far, we see two ways that NMES may be deleterious to denervated muscle: (1) it may cause fiber degeneration, excessive fibrosis, or both; or (2) it may retard re-innervation. The question then is, are these effects due to the electricity itself or are they secondary to the "exercise" the stimulations produce?

With respect to both muscle fiber degeneration (with or without associated fibrosis) and retardation of re-innervation, the answer seems to lie with the exercise. For example, as far back as 1915, Lovett[71] reported that unaccustomed or over-use of paretic muscles frequently caused polio patients to lose strength instead of gaining it. Lundervold and Seyffarth[72] confirmed this, not only in polio patients but in normal subjects who underwent compression of their peroneal nerves for 20 to 30 minutes. In this latter situation, subjects who did not walk until some hours had passed after the compression was released showed full return of function by day's end; but those who walked immediately after release of the compression took 3 to 4 days before their normal strength and endurance returned.

Similarly, Bennett and Knowlton[73] described four patients with poliomyelitis and one with C5-6 quadriplegia in whom "excessive" exercise of weak muscles was followed by considerable clinical deterioration.

Although the exact cause of these strength decreases has not been ascertained, it is reasonable to surmise either that remaining motor units in a partially denervated muscle can be damaged by overuse, that use of recently reinnervated units causes immature neuromuscular junctions to "detach" and thereby re-denervate the muscle fibers, or both.

If these clinical observations are valid, perhaps strong NMES of denervated muscles, carried out day after day, causes so much muscle fiber damage that after a while degeneration and fibrosis ensue. And this could occur regardless of whether the muscle is completely or partially denervated.

With respect to the second possible deleterious effect of NMES (retarding re-innervation), a number of animal studies have reported this. But here too the situation is complicated because some types of re-innervation are affected more than others. For example, when muscles are partially denervated by cutting one of their motor roots, NMES suppresses re-innervation by terminal sprouting but not by nodal sprouting.[74,75] However, in muscles completely denervated by crushing their nerves not too far proximally, NMES suppresses re-innervation by a "foreign" nerve (eg, re-innervation of the soleus muscle by the peroneal nerve,[69]) but not the appropriate nerve.[75,76] It should be noted, though, that in these two studies, the "appropriate" and "foreign" nerves had to regenerate following different types of injuries. The former had simply been crushed, but the latter had been cut and then rerouted and implanted into the new target muscle. Since nerves damaged by crushing generally regenerate better and faster than nerves damaged by cutting anyway, finding that NMES in these cases did not suppress re-innervation by the appropriate nerve may not be relevant to the clinical situations we are considering. What might be more important is that re-innervation by the *cut* nerve *was* suppressed.

But as stated in the first part of this chapter, for just about every report concerning the effects of NMES on denervated muscle, a contradictory one has also appeared (and if it hasn't, history teaches us that it soon will!). Therefore, for the sake of fairness and objectivity with respect to the deleterious effects just mentioned, the reader should be aware that Herbison, Teng, and Gordon[77] found no histological or weight differences between stimulated and non-stimulated rat muscles 6 to 7 weeks after re-innervation had occurred following crush of their sciatic nerves, although treatment was given daily until the time of sacrifice (ie, well into the re-innervation period); that Harada, Nakano, and Fujiwara[78] found neuromuscular electrical stimulation suppressed atrophy of Type I fibers in crush-denervated rat extensor digitorum longus muscle (opposite to the findings of Girlander and associates[70]); and that Pachter, Eberstein, and Goodgold[10] found that NMES retarded atrophy in both Type I and II fibers 28 days after excising a segment of sciatic nerve in rats, but with more effect on Type II fibers.

OTHER PROBLEMS ASSOCIATED WITH STIMULATION

Let's assume for the moment that NMES does benefit denervated muscle from the viewpoint of retarding atrophy and subsequent degeneration. But since retardation of atrophy is not the same as prevention (and there have been very few reports of absolute prevention), stimulation is at best only a delaying action, and if enough time goes by, treated muscle will still become as atrophic as non-treated muscle. Furthermore, this raises the question as to why stimulation does not substitute entirely for normal activation? One can think of at least two possibilities:

1. The quality and quantity of stimulation that has been employed in all the different studies still does not approach the exercise that a normally innervated muscle undergoes.
2. Denervation results not only in relative inactivity of muscle (for which stimulation hopes to substitute), but also in muscles being deprived of chemical trophic influences secreted into the muscle fibers by their

motor nerves. Stimulation cannot substitute for this. In other words, certain aspects of muscle metabolism may be regulated by muscle activity while other aspects possibly depend on neurosecretory functions of anterior horn cells mediated via axonal transport mechanisms.[1,37,44–47,79–81] The most direct confirmatory evidence for this latter possibility comes from the studies by Davis and associates.[44,45] In the first of these papers, it was reported that denervated extensor digitorum longus muscles of rats, injected twice daily for 1 week with an extract of peripheral nerves, lost less weight and total protein than denervated muscles injected with saline or heat-inactivated extract or not injected at all. These differences were associated histologically with 16 percent less atrophy of Type IIB fibers. Type IIA fibers, however, were not affected, atrophying by the same amount as control muscles. Type I fibers had not changed during the short time of the study (only 7 days), so no conclusions were reached concerning whether the extract had any affect on them (Type I fibers are known to undergo denervation atrophy much slower than Type II fibers). The second paper reported that the factor in the extract that retards the Type IIB atrophy was a glycoprotein of approximately 100,000 molecular weight. Therefore, if denervation changes result from both inactivity and deprivation of trophic factors, the inability of NMES to maintain these muscles fully and indefinitely becomes more understandable.

So where do we stand at this point in time? First, we know that there is no unanimity of opinion concerning how well NMES affects denervated muscle. One cannot, therefore, be convicted of malpractice or negligence for not using it. Second, there is some evidence that NMES may actually be deleterious to denervated muscle, and while this is also questioned, the reports cast a further pall over using the technique. Third, if the site of a lesion is such that re-innervation can be reasonably expected within, say, 12 to 18 months (assuming the classical concept that nerve regeneration proceeds at the average rate of 1 inch per month), stimulation to retard degeneration is not necessary because human muscle does not degenerate that fast anyway.[27] And fourth, at least two studies on humans have reported that recovery of non-stimulated muscles can indeed equal that of stimulated muscles over this period of time (ie, up to 18 months) as long as other appropriate care is given.[50,53] (It should be noted, however, that in the second report[53] very little information is given to substantiate the claim of ineffectiveness. Furthermore, I suggest reading the free discussion that follows this paper. Some interesting opinions are expressed.)

But what about patients in whom the first signs of regeneration are not reasonably expected before 24 months or more? It is these people who are most at risk for irreversible fibrosis of muscles and it is therefore they who require the most maintenance, so the question arises: Should electrical stimulation be included as part of their overall treatment program? Ignoring for the moment the issues we have been discussing regarding the dubious efficacy of NMES, these cases raise even further problems, namely those introduced by the mundane world of finances and of patient compliance. Putting it bluntly, how much extra will it cost, either the patient or third parties, if these controversial treatments are now added to an already extensive and intense rehabilitation schedule? And as mentioned earlier, if stimulation to be effective has to be given two or three times daily, not much spare time will remain during the rest of the day for the patient to do anything else? And this brings us face to face with the problem of patient compliance alluded to earlier by Osborne.[62] How many patients are going to be willing and able to faithfully participate in these daily treatments over these many years? And how much will they lose if they miss some treatments due to sickness, holidays, and vacation time? These are the realistic questions of life, and we do not know the answers to them.

Of course, if NMES was unequivocally useful, these last points would probably be mentioned only in passing. But in view of the facts at hand, they too must weigh heavily when deciding whether or not to include NMES in the long-term treatment of peripheral nerve injury.

SUMMARY

There was a time some years ago when the general consensus held that NMES was beneficial to denervated muscle but had no effect on innervated muscle. Today the climate has changed. The latest buzz words include "Russian technique" and "functional electric stimulation," both of which describe electrical methods for improving strength and endurance of normal muscles in humans. Equally intriguing is that in intact animals, NMES with appropriate parameters can actually convert fast muscles into slow (although all changes reverse soon after cessation of NMES treatment.)[82] Thus the pendulum swings. It now seems that NMES can indeed be used safely and effectively to influence innervated muscle.

With denervated muscle, however, the current picture is less optimistic. Although many investigators have reported that NMES is beneficial with respect to retarding denervation atrophy, few if any have claimed total prevention. As described, this may reflect the inability of NMES to substitute for possible chemical trophic effects of innervation. Furthermore, since many of these positive reports were based on animal studies carried out over relatively short time spans, their findings may not even be applicable to the realities of human nerve injuries that may require years to regenerate. And finally, there is the question of whether it is worth the time, effort, and money to give years of controversial treatments. In my opinion, the answer is no; but I am sure there are those who disagree!

REFERENCES

1. Davis HL. Is electrostimulation beneficial to denervated muscle? A review of results from basic research. *Physiother Can.* 35:306, 1983
2. Jacobs SR, Jaweed MM, Herbison GJ, Stillwell GK. Electrical stimulation of muscle. In: Stillwell GK, ed. *Therapeutic Electricity and Ultraviolet Radiation*, 3rd ed. Baltimore, Williams & Wilkins, 1983
3. Sunderland S. *Nerves and Nerve Injuries*, 2nd ed. Edinburgh, Churchill Livingston, 1978
4. Knowlton GC, Hines HM. Kinetics of muscle atrophy in different species. *Proc Soc Exp Biol Med.* 35:394, 1936
5. Weiss P, Edds MV Jr. Spontaneous recovery of muscle following partial denervation. *Am J Physiol.* 145:587, 1946
6. Bajusz E. "Red" skeletal muscle fibers: Relative independence of neural control. *Science.* 145:938, 1964
7. Engel WK, Brooke MH, Nelson PH. Histochemical studies of denervated or tenotomized cat muscle: Illustrating difficulties in relating experimental animal conditions to human neuromuscular disease. *Ann NY Acad Sci.* 138:160, 1965
8. Karpati G, Engel WK. Histochemical investigation of fiber type ratios with myofibrillar ATP-ase reaction in normal and denervated skeletal muscles of guinea pig. *Am J Anat.* 122:145, 1968
9. Melichna J, Gutmann E. Stimulation and immobilization effects on contractile and histochemical properties of denervated muscle. *Eur J Physiol.* 352:165, 1974
10. Pachter BR, Eberstein A, Goodgold J. Electrical stimulation effect on denervated skeletal myofibers in rats: A light and electron microscopic study. *Arch Phys Med Rehabil.* 63:427, 1982
11. Boyes G, Johnston I. Muscle fiber composition of rat vastus intermedius following immobilization at different muscle lengths. *Eur J Physiol.* 381:195, 1979
12. Jaweed MM, Herbison GJ, DiTunno JF. Denervation and reinervation of fast and slow muscles: A histochemical study in rats. *J Histochem Cytochem.* 23:808, 1975
13. Booth FW. Effect of limb immobilization on skeletal muscle. *J Appl Physiol.* 52:1113, 1982
14. Wills CA, Caiozzo MS, Yasukawa DI, et al. Effects of immobilization on human skeletal muscle. *Ortho Rev.* 11:57, 1982
15. Booth FW. Time course of muscular atrophy during immobilization of hindlimbs in rats. *J Appl Physiol.* 43:656, 1977
16. Thompsen P, Luco JV. Changes of weight and neuromuscular transmission in muscles of immobilized joints. *J Neurophysiol.* 7:246, 1944
17. Williams PE, Goldspink G. Longitudinal growth of striated muscle fibers. *J Cell Sci.* 9:751, 1971
18. McMinn RMH, Vrbova G. Morphological changes in red and pale muscles following tenotomy. *Nature.* 195:509, 1962
19. Herbison GJ, Jaweed MM, DiTunno JF. Muscle atrophy in rats following denervation, casting, inflammation, and tenotomy. *Arch Phys Med Rehabil.* 60:401, 1979
20. Edstrom L. Selective changes in the sizes of red and white muscle fibers in upper motor lesions and Parkinsonism. *J Neurol Sci.* 11:537, 1970
21. Edstrom L. Selective atrophy of red muscle fibers in the quadriceps in long-

standing knee-joint dysfunction: Injuries to the anterior cruciate ligament. *J Neurol Sci.* 11:551, 1970

22. Gutmann E, Guttmann L. The effect of galvanic exercise on denervated and re-innervated muscles in the rabbit. *J Neurol Neurosurg Psychiat.* 7:7, 1944
23. Aird RB, Nafziger HC: The pathology of human striated muscle following denervation. *J Neurosurg.* 10:216, 1953
24. Altschul R. Atrophy, degeneration and metaplasia in denervated skeletal muscle. *Arch Path.* 34:982, 1942
25. Chor H, Cleveland D, Davenport HA, et al. Atrophy and regeneration of the gastrocnemius-soleus muscles. *JAMA.* 113:1029, 1939
26. Tower SS. Atrophy and degeneration in skeletal muscle. *Am J Anat.* 56:1, 1935
27. Bowden REM, Gutmann E. Denervation and re-innervation of human voluntary muscle. *Brain.* 67:273, 1944
28. Reid GA. A comparison of the effects of disuse and denervation upon skeletal muscle. *Med J Aust.* 2:165, 1941
29. Sunderland S, Ray LJ. Denervation changes in mammalian striated muscle. *J Neurol Neurosurg Psychiat.* 13:159, 1950
30. Willard WA, Grau EC. Some histological changes in striate muscle following nerve section. *Anat Rec.* 27:192, 1924
31. Adams RD, Denny-Brown D, Pearson CM. *Diseases of Muscle.* London, Cassell, 1962
32. Denny-Brown D. The influence of tension and innervation on the regeneration of skeletal muscle. *J Neuropath Exp Neurol.* 10:94, 1951
33. Schiff M. Ueber motorische Lähmung der Zunge. *Arch Physiol Heilkunde.* 10:579, 1851
34. Cannon WB, Rosenblueth A. *The Supersensitivity of Denervated Structures.* New York, Macmillan, 1949
35. Axelsson J, Thesleff S. A study of supersensitivity in denervated mammalian skeletal muscle. *J Physiol.* 147:178, 1959
36. Albuquerque EX, McIsaac RJ. Fast and slow mammalian muscles after denervation. *Exp Neurol.* 26:183, 1970
37. Guth L, Kemerer VF, Samaras TA, et al. The roles of disuse and loss of neurotrophic function in denervation atrophy of skeletal muscle. *Exp. Neurol.* 73:20, 1981
38. Ware F, Bennett AL, McIntyre AR. Membrane resting potential of denervated mammalian skeletal muscle measured in vivo. *Am J Physiol.* 177:115, 1954
39. Belmar J, Eyzaguirre C. Pacemaker site of fibrillation potentials in denervated mammalian muscle. *J Neurophysiol.* 29:425, 1966
40. Purves D, Sakmann B. Membrane properties underlying spontaneous activity of denervated muscle fibers. *J Physiol.* 239:125, 1974
41. Brown MC, Holland RL, Hopkins WG. Motor nerve sprouting. *Ann Rev Neurosci.* 4:17, 1981
42. Reid J. On relation between muscular contractility and the nervous system. *Lond Edinb Mon J Sci.* 1:320, 1841.
43. Langley JN, Kato T. The rate of loss of weight in skeletal muscle after nerve section with some observations on the effect of stimulation and other treatment. *J Physiol.* 49:432, 1915
44. Davis HL, Kiernan JA. Neurotrophic effects of sciatic nerve extract on denervated extensor digitorum longus muscle in the rat. *Exp Neurol.* 69:124, 1980

45. Davis HL, Heinicke EA, Cook RA, Kiernan JA. Partial purification from mammalian peripheral nerve of a trophic factor that ameliorates atrophy of denervated muscle. *Exp Neurol.* 89:159, 1985

46. Luco, JV, Eyzaguirre C. Fibrillation and hypersensitivity to ACh in denervated muscle: Effect of length of degenerating nerve fibers. *J Neurophysiol.* 18:65, 1955

47. Spielholz NI, Sell GH, Goodgold J, et al. Electrophysiological studies in patients with spinal cord lesions. *Arch Phys Med Rehabil.* 53:558, 1972

48. Langley JN. Observations on denervated muscle. *J Physiol.* 50:335, 1916

49. Solandt DY, Magladery JW. The relation of atrophy to fibrillation in denervated muscle. *Brain.* 63:255, 1940

50. Doupe J, Barnes R, Kerr AS. Studies in denervation: H. The effect of electrical stimulation on the circulation and recovery of denervated muscle. *J Neurol Psych.* 6:136, 1943

51. Hartman FA, Blatz WE. Studies in the regeneration of denervated mammalian muscle. III. Effects of massage and electrical treatment. *J Physiol.* 53:290, 1920

52. Molander CO, Steinitz FS, Asher R. Effect of the galvanic current on paralyzed muscle: An experimental study on the dog. *Arch Phys Ther.* 22:154, 1941

53. Newman WK, Berris JM, Bohn SS. Management of facial paralysis by physical methods. *Arch Phys Ther.* 21:270, 1940

54. Pollock LJ, Arieff AJ, Sherman IC, et al. Electrotherapy in experimentally produced lesions of peripheral nerves. *Arch Phys Med Rehabil.* 32:377, 1951

55. Cook DD, Gerard RW. The effect of stimulation on the degeneration of a severed peripheral nerve. *Am J Physiol.* 97:412, 1931

56. Fischer E. The effect of faradic and galvanic stimulation upon the course of atrophy in denervated skeletal muscles. *Am J Physiol.* 127:605, 1939

57. Herbison GJ, Teng C-S, Reyes T, Reyes O. Effect of electrical stimulation on denervated muscle of rat. *Arch Phys Med Rehabil.* 52:516, 1971

58. Kosman AJ, Osborne SL, Ivy AC. The effect of electrical stimulation upon the course of atrophy and recovery of the gastrocnemius of the rat. *Am J Physiol.* 145:447, 1946

59. Kosman AJ, Osborne SL, Ivy AC. The comparative effectiveness of various electrical currents in preventing muscle atrophy in the rat. *Arch Phys Med.* 28:7, 1947

60. Kosman AJ, Osborne SL, Ivy AC. The influence of duration and frequency of treatment in electrical stimulation of paralyzed muscle. *Arch Phys Med.* 28:12, 1947

61. Kosman AJ, Wood EC, Osborne SL. Effect of electrical stimulation upon atrophy of partially denervated skeletal muscle of the rat. *Am J Physiol.* 154:451, 1948

62. Osborne SL. The retardation of atrophy in man by electrical stimulation of muscles. *Arch Phys Med Rehabil.* 32:523, 1951

63. Solandt DY, DeLury DB, Hunter J. Effect of electrical stimulation on atrophy of denervated skeletal muscle. *Arch Neurol Psych.* 49:802, 1943

64. Wakim KG, Krusen FH. The influence of electrical stimulation on the work output and endurance of denervated muscle. *Arch Phys Med Rehabil.* 36:370, 1955

65. Wehrmacher WT, Thomson JD, Hines HM. Effects of electrical stimulation on denervated skeletal muscle. *Arch Phys Med.* 26:261, 1945

66. Nix WA. The effect of low-frequency electrical stimulation on the denervated extensor digitorum longus muscle of the rabbit. *Acta Neurol Scand.* 66:521, 1982

67. Nix WA, Dahm M. The effect of isometric short-term electrical stimulation on denervated muscle. *Muscle Nerve.* 10:136, 1987

68. Schimrigk K, McLaughlin J, Gruninger W. The effect of electrical stimulation on the experimentally denervated rat muscle. *Scand J Rehab Med.* 9:55, 1977

69. Jansen JKS, Lomo T, Nicolaysen K, Westgaard RH. Hyperinnervation of skeletal muscle fibers: Dependence on muscle activity. *Science.* 559, 1973

70. Girlanda R, Dattola R, Vita G, et al. Effect of electrotherapy on denervated muscles in rabbits: An electrophysiological and morphological study. *Exp Neurol.* 77:483, 1982

71. Lovett RW. The treatment of infantile paralysis. *JAMA.* 64:2118, 1915

72. Lundervold A, Seyffarth H. Electromyographic investigations of poliomyelitic paresis during the training up of the affected muscles, and some remarks regarding the treatment of paretic muscles. *Acta Psychiat Neurol.* 17:69, 1942

73. Bennett RL, Knowlton GC. Overwork weakness in partially denervated skeletal muscle. *Clin Orthop.* 12:22, 1958

74. Brown MC, Holland RL, Ironton R. Nodal and terminal sprouting from motor nerves in fast and slow muscles of the mouse. *J Physiol.* 306:493, 1980

75. Ironton R, Brown MC, Holland RL. Stimuli to intramuscular nerve growth. *Brain Res.* 156:351, 1978

76. Brown MC, Ironton R. Suppression of motor nerve terminal sprouting in partially denervated mouse muscles. *J Physiol.* 272:70, 1977

77. Herbison GJ, Teng C-S, Gordon EE. Electrical stimulation of reinnervating rat muscle. *Arch Phys Med Rehabil.* 54:156, 1973

78. Harada Y, Nakano K, Fujiwara M. Effects of electrical stimulation on the denervated rat muscle. *Acta Med Hypogoensia.* 4:129, 1979

79. Buller AJ, Eccles JC, Eccles RM. Interactions between motoneurones and muscles in respect of the characteristic speeds of their responses. *J Physiol.* 150:417, 1960

80. Drachman DB, Witzke F. Trophic regulation of acetylcholine sensitivity of muscle: Effect of electrical stimulation. *Science.* 176:514, 1972

81. Gutmann E. Neurotrophic regulation. *Ann Rev Physiol.* 38:177, 1976

82. Salmons S, Henriksson J. The adaptive response of skeletal muscle to increased use. *Muscle Nerve.* 4:94, 1981

CHAPTER 6

Clinical Uses of Neuromuscular Electrical Stimulation

Lucinda L. Baker

Electrical stimulation has been used to create muscular contractions for many years, dating back to the pioneering work of Duchenne.[1,2] Neuromuscular electrical stimulation (NMES) is the actuation of muscular tissue through the intact peripheral nervous system. The popularity of NMES for management of a variety of patient problems has waxed and waned throughout the years. Today it is recognized that many of the NMES programs previously deemed ineffective were thought to be so because of inadequacies of both treatment management and stimulation parameters. The purpose of this chapter is to identify the treatment paradigms necessary to ensure success of NMES treatment programs in a wide variety of practice settings.

There are five major categories of treatment programs that use NMES.[3–5] The categories are grouped accordingly to treatment goals. They include the use of NMES to (1) strengthen or maintain muscle mass or both during or following periods of enforced inactivity; (2) maintain or gain range of motion; (3) facilitate voluntary motor control; (4) temporarily reduce the effects of spasticity; and (5) temporarily provide for orthotic substitution. Stimulation programs designed to maintain muscle strength during immobilization or to strengthen normal muscle are described in Chapter 7. The present chapter will focus on the last four treatment goals.

MAINTAINING RANGE OF MOTION

Maintaining range of motion can be of major concern in some patients with central nervous system lesions that result in spasticity. Depending on the patient's activity level, range of motion (ROM) techniques may be self-administered or taught to family members. For the patient with minimal spastic tone, self-administered ROM techniques are often successful. The patient who demonstrates moderate to severe spasticity frequently has difficulty completing self-administered home programs. When the decreased ROM interferes with function, basic hygiene, and positioning of the spastic limb, surgical intervention is frequently the treatment of choice. To avoid costly and potentially dangerous surgical procedures, NMES can be used as a means of prophylactically maintaining joint ROM for those high-risk patients.

In a study reported by Baker and co-workers, nine hemiplegic patients who demonstrated full passive ROM but also exhibited moderate wrist and finger flexor spasticity were treated exclusively with NMES for the purpose of maintaining wrist extension ROM.[6] A slight increase in extension ROM was obtained (Fig. 6–1). The treatment protocol was replicated in five physical therapy clinics across the country.[7] Two centers had minimal exposure, and the other three clinics had no experience with the use of NMES for maintenance of ROM prior to the study. During a 9-month data-collection period, these five centers treated 68 patients with spasticity and minimal ROM limitations at the wrist and fingers. The use of NMES was as effective in maintaining ROM in the multi site study as it was in the single-treatments setting.[6,7]

A further observation made by Baker and co-workers was that patients who had been using NMES at home for their ROM programs demonstrated a decrease in available range *after* the stimulation was discontinued and the traditional, passive ROM treatment protocol was reinstituted.[6] Thus, at least at the wrist and fingers, the patients were more successful in maintaining ROM at home when the treatment consisted of electrically induced ranging techniques rather then the traditional, self-administered passive programs. Initially, it may be difficult to justify the cost of a cyclical electrical stimulator for home use compared to the cost of manual ROM techniques. But NMES compares favorably both in terms of cost and human suffering if even a relatively minor surgical procedure is avoided. Thus, for the patient who has spasticity that interferes with function, hygiene, or positioning, an NMES home-treatment program may be an effective means of avoiding both the physical and financial costs associated with limited ROM.

Since the patient most likely to benefit from this NMES treatment program is one who demonstrates moderate to severe spasticity, care must be taken to ensure that appropriate stimulus parameters and positioning techniques are used. Full ROM without a quick jerking response is desired. A long, slow approach to maximum stimulus amplitude is a critical feature to the success of an NMES program designed to activate either a spastic muscle or its antagonist.

In addition, the anatomical characteristics of the muscles being stimulated and of other muscles surrounding the treated joint must be considered. Baker and co-workers noted that to ensure full extension of the interphalangeal joints in a patient with severe spasticity of the wrist or finger flexors, the electrically

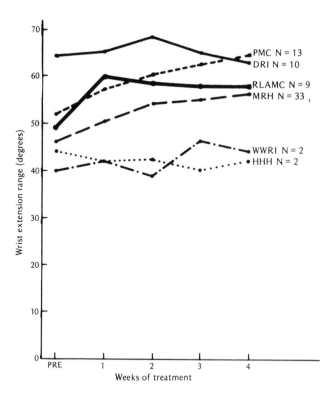

	Pre	1	2	3	4
RLAMC	47.8 ± 4.3	56.7 ± 3.6	55.6 ± 3.9	56.2 ± 3.9	57.9 ± 4.1
DRI	64.4 ± 2.6	65.2 ± 3.3	68 ± 3.3	65.2 ± 3.2	63 ± 3.5
MRH	46.2 ± 1.7	50.4 ± 1.2	53.6 ± 2.3	54.9 ± 2.4	56.0 ± 2.3
PMC	51.5 ± 3.5	56.9 ± 4	60 ± 3.8	62.2 ± 3.8	63.8 ± 3.6
WWRI	40 ± 9	42.5 ± 6.5	39 ± 1	46 ± 4	44 (1 and 2)
HHH	43.5 ± 1.5	42 ± 2	41.5 ± 6.5	40.5 ± 2.5	42 ± 1

Figure 6–1. Effect of an NMES range-of-motion program in hemiparetic patients with finger and wrist flexor spasticity but no significant range limitations. Data supplied by six different clinics, including those from a previously reported study (*Phys Ther* 59:1495, 1979). Means and standard error of the means are represented.

stimulated range allowed at the wrist and at the metacarpal-phalangeal joints had to be limited.[6] The pattern of activity of multijoint stimulated muscles or a spastic muscle may dictate alteration of a patient's position or the extent of stimulated range allowed.

The rationale for the use of NMES in the maintenance of ROM is based on the same concepts as a passive range of motion program. As long as the joints and surrounding muscles can be taken through full ROM several times daily, the likelihood of a spontaneous reduction of that range is minimal. The addition of the NMES provides an automatic means of achieving full ROM multiple times and temporarily decreases tone in spastic muscles. The decrease in spasticity is discussed later in the chapter.

A NMES program potentially provides an efficient means of carrying out either therapist- or patient-controlled treatment programs. Most therapists or patients have neither the time nor the perserverance to put a single joint or constellation of joints through full ROM 50 to 100 times each treatment session. When cycled NMES is used to do the ROM program the extended treatment time is possible. Obviously the patient cannot be left totally unsupervised during this type of program, since changes in spastic tone may necessitate modifications in stimulus parameters, electrode placements, or both. The level of direct therapist supervision however, is reduced, and the effectiveness of the ROM treatment program is potentially increased. For the patient using stimulation at home to maintain ROM, the addition of a timer to the cycled NMES program will ensure the patient receives adequate treatment and does not give up after one or two repetitions of a passive ROM program. NMES for maintenance of ROM uses the same rationale for its therapeutic effect as does conventional passive ROM. In addition, it provides a means of carrying out the treatment program in a therapist-efficient manner. Home use may be effective because of its consistent and controlled treatment duration.

CORRECTION OF CONTRACTURES

Reduction of joint limitations using any nonsurgical treatment technique is possible only if the restriction is due to intrinsic soft-tissue shortening and not to bony obstruction of the joint. The shortening usually includes both the connective tissue surrounding the joint and the muscles acting across the joint on the shortened side.[8–11]

One of the first reports of the use of NMES in reducing ROM limitation was presented by Munsat and associates, who reported that implanted electrodes on the femoral nerve provided activation of the quadriceps femoris muscle group sufficient to decrease long-standing knee flexion deformities in five semicomatose patients.[12] The treatment program that was used was extremely aggressive (6 hr cyclical stimulation daily). In addition, the deforming force of the spastic hamstring muscles had been reduced by surgical lengthening of the hamstring tendons prior to the inception of the stimulation program. Under these conditions, two patients demonstrated complete reduction of knee flexion contractures and two others had a reduction of their contractures to noninterfering levels. The fifth patient showed a failure of the implanted electrode before full reduction of the knee flexion contracture was attained. Thus, although Munsat and associates were able to demonstrate a degree of effectiveness in the management of joint contractures by NMES, their study also raised many questions.[12]

Baker and co-workers evaluated seven chronic hemiplegic patients with moderate spasticity in the wrist and finger flexors, as well as some joint limitation at the wrist and metacarpophalangeal (MP) joints.[6] Using NMES as the exclusive means of gaining ROM, these authors reported a 36-degree increase in wrist extension and a 27-degree increase in MP extension after a 4-week treatment program. In contrast to the study reported by Munsat and associates,[6] Baker and co-workers used a less aggressive stimulation treatment program (90 min cyclical stimulation) and their patients had not previously undergone any surgical procedure to reduce the deforming force (ie, wrist and finger flexors).[7] In addition, several of these patients carried out the NMES treatment program at home, after an initial orientation program in the hospital.

Therapists at the five clinics mentioned earlier were also instructed in the use of NMES for contracture reduction in the wrist and fingers.[7] They used the NMES treatment program as the means of managing soft tissue contractures for the 9-month data collection period. During that time the five centers treated only 16 patients with wrist extension ranges of less than 30 degrees. The progress of the contracture correction programs carried out in each clinic is demonstrated in Figure 6–2. Therapists at one center saw no patients with limited wrist extension ROM. Therapists at some centers were more successful in the contracture management program than others.[7]

The one patient with limited wrist extension who was treated at the center designated HHH was unsuccessful in increasing his ROM. However, therapists at this center treated only three patients with NMES programs during the entire 9-month data collection period. While the treatment program was fixed for all centers (60 to 90 min cyclical NMES daily), the therapists at this clinic were apparently never able to achieve an adequate level of confidence employing the NMES treatment programs because of the small number of patients being treated with the technique. An inability to advance the treatment program (to increase amplitude as range of motion increased) may have contributed to the lack of success with this patient.[7]

Therapists at the center designated WWRI were able to demonstrate increased ROM but only after 2 weeks of treatment. This treatment outcome is in contrast to that of the original study (designated RLAMC). Further investigation of the data demonstrated a significant difference in the time since the onset of a cerebrovascular accident (CVA) for patients treated at WWRI. The patients treated at WWRI had experienced a CVA an average of 9 years earlier and thus could be presumed to have long-standing flexion deformities. The fact that these joint limitations yielded to NMES treatment programs at all is evidence of the program effectiveness. If a more aggressive treatment program had been used with these patients, or if the study period had extended beyond the 4 weeks of data collection, then greater ROM increases probably would have been observed.[7]

The patients seen at the centers designated as MRH and PMC were similar

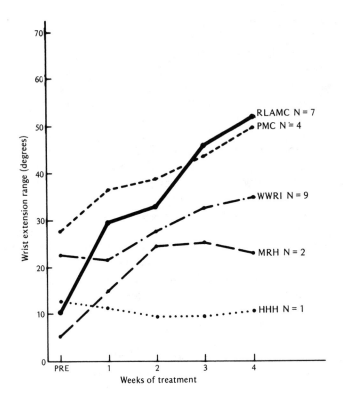

	Pre	**1**	**2**	**3**	**4**
RLAMC	16.4 ± 10.4	30 ± 9.1	36.4 ± 7.3	42.1 ± 7.5	48 ± 6.8
MRH	5.5 ± 21.5	16.5 ± 16.5	25 ± 5	26.5 ± 6.5	24.5 ± 10.5
PMC	28 ± 1	37 ± 8.4	39 ± 3.1	43.8 ± 2.6	49.5 ± 3.7
WWRI	23.3 ± 3.0	22.8 ± 4.3	28.2 ± 2.7	33.1 ± 3.0	35.4 ± 2.9
HHH	13	12	10	10	11

Figure 6–2. Effect of an NMES range-of-motion program in hemiparetic patients with finger and wrist flexor spasticity and passive wrist extension range of less than 30 degrees. Data supplied by five different clinics, including those from a previously reported study (*Phys Ther* 59:1495, 1979). Means and standard error of the means are represented.

to those seen by Baker and associates.[6] Although therapists at these two centers were not quite as successful as those in the original study, they did demonstrate significant ROM increases in their patients.[7] Other centers have independently reported success with NMES in contracture management programs.[1,13]

The success of the NMES treatment program in increasing joint ROM appears to be dependent upon matching the aggressiveness of the treatment program to the duration and severity of the joint limitation. In addition, the program is equally dependent upon the ease with which the therapist can handle the parameters of NMES and their modification, so as to ensure an optimal treatment for each patient.

The technique of NMES to gain range of motion is something of a cross between the traditional high-load, brief-stretching method and the more recently described low-load, prolonged-stretching systems.[14] The amplitude of NMES must always be maintained at levels low enough to avoid a "jamming" effect of the joint at the end of range, which is often painful and may lead to swelling and effusion of the joint. The quality of the stretch placed on the shortened tissues must be a relatively low intensity. Although each stimulated contraction is maintained for a matter of seconds, the number of repetitions inherent in a 60- to 90-min treatment program provides an accumulation of time on stretch that is substantial. In addition to providing stretch, a ROM program incorporating NMES also encourages facilitation and strengthening in the muscles that oppose the contracture.[15,16] These latter benefits are not provided by any other stretching techniques.

NMES may be used as an adjunct to other treatment programs designed to increase ROM. Combining NMES with serial casting or dropout casts has been effective.[17] When casting is used to manage joint limitations, electrode placements can be identified before applying the cast. Windows over the appropriate areas can be cut to allow access for electrode placement. Since an increase in pressure over bony prominences will occur during the stimulation cycle, great care must be taken with casting techniques before combining a stimulation procedure with a casting program, so that the integrity of the patient's skin is not compromised. The combination of stimulation and casting is especially effective in reducing plantar flexion contractures, which are frequently difficult to reduce by either technique separately. The combined effectiveness of the two techniques appears to be significantly better than either treatment alone.[17] Stimulation of the hip extensors, coupled with positioning for reduction of hip flexion contractures, is also frequently an efficacious combination.

FACILITATION AND RE-EDUCATION

Almost since its rediscovery in modern medical practice, muscle re-education and facilitation capabilities have been attributed to NMES.[6,15,18–21] Muscle re-education has been documented in both the neurologically impaired patient,[21–26] and the orthopedic patient recovering from trauma or surgery.[27–29] Although the neurophysiologic progress involved in muscle facilitation and re-education treatment programs is not well understood, some characteristics of the phenomenon have been recorded.

In 1951, Weinstein and Gordon reported that the addition of "faradism" to the rehabilitation program of hemiplegic patients improved the functional outcome of the treatment.[30] The authors, however, failed to report the effects of a traditional therapy program exclusive of NMES.[30] In 1977 Cranstam and co-workers reported that seven hemiparetic patients demonstrated increased electromyographic (EMG) and maximal voluntary torque levels of the dorsiflexors, plantar flexors, and knee flexors after 10 minutes of NMES to the dorsiflexors.[18] These values were compared to prestimulation levels and were found to be significantly greater after the treatment intervention than before treatment. However, the investigators evaluated the patients for only 1 hr after a stimulation session and had no control group.[18] Merletti and associates reported that 24 patients receiving 20 min peroneal nerve stimulation daily for 5 weeks had significantly stronger voluntary dorsiflexion than did 25 patients who had not received the treatment.[22] Stimulation was given daily throughout the assessment period, however, and few data were available concerning the effect of the program after termination of the stimulation. In a more recent study, Merletti and co-workers identified therapeutic gains in 38 (76 percent) of 50 hemiparetic patients when peroneal NMES was used.[31] Once again, follow-up data after the termination of the program were not available. Similar effects, though less well documented, have been reported for patients with multiple sclerosis and for children with cerebral palsy.[20,23] Additionally, not all investigators have been able to document significant changes in muscle control or function in the neurologically involved patients once the NMES is discontinued.[32,33]

The treatment outcome of the neurologically involved patient contrasts with the orthopedically involved patient. The addition of NMES to traditional postoperative or nonoperative rehabilitation programs has demonstrated significant changes in the quality of a voluntary muscle contraction and in the timing of synergistic muscles.[27–29] In one report, patients treated with NMES added to the rehabilitation process improved by 75 percent during the first 2-week postoperative period.[34] These gains, both in appropriate timing of muscle contractions and in the quality of the voluntary contractions, are undoubtedly re-educational in nature. Moritani and DeVries were able to demonstrate that in healthy young subjects undergoing voluntary weight training, the strength gains made in the first 3 weeks of the program were due mainly to increased efficiency in recruiting motor units, with only minor changes in the tension output of the available motor units.[35] Considering the quality of the sensory excitation inherent in the use of surface NMES, the findings of the authors appear to be equally applicable to most of the NMES strengthening programs.

At least two attempts have been made to evaluate the effects of NMES on the re-education and facilitation of healthy subjects. Fleury and Lagasse reported the use of NMES during a reaction-time training program in 62 healthy subjects.[36] They found that the 42 subjects receiving NMES were able to reduce their reaction times significantly in comparison with the 20 subjects who carried out their training without the addition of NMES. Although the times associated with actual movement were no different between the groups, central latency (the time needed to begin the response to the trigger signal) was significantly reduced in the stimulated group. There appeared to be no change in the muscle response to the task, but the processing time needed to initiate the desired response was enhanced in those subjects receiving NMES.[36]

In a similar manner, LeDoux and Quinones reported the use of NMES as an education assist in healthy subjects who were attempting to learn great-toe abduction.[15] Stimulation was applied to the abductor hallicus during voluntary abduction of the great toe in one group of subjects, while a second group of subjects received verbal encouragement from a therapist during attempted abduction of the great toe. After 3 weeks of training, active ROM into abduction was carried out and was compared with pretreatment measurements. The authors found a significant increase in abduction capabilities in those subjects who had received NMES, when compared with those subjects receiving treatment without NMES.[16] Thus, even normal subjects have demonstrated increased quality and timing of muscle contractions after application of NMES for muscle facilitation and re-education.

The potential of NMES as a facilitation or re-education technique might be increased, especially for the neurologically involved patient, if a structured program involving the patient's direct participation were augmented with some form of feedback. Electromyographic (EMG) feedback treatment programs have been very successful in augmenting the treatment of the neurologically involved patient.[37–39] The addition of NMES to an EMG feedback program requires special equipment.[40] While such equipment has recently become generally available, no studies to date have reported the effectiveness of such a combined treatment program. An alternative to the combination of NMES and EMG is the use of position or motion feedback with NMES. Several forms of position or motion feedback devices have been reported,[41–43] and a few of these have been combined with NMES to further enhance the effectiveness of facilitation treatment programs.[44,45]

A positional feedback stimulation training device was described by Bowman and associates in their report on the effects of a 4-week treatment program with a group of hemiparetic patients.[44] The treatment paradigm consisted of a patient's initiation of voluntary wrist extension, during which he received several forms of audio and visual feedback concerning actual wrist movement. As the patient approached a maximal extension range, NMES was triggered, which augmented the voluntary contraction, allowing full extension of the wrist. Twice-daily treatment with the combined feedback-stimulation program has been reported to increase both voluntary wrist-extension torque and selective ROM in hemiparetic patients.[44] Follow-up studies of these patients at 6-month and 1-year intervals have demonstrated a maintenance of the active ROM and of the torque attained during the treatment program (Fig. 6–3). A similar program has been reported using feedback stimulation to enhance voluntary knee extension in hemiparetic patients. This study identified signifi-

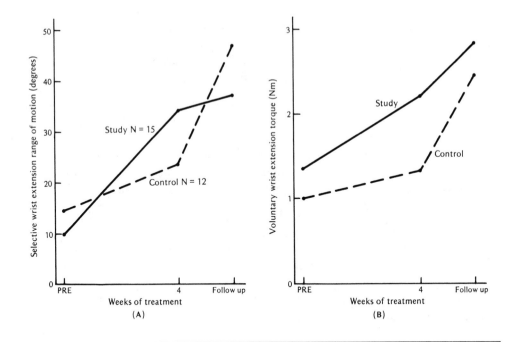

A. Selective Range of Motion

	Pre	4	Follow-up	
Study	9.7 ± 3.3	34.8 ± 7.9	37.7 ± 5.2	N = 15
Control	14.4 ± 5.6	24.3 ± 7.2	47.4 ± 6.8	N = 12

B. Torque

	Pre	4	Follow-up	
Study	1.33 ± 0.42	2.23 ± 0.55	2.89 ± 0.62	N = 15
Control	1.01 ± 0.23	1.38 ± 0.34	2.51 ± 0.49	N = 12

Figure 6–3. Effects of a feedback stimulation treatment program on selective range of motion (**A**) and torque (**B**) at the wrist in hemiparetic patients. Control subjects were treated with traditional facilitation techniques. Measurements were taken prior to the initiation of treatment, after 4 weeks of treatment, and 6 months to 1 year after termination of treatment. Means and standard error of the means are represented.

cantly greater improvements in knee extension torque in those patients receiving NMES with biofeedback, when compared to patients receiving only conventional physical therapy.[45]

In addition to the use of NMES with specific feedback treatment techniques, the incorporation of NMES into a variety of functional or craft activities can assist the neurologically involved patient with the integrated use of specific muscle groups or whole body parts.[17,46-48] Examples of this might include: (1) the addition of NMES to balancing activities, to enhance proximal stability; (2) short cycles of NMES to either flexor or extensor muscle groups, practicing smooth reciprocal weight shifting; (3) submotor NMES used as a reminder to integrate an involved extremity into a bilateral task; and (4) therapist-controlled externally triggered NMES, augmenting a proprioceptive neuromuscular facilitation or "Brunstrom" pattern, or providing an additional point of control during a neurodevelopmental treatment program. The creative incorporation of NMES into multiple facilitation treatment programs is dependent only upon the therapist's ability to quickly and competently make adjustments to stimulus parameters and to create the best possible sensory or motor stimulation program for the individual patient.

The basis of the facilitation and re-education treatment programs, in healthy individuals as well as in orthopedically or neurologically involved patients, is the bombardment of the central nervous system (CNS) with sensory information. The use of NMES on the surface of the body results in a tremendous amount of cutaneous afferent influx to the CNS.[69] This can be an impeding factor in those treatment programs aimed at creating strong muscle contractions, because subjects and patients frequently cannot tolerate the massive cutaneous afferent activity and therefore interpret the sensory barrage as being noxious or painful.[3,49-51] Careful training programs are necessary before most subjects will tolerate truly supramaximal electrically stimulated muscle contractions.[3,51] This profound cutaneous afferent activity is undoubtedly a major factor in the effectiveness of facilitation and re-education treatment programs.

In addition to cutaneous information, as NMES is increased in amplitude (to create a stronger muscle contraction) kinesthetic and (when the joint is allowed to move) proprioceptive information also ascend to the CNS. Since these various afferent systems travel through different pathways and to different destinations within the neuraxis, NMES provides the clinician with a very powerful tool by which to affect both automatic and cognitive levels of the CNS. For the neurologically involved patient with deficits in either transmission or integration of sensorimotor information, NMES provides a multiplicity of both sensory pathways and potential integrative centers, enhancing the probability that some part of the afferent message will reach appropriate centers. The orthopedically involved patient is frequently dealing with a sensorimotor alienation (due to pain or trauma) and may have difficulty recruiting a motor contraction due to neural inhibition.[3] The addition of NMES to the treatment program for this patient increases the ease of recruitment on two levels: (1) a direct excitation onto the alpha motoneuron, through peripheral stimulation of the Ia myotatic sensory system; and (2) ascending afferent information, which will be integrated at conscious and subconscious levels of the CNS and which may result in central modulation of the alpha motoneuron. Eccles and McIntyre have theorized that synaptic contacts that remain unused for prolonged periods of time may atrophy, much as muscle does with disuse.[52] Vodovnik has incorporated this concept into his theory of how NMES can both increase the quality of motor control in some patients and seemingly reduce inappropriate muscle activity in others.[53] In either case, some set of synapses is abnormally inactive, whether it is the excitatory control taking place directly onto the motoneuron or the inhibitory influence of an interneuron. The addition of NMES to an appropriate muscle or afferent pathway may provide an artificial drive of the inactive synapse, reducing the effects of synaptic atrophy and restoring a more normal balance to the system. Although extremely simplistic in nature, this concept may be useful in anticipating the therapeutic effects of NMES and in deciding what muscles or sensory pathways might provide the most effective treatment for individual patients.

SPASTICITY MANAGEMENT

NMES has been used in a variety of ways to decrease spasticity.[54–56] Three programs have been described in the literature over the past several years, and all three have reported variable success in controlling spastic muscle tone. Unlike other treatment programs using NMES techniques, assessment of the effects of NMES on spasticity remain elusive, due mainly to the variable nature of spasticity itself. In reality, spasticity is a constellation of symptoms that may be caused by any number of sources and different types of pathology. Although the outward signs of the spastic multiple sclerosis patient may resemble the spasticity of a patient with a spinal cord injury, the source of the abnormal muscle tone may be very different in the two patients. The effectiveness of NMES treatments will vary according to (1) which structures of the CNS are most sensitive to the particular characteristics of the specific NMES program used; and (2) the source of the spasticity itself. Because the site of action of most NMES programs designed to affect spasticity is speculative at best, and because the source of the spastic drive in any given patient is also largely unknown, the effectiveness of NMES in the treatment of spasticity is frequently unpredictable.

A further complication is the inability to assess spasticity accurately and objectively. In fact, many neurologists and neurophysiologists cannot agree on a specific definition of spasticity or on whether spasticity is truly a major impediment to function for most patients.[57] For purposes of this discussion, however, I use a definition of spasticity that encompasses both hyperactive stretch reflexes and cutaneous reflexes. The responses of these hyperexcitable reflexes do in fact interfere with function in many patients.

Since spasticity is usually associated with motoneuron excitability elicited by some abnormal drive, the only way to affect long-term or permanent control of spasticity is to alter the drive onto the motoneuron. Most treatment programs, including those incorporating NMES, provide some means of temporary interruption or balancing of this abnormal drive, either at the source of the drive or at the level of the motoneuron itself. Since the interruption is temporary, the effects of treatment are usually seen as temporary. Long-lasting carry-over, as reported in some cases of facilitation, is usually not seen in the area of spasticity management by NMES techniques.

Antagonist Muscle Stimulation

One of the earliest reports of decreased spasticity after NMES of the antagonist muscle groups came from Vallejo in 1952.[58] Levine and co-workers reported that stimulation of the antagonist to a spastic muscle, followed by vigorous ROM exercises, led to dramatic decreases in muscle tone. The authors emphasized the need to evaluate each patient but found that, when spasticity impeded volitional control, the addition of NMES to the treatment program provided significant increases in muscle-tone management.[58] These same observations have been made more recently by Alfieri, who reported that 90 percent of some 96 hemiparetic patients evidenced decreased muscle tone after multiple treatment sessions of NMES to the antagonists of spastic muscles.[59] Although the immediate effects of the treatment were reportedly decreased within 1 hr after stimulation, Alfieri stated that spasticity tended to decrease and was maintained at a lower level after varying numbers of treatment sessions. Although the follow-up on those patients who received NMES treatments did demonstrate long-term reduction of muscle tone in this study, the author did not report the effects of any other treatment, or the effects of no treatment at all, on the long-term spasticity of similar hemiplegic patients.[59]

Thus, it is difficult to determine whether NMES was more effective than other treatment programs designed to reduce muscle tone, or is any different from no treatment intervention, in the chronic hemiparetic patient. Cranstam and Larsson attribute the long-lasting effects of NMES to an increase in voluntary control, which may potentially overcome the spastic muscle after the initial inhibitory period.[55] Not all authors have reported an effect once stimulation has been discontinued, although a decrease in tone is nearly always seen during the stimulation period.[60]

The neurophysiologic rationale for the effectiveness of NMES to the antagonist of the spastic muscle seems to rest on the principle of reciprocal inhibition. However, the time course of reciprocal inhibition, a disynaptic system, is very short, measurable in milliseconds. How, then, do clinicians report therapeutic decreases in muscle tone for up to 1 hr after a treatment program? The phenomenon known as post-tetanic potentiation (PTP) may account for some of the therapeutic effects that exceed the length of the treatment program. Although usually described as a prolonged activation of an excitatory reflex pathway, Tan and colleagues have evaluated the effects of tetanization of an antagonist reflex pathway and have reported a decrease in the normal PTP response.[61] The authors refer to this as post-tetanic depression and, although they were not evaluating spasticity per se, this may be a significant factor in the effectiveness of NMES in reducing muscle tone in antagonist muscle groups.

The effectiveness of this treatment technique, even in subjects with normal muscle tone, was demonstrated by Liberson and can be evaluated by self-stimulation. Liberson used NMES to establish a contraction of the finger extensors that a healthy subject could not voluntarily overcome using the finger flexor muscles.[62] The quality of the stimulated muscle contraction was then graded in a standard manual muscle test manner. The subject was unable to effectively flex against a "fair-level" stimulated finger extension contraction. That the normal finger flexors were unable to counter a fair-level stimulated extensor contraction can be attributed to the effects of reciprocal inhibition from the Ia myotatic receptors of the extensors onto the flexor musculature.[62] There has been no documentation of the more prolonged effects of this type of NMES in normal subjects.

Agonist Muscle Stimulation

In 1950, Lee and colleagues reported that NMES of spastic muscle with a frequency of 100 to 350 Hz resulted in a "fair" reduction of the spastic tone that lasted for several hours.[63] Several problems were noted by the authors, however, not the least of which included blistering and burns in 5 of the 19 patients. The use of NMES to the spastic muscle for the management of spasticity continued sporadically over the next several years, but no reports of the long-lasting and generalized effects seen by Lee and co-workers were made.[63] With the rediscovery of the use of NMES for facilitation and re-education treatment programs and of NMES strengthening programs, some concern about the use of stimulation with spastic muscles was voiced.

Two reports were published on the effects of NMES using frequencies to produce tetany in a total of 17 spinal-cord-injured (SCI) patients. In one study, Bowman and Bajd stimulated the spastic quadriceps muscles in ten SCI patients and recorded the change in resting muscle tone immediately after the stimulation program and 30 min later.[64] Four patients demonstrated a slight decrease in spasticity levels after the NMES program, while two more patients had an immediate slight increase in tone but showed a measurable decrease at the 30-min assessment period. One patient demonstrated a slight increase in tone that continued through the 30 minute posttest, and three patients failed to demonstrate any consistent change in spastic muscle tone after the NMES program.[64]

In the second study, Vodovnik and associates evaluated the effect of rhythmical NMES of bilateral knee extensor and knee flexor musculature in seven

SCI patients. Only two patients showed objectively measurable decreases in spasticity, three reported subjective improvement, and the remaining two experienced no change after the NMES program.[65]

These studies have largely allayed fears that NMES programs may actually increase spasticity in muscles that demonstrate hypertonia. The effectiveness of NMES activation of the spastic muscle for the purpose of decreasing abnormal tone appears to be unpredictable, at least in SCI patients. In all, 8 of the 17 patients were reported to have a measurable decrease in spasticity after the NMES treatment. This decrease in tone persisted for a minimum of 30 min.[64,65] No specific characteristics could be found that distinguished these eight patients from those who showed no significant or consistent response to NMES treatments. Thus, the use of NMES to activate a spastic muscle for some specific therapeutic goal, such as ROM or facilitation of voluntary motor control, would seem merited for most patients. The effectiveness of the program for management of spasticity is somewhat less predictable, and each patient must be evaluated individually before the appropriateness of NMES treatment can be determined. In addition, further evaluation of the technique must be made in patients with spasticity due to different types of neuropathology, in order to determine if the therapeutic effects are the same, enhanced, or nonexistent under various sources of spastic drive.

The neurophysiological rationale for the effectiveness of NMES activation of the spastic muscle may be two-fold. Electrical stimulation of the neuromuscular system at frequencies of 100 to 350 Hz, such as Lee and associates employed, may lead to fatigue of the peripheral system.[63] In experimental animal research, Solomonow and co-workers reported a 95-percent reduction in muscle tension after an electrical signal with a frequency of 600 Hz was applied. They theorized that either neuromuscular junction fatigue or a possible depletion of Ca^{++} release at the postsynaptic binding sites might have been responsible for the reduction in muscle tension.[66] Bowman and McNeal performed a similar study, but they recorded a complete block of nerve conduction past an electrode that was being stimulated at frequencies of 2000 Hz or more. This conduction block was reversible, usually within 1 sec after the stimulation was discontinued.[54] Both of these studies have demonstrated that NMES can potentially create a peripherally mediated reduction in spastic tone. Both experiments were conducted under laboratory conditions, with electrodes placed directly on the exposed nerves. How effective these higher-frequency techniques might be with regard to surface nerve-stimulation techniques is unknown at this time.

A second possible neurophysiological mechanism by which NMES of the spastic muscle might affect a reduction of muscle tone rests in the antidromic activation of the alpha motoneuron axon. With peripherally applied NMES, the electrically elicited action potential is propagated in both directions: orthodromically, toward the motor end place, and antidromically, toward the spinal cord. Although orthodromic propagation provides the immediately visible muscle contraction, antidromic propagation may provide a spinal-level response that could lead to a longer-lasting modulation of the spastic tone. With each voluntary and stimulated action potential, the alpha motoneuron activates the motor unit and excites a pool of Renshaw cells through recurrent collaterals. The Renshaw cells inhibit the alpha motoneurons of the activated pool and the motoneurons of synergistic muscles.[67] The function of the Renshaw system is to serve as modulators and stabilizers of motoneuron firing frequencies. There is some evidence that spastic patients may not have normal supraspinal modulation of the Renshaw cells, especially during voluntary activation. Although the majority of this evidence has been developed with either hemiparetic stroke patients or multiple sclerosis patients, a similar pattern appears to be present in the SCI population as well.[68] Again invoking Eccle's theory of synaptic disuse, and coupling it with Vodovnik's theory of NMES providing an artificial drive to essentially strengthen synaptic contacts, the effects of NMES on the spastic muscle group may lead to a reduction in tone if a major source of the unbridled alpha motoneuron activity is a lack of control from the Renshaw system.[53,68] If antidromic activation of the alpha motoneuron acts as a source of posttetanic potentiation onto the Renshaw cells, the therapeutic effect might be expected to follow a time course similar to that seen in NMES programs using activation of the antagonist to the spastic muscle. Unfortunately, we do not have adequate information on which types of spasticity may be due to inappropriate Renshaw cell activity. This may contribute to the variability in the responses to NMES programs activating the spastic muscle reported by Bowman and Bajd and by Vodovnik and colleagues.[64,65]

Sensory Habituation

In the early 1970s, Dimitrijevic and Nathan reported a series of studies with complete SCI patients.[56,69,70] This research indicated that relatively low-frequency, low-amplitude sensory stimulation could lead to an habituation response that, after several hours of treatment, might be generalized to include a large part of the functionally isolated spinal cord.[56] Although habituation of specific cutaneous, polysynaptic pathways and of the monosynaptic myotatic reflex has been well documented, the generalized desensitization of the spinal interneuron networks has remained elusive.[13,71,72] The time course of the generalized habituation is reported to be several hours instead of several seconds or minutes.[56,70] The characteristics that establish an all-inclusive interneuron suppression are less well documented, but stimulus regularity appears to be a key ingredient.[69,70,73]

A similar, more recent report by Walker described a 20-Hz stimulation of median, radial, and saphenus nerves for 1 hr, resulting in up to 3 hr reduced clonus and rigidity.[74] Although unilateral stimulation reportedly affected clonus bilaterally, the time course of the effect was different for each extremity. These differences included an immediate but incomplete reduction of clonus on the side contralateral to the stimulation, with a further reduction noted during the next 90 min. A decrease in the severity of clonus on the side ipsilateral to stimulation was not noted for the first 90 min after the treatment (in most patients) but was reported after 2 hr. The mechanisms by which this suppression is mediated are unknown, but the time delays in the therapeutic bilateral and distal effects (ie, upper-extremity stimulation affected lower-extremity clonus), implicate supraspinal mechanisms. The majority of the patients treated in the study were diagnosed as having multiple sclerosis, and no specific information as to the site of their lesions was presented. Walker also stated that the stimulation did not cause hyperreflexia, scissoring, or abnormal Babinski sign.[74]

Sensory habituation is an extremely tenuous treatment program at this time, with insufficient documentation to determine what NMES parameters are most important to ensure the therapeutic effect. The few areas of agreement seem to rest in the repetitive, consistent nature of the stimulus and in the rather prolonged stimulation program required to create an observable reduction in muscle tone. NMES at sensory levels, with minimal motor-evoked responses, also appears to be a consistent characteristic of the successful program. Although most authors agree that the habituation of a specific reflex (eg, the flexion reflex) occurs in the interneuron network at the spinal cord level,[71,72] the more generalized interneuron suppression described by Dimitrijevic and Nathan[56] and by Walker[74] may require a more prolonged treatment program, with multiple sites of stimulation, and may be potentiated by some supraspinal control. A great deal of work remains to be done before this form of NMES can be effectively harnessed for use in the therapist's armamentarium of therapeutic programs for the reduction of spasticity.

ORTHOTIC SUBSTITUTION

The use of NMES as a substitute for conventional orthoses provides both therapists and patients with a degree of flexibility previously unavailable. A patient wearing a knee/ankle/foot orthosis (KAFO) is obliged to walk with a "pegleg" throughout his or her gait-training program. In contrast, the same patient, using an ankle/foot orthosis and receiving NMES to control knee extension, now has the capability of attaining both stance stability and more appropriate knee and hip flexion during the swing phase of gait. In a similar manner, NMES can be used in both the upper and lower extremities in place of conventional bracing, or as an adjunct to bracing, during functional training programs. The goal in most of these NMES programs is to increase the patient's motor control, with an eye to reducing the patient's dependence on the external control provided by the stimulation.[3,4] Thus, in reality this type of treatment program is a form of facilitation re-education. At the present time, two NMES programs of orthotic substitution are used as semipermanent replacements for conventional bracing. Because these uses of NMES have been developed with truly functional goals in mind, this type of stimulation program is referred to as functional electrical stimulation (FES).

The first of these FES programs includes the use of stimulation to gain normal shoulder alignment in the hemiparetic patient who demonstrates shoulder subluxation. Many hemiparetic patients demonstrate shoulder subluxation during the flaccid phase of recovery from a cerebral vascular accident (CVA).[75] If the shoulder joint is not protected during this phase of recovery, stretch of the shoulder capsule can occur. Basmajain has demonstrated that, at rest, the passive shoulder capsule provides appropriate glenohumeral alignment and that the supraspinatus and posterior deltoid muscles serve as the first line of muscular protection for the joint under stress.[76] In the hemiplegic patient, however, if the shoulder joint is stressed (as it is continually by gravity while the patient is in an upright posture), there may be no immediate source of protection. The result is a stretch of the ligamentous capsule. As the patient regains muscle tone and voluntary control at the shoulder joint, if the capsule is stretched, normal glenohumeral alignment may or may not recur. In many hemiparetic patients, the joint capsule is stretched to such a degree that the resting muscle tone cannot correct for the ligamentous laxity, and shoulder subluxation persists. This stretching of the joint capsule may contribute to pain[77,78] as well as to dysfunction in the paretic limb and, in extreme cases, may lead to peripheral nerve damage.[79] Shoulder slings are commonly used to help avoid further shoulder subluxation but cannot always assist in re-establishing glenohumeral alignment. Electrical stimulation of the posterior deltoid and supraspinatus muscles provides a means of attaining normal shoulder integrity and, with a proper FES training program, can be used for most of the patient's waking and active hours (Fig. 6–4).[80]

Most patients demonstrate adequate return of muscle tone in the surrounding shoulder muscles and can discard the protection of either sling or stimulation, as long as the shoulder capsule has been maintained.[80] For those patients who demonstrate significant residual subluxation (usually more than 5 mm by radiograph), FES can be continued as a means of long-term protection for the shoulder joint, while maintaining a degree of cosmesis unattainable with any sling. Aside from the cosmetic aspect, long-term use of FES has the added advantage of affording nearly normal shoulder integrity for prolonged periods of time, while the average sling allows a significant degree of subluxation to persist. In addition, if the patient has recovered distal function of the extremity, the FES orthotic substitute allows a degree of freedom of movement unattainable with a sling.

The second semipermanent use of FES for orthotic substitution is the dorsiflexion gait-assist program for both hemiparetic and SCI patients.[20,31,81,82] Externally triggered FES, usually activated by a switch in the shoe of the involved extremity, can be used to enhance dorsiflexion in the stroke patient or to create a lower-extremity flexion reflex in the SCI patient. Follow-up, continuing for nearly 12 years, of seven hemiparetic patients using FES for dorsiflexion assist showed that four patients no longer required stimulation to attain dorsiflexion during the swing phase of gait and that three patients still used the FES orthotic substitute for *all* gait activities.[83] Although similar treatment programs have been described for paraparetic patients (both SCI and

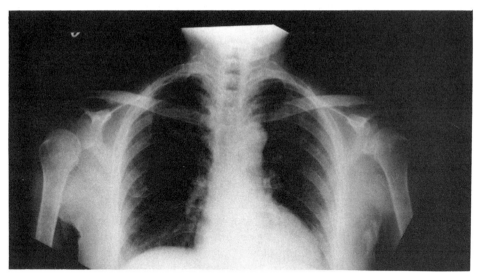

A

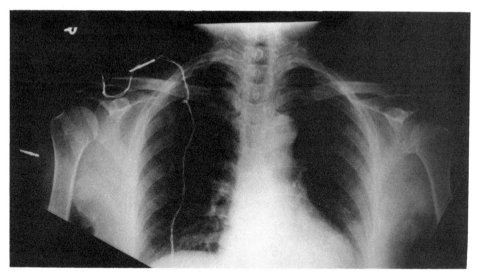

B

Figure 6–4. Example of a hemiparetic patient with a subluxed shoulder (**A**) (right shoulder). Effect of electrical stimulation of the posterior deltoid and supraspinatus muscles is shown in **B** (electrode wires can be seen).

multiple sclerosis patients), no long-term follow-up reports have been found in the literature.[56,81,82]

In both flexion-reflex and dorsiflexion-assist applications, patients receiving FES for the enhancement of the swing phase of gait must first demonstrate adequate stance stability. For hemiparetic patients, that includes adequate gastroc-soleus control to ensure smooth, stable tibial advancement during the final stages of stance. In paraparetic patients, the effect of peroneal nerve stimulation must be assessed against the patients' voluntary control of hip and knee extensor musculature. Patients in whom the activation of a flexion reflex is a powerful inhibition to the extensor muscles may lose stability if the transition between extension and flexion is too abrupt.

Although FES treatment programs can be performed at home by the patient, allowing long-term independent use, they are considered to be semipermanent in that surface electrodes are used. Although surface NMES is desirable in most therapeutic treatment programs, orthotic use of FES will not be truly permanent until adequate implant electrode technology is available. In addition to the two programs presently available, numerous multichannel, fully implanted stimulation systems are in the research stage and should become available to physicians, therapists, and patients alike within the next few years. The goal of the new technology is to provide multichannel, functional gait-assist capabilities to paraparetic patients and, eventually, to paraplegic patients. Despite a good deal of enthusiastic reporting by the nonmedical press, by late 1989 no system was capable of providing a paraplegic subject truly functional gait in an independent environment.

The challenges of multifaceted implant systems are many.[84] Control sequences and mechanisms remain of prime concern at this time.[85–91] It is not enough to allow a user to go from point A to point B if all conscious effort must be put into controlling the sequence of triggering stimulation on and off during the process of ambulation. Thus, semiautomatic trigger sources that allow appropriate timing of specific muscle patterns are under investigation. In addition, different patterns of muscle activity may be necessary for fully functional independence; for example, a single set of controls to activate level walking may not be adequate if there is a need to ascend or descend an incline or to step up a curb. Control of a multijoint extremity may not be easily accomplished in the presence of spasticity, as it may vary in quality and intensity depending upon the effort and the environmental factors involved. Some form of sensory feedback is necessary; few users will be comfortable floating 3 feet above the ground with no awareness of upright support. Mechanisms for providing lateral and anterior–posterior balance are essential, as is a means of enhancing trunk stability for the patient with poor axial control. Although coming-to-standing and primitive stepping patterns are currently available by using two-, four-, or even six-channel FES, at this time, the concerns mentioned limit the usefulness of these gait activities primarily to the laboratory.[47,82,90,92–97]

Although much research effort has been directed at increasing the ambulatory capability of paraparetic patients, other investigators are developing upper-extremity FES orthoses for use by quadriparetic patients.[82,87,89,98,99] Many of the problems found in upper extremity stimulation are similar to those encountered in ambulation programs. Although balance is not a concern with regard to the upper extremities, fine motor control demands even more sophisticated sequencing of FES, and feedback becomes essential to adequate functioning of the extremities. While gait activities can be controlled through gross motor activation, function of the hand and upper arm demands precise timing and muscle balance. There has been progress in these areas, and presently several centers are evaluating semipermanent FES systems to enhance hand function in quadriplegic subjects.[100] One eight-channel stimulator system has been fully implanted into a quadriplegic subject to enhance hand function.[101] These systems are still developmental in nature, but may be more widely available in the future.

Another area of involvement for the rehabilitation practitioner is the use of NMES to enhance exercise in the paretic or paraletic patient. Although the benefits of exercise are obvious, there still remains little objective documentation of long-term or generalized NMES benefits to date.[102–104] Areas that concern the rehabilitation practitioner include both the user's ability to demonstrate adequate cardiovascular response to an electrically induced exercise demand, and the safety of insensate extremities during the exercise activity. When multichannel gait-assist and upper-extremity orthoses become available, some form of conditioning exercise will be necessary to ensure adequate quality of muscle contraction, in order to meet the demands placed on the extremities by the increased functional capabilities. Questions remain, however, as to the need for continuous exercise from the time of injury until the patient (or technology) is ready for functional intervention. Research has demonstrated that even muscles subjected to years of disuse atrophy can be adequately strengthened for function within a few months.[12,16,105–107] The question, then, becomes: Is there justification for the time, expense, and (not least of all) risk to the user of a long-term exercise program? While some investigators report general health benefits from particular types of NMES programs,[104] others are more cautious in their assessment of long-term benefits.[108–110] Obviously, a tremendous amount of research remains to be done. Until the effects of exercise are objectively assessed, the rehabilitation practitioner must temper the natural enthusiasm of the potential user with up-to-date information regarding both risks and benefits of long- and short-term NMES use.

SUMMARY

Evidence has been presented that neuromuscular electrical stimulation can be effective in several broad therapeutic applications. NMES has been found to effectively maintain joint ROM in the presence of spasticity and, under some circumstances may be more efficient in doing so than the traditional passive programs. NMES has also been found to be an effective tool in treatment programs aimed at reducing soft tissue joint contractures. The NMES treatment programs incorporate some aspects of both low-load, prolonged stretching techniques and high-load, brief stretching techniques, while maintaining the efficient use of therapist time.

Stimulation for the enhancement of motor control, whether it is called a facilitation technique or a muscle re-education program, provides a tremendous amount of sensory information to the CNS through a variety of sensory modalities and afferent pathways, for both automatic and conscious processing. As such, NMES is an extremely powerful tool in programs designed to enhance voluntary control. In addition, NMES can be incorporated into almost any traditional facilitation technique to further enhance a patient's motor control.

The application of NMES to spasticity-management programs is the least understood of the treatment programs enhanced by its addition. Due to the lack of clear neurophysiological rationale, no specific parameters of NMES will ensure success with any given patient. However, several alternative treatments have been presented, and many patients will demonstrate an appropriate response to some form of NMES intervention.

The final, and most volatile, use of NMES includes the orthotic substitution capability of stimulation—true functional electrical stimulation. Orthotic substitution by NMES is an extremely active research area. Advances in independent ambulation for paraparetic and paraplegic patients, and increased upper-extremity functioning for quadriparetic patients, will place new demands on the rehabilitation practitioner in both training and strengthening patients for truly independent activities of daily living.

REFERENCES

1. McNeal DR. 2000 years of electrical stimulation. In Hambrecht FT, Reswick JB, eds. *Functional Electrical Stimulation: Applications in Neural Prosthetics*. New York, Marcel Dekker, 1977: 3–35
2. Reswick JB. A brief history of functional electrical stimulation. In Fields WS, Leavitt LA, eds. *Neural Organization and Its Relevance to Prosthetics*. New York, Intercontinental, 1973: 3–13
3. Benton LA, Baker LL, Bowman BR, Waters RL. *Functional Electrical Stimulation—A Practical Clinical Guide*, 2nd ed. Downey, CA, Professional Staff Association of Rancho Los Amigos Medical Center, 1981
4. Baker LL. Neuromuscular electrical stimulation in the restoration of purposeful limb movements. In: Wolf SL, ed. *Electrotherapy—Clinics in Physical Therapy*. New York, Churchill Livingstone, 1981: 25–48
5. McNeal DR, Bowman BR. Peripheral neuromuscular stimulation. In: Myklebust JB, et al, eds. *Neural Stimulation*. Boca Raton, CRC Press, 1985; 2:95–118
6. Baker LL, Yeh C, Wilson D, Waters RL. Electrical stimulation of wrist and fingers for hemiplegic patients. *Phys Ther*. 59:1495, 1979
7. Waters RL, Bowman BR. *Multicenter Functional Electrical Stimulation Evaluation*

for Contracture Prevention and Correction. Final report to the Veterans Administration no. V790p1441, Washington, DC, 1981

8. Akeson W, Amiel D, Woo S. Immobility effects on synovial joints: The pathomechanics of joint contracture. *Biorheology.* 17:95, 1980

9. Johns RJ, Wright V. Relative importance of various tissues in joint stiffness. *J Appl Physiol.* 17:824, 1962

10. Sapega AA, Quedenfeld TC, Moyer RA, Butler RA. Biophysical factors in range-of-motion exercise. *Phys Sports Med.* 9:57, 1981

11. Tabary JC, Tabary C, Tardieu C, et al. Physiological and structural changes in the cat's soleus muscle due to immobilization at different lengths by plaster casts. *J Physiol.* (Lond). 224:231, 1972

12. Munsat TL, McNeal DR, Waters RL. Preliminary observations on prolonged stimulation of peripheral nerve in man. *Arch Neurol.* 33:608, 1976

13. Mazliah J, Naumann S, White C, et al. Electrostimulation as a means of decreasing knee flexion contractures in children with spina bifida. *Proc Rehabil Eng Soc North Am.* 6:63, 1983

14. Light KE, Nuxik S, Personius W, Barstrom A. Low-load prolonged stretch vs. high-load brief stretch in treating knee contractures. *Phys Ther.* 64:330, 1984

15. LeDoux J, Quinones MA. An investigation of the use of percutaneous electrical stimulation in muscle reeducation. *Phys Ther.* 61:678, 1981

16. Peckham PH, Mortimer JT, Marsolais EB. Alteration in the force and fatigability of skeletal muscle in quadriplegic humans following exercise induced by chronic electrical stimulation. *Clin Orthop.* 114:326, 1976

17. Baker LL, Parker K, Sanderson D. Neuromuscular electrical stimulation for the head-injured patient. *Phys Ther.* 63:1967, 1983

18. Cranstam B, Larsson L-E, Prevec TS. Improvement of gait following functional electrical stimulation. *Scand J Rehabil Med.* 9:7, 1977

19. Gracanin F. Functional electrical stimulation in external control of motor activity and movements of paralyzed extremities. *Int Rehabil Med.* 6:25, 1984

20. Ship G, Mayer N. Clinical usage of functional electrical stimulation in upper motor neuron syndromes. In: Hambrecht FT, Reswick JB, ed. *Functional Electrical Stimulation: Applications in Neural Prostheses.* New York, Marcel Dekker, 1977: 65–82

21. Vodovnik L. Information processing in the central nervous system during functional electrical stimulation. *Med Biol Eng.* 9:675, 1971

22. Merletti R, Zelaschi F, Latella D, et al. A control study of muscle force recovery in hemiparetic patients during treatment with functional electrical stimulation. *Scand J Rehabil Med.* 10:147, 1978

23. Riso RR, Crago PE, Sutin K, et al. An investigation of the carry-over or therapeutic effects of FES in the correction of drop foot in the cerebral palsy child. *Proc Int Conf Rehabil Eng.* 1:220, 1980

24. Vodovnik L. Therapeutic effects of functional electrical stimulation of extremities. *Med Biol Eng Comput.* 19:470, 1981

25. Vodovnik L, Rebersek S. Improvements in voluntary control of paretic muscles due to electrical stimulation. In: Fields WS, Leavitt LA, eds. *Neural Organization and Its Relevance to Prosthetics.* New York, Intercontinental, 1973: 101–116

26. Waters RL. The enigma of "carry-over." *Int Rehabil Med.* 6:9, 1984

27. Ericksson E, Haggmark T. Comparison of isometric muscle training and electrical

stimulation supplementing isometric muscle training in the recovery after major knee ligament surgery—A preliminary report. *Am J Sports Med.* 7:169, 1979

28. Johnson DH, Thurston P, Ascroft PJ. The Russian technique of faradism in the treatment of chrondromalacia patellae—Clinical study. *Physiother Can.* 29:266, 1977

29. Williams JGP, Street M. Sequential faradism in quadriceps rehabilitation. *Physiology.* 62:252, 1976

30. Weinstein MV, Gordon A. The use of faradism in the rehabilitation of hemiplegics. *Phys Ther Rev.* 31:515, 1951

31. Merletti R, Andina A, Galante M, et al. Clinical experience of electronic peroneal stimulators in 50 hemiparetic patients. *Scand J Rehabil Med.* 11:111, 1979

32. Mifsud M, Literowich W, Naumann S, et al. Transcutaneous muscle stimulator with two independent channels for use by cerebral palsied children with spastic diplegia. *Digest Can Med Biol Eng Conf.* 9:31, 1982

33. Teng EL, McNeal DR, Kralj A, et al. Electrical stimulation and feedback training: Effects on the voluntary control of paretic muscles. *Arch Phys Med Rehabil.* 57:228, 1976

34. Godfrey CM, Jayawardena H, Quance TA, Welsh P. Comparison of electro-stimulation and isometric exercise in strengthening the quadriceps muscle. *Physiother Can.* 31:265, 1979

35. Moritani T, DeVries HA. Neural factors versus hypertrophy in the time course of muscle strength gain. *Am J Phys Med* 58:115, 1979

36. Fleury M, Lagasse P. Influence of functional electrical stimulation training on premotor and motor reaction time. *Percept Motor Skills.* 48:387, 1979

37. Basmajian JV, Kukulka CG, Narayan MG, et al. Biofeedback treatment of foot-drop after stroke compared with standard rehabilitation technique: Effects on voluntary control and strength. *Arch Phys Med Rehabil.* 56:231, 1975

38. Hurd WW, Pegram V, Nepomuceno. Comparison of actual and simulated EMG biofeedback in the treatment of hemiplegic patients. *Am J Phys Med.* 59:73, 1980

39. Takebe K, Kukulka CG, Narayan MG, et al. Biofeedback treatment of foot drop after stroke compared with standard rehabilitation technique, part 2: Effects on nerve conduction velocity and spasticity. *Arch Phys Med Rehabil.* 57:9, 1976

40. Solomonow M, Baratte R, Miwa T, et al. A technique for recording the EMG for electrically stimulated skeletal muscle. *Orthopedics* 8:492, 1985

41. Brudny J, Korein J, Grybnbaum BB, et al. Helping hemiparetics to help themselves—Sensory feedback therapy. *JAMA.* 241:814, 1979

42. Harris FA. Treatment with a position feedback-controlled head stabilizer. *Am J Phys Med.* 58:169, 1979

43. Koheil R, Mandel AR. Joint position biofeedback facilitation of physical therapy in gait training. *Am J Phys Med.* 59:288, 1980

44. Bowman BR, Baker LL, Waters RL. Positional feedback and electrical stimulation: An automated treatment for the hemiplegic wrist. *Arch Phys Med Rehabil.* 60:497, 1979

45. Winchester P, Montgomery J, Bowman B, Hislop H. Effects of feedback stimulation training and cyclical electrical stimulation on knee extension in hemiparetic patients. *Phys Ther.* 63:1096, 1983

46. Craik RL, Cozzens B, Miyazaki S. Enhancement of swing phase clearance through sensory stimulation. *Ann Conf Rehabil Eng.* 4:217, 1981

47. Malezic M, Stanic U, Kljajic M, et al. Multichannel electrical stimulation of gait in motor disabled patients. *Orthopedics* 7:1187, 1984

48. Bajd T, Kralj A, Turk R, et al. Standing-up for a healthy subject and a paraplegic patient. *J Biomechanics.* 15:1, 1982

49. Currier DP, Mann R. Muscular strength development by electrical stimulation in healthy individuals. *Phys Ther.* 63:915, 1985

50. Mohr T, Carlson B, Sulentic C, Landry R. Comparison of isometric exercise and high volt galvanic stimulation on quadriceps femoris muscle strength. *Phys Ther.* 65:606, 1985

51. Selkowitz DM. Improvement in isometric strength of the quadriceps femoris muscle after training with electrical stimulation. *Phys Ther.* 65:186, 1985

52. Eccles JC, McIntyre AK. The effects of disuse and of activity on mammalian spinal reflexes. *J Physiol (Lond).* 121:492, 1953

53. Vodovnik L. Indirect spinal cord stimulation—Some engineering viewpoints. *Appl Neurophysiol.* 44:97, 1981

54. Bowman BR, McNeal DR. Response of single alpha motoneurons to high frequency pulse trains—Firing behavior and conduction block phenomenon. *Appl Neurophysiol.* 49:121, 1986

55. Cranstam B, Larsson LE. Electrical stimulation in patients with spasticity. *Electroencephalogr Clin Neurophysiol Soc Proc.* 38:214, 1975

56. Dimitrijevic MR, Nathan PW. Studies of spasticity in man. 4. Changes in flexion reflex with repetitive cutaneous stimulation in spinal man. *Brain.* 93:743, 1970

57. Landau WM. Spasticity: What is it? What is it not? In: Feldman RG, Young RR, Koella WP, ed. *Spasticity: Disordered Motor Control.* Chicago, Year Book, 1980; 17–24

58. Levine MG, Knott M, Kabat H. Relaxation of spasticity by electrical stimulation of antagonist muscles. *Arch Phys Med.* 33:668, 1952

59. Alfieri V. Electrical treatment of spasticity—Reflex tonic activity in hemiplegic patients and selected specific electrostimulation. *Scand J Rehab Med.* 14:117, 1982

60. Fulbright JS. Electrical stimulation to reduce chronic toe-flexor hypertonicity—A case report. *Phys Ther.* 64:523, 1984

61. Tan W, Agar A, Marangoz C. Decreased post-tetanic potentiation of monosynaptic reflexes by simultaneous tetanization of antagonist nerves. *Exp Brain Res.* 31:499, 1978

62. Liberson WT. Experiment concerning reciprocal inhibitions of antagonists elicited by electrical stimulation of agonists in a normal individual. *Am J Phys Med.* 44:306, 1965

63. Lee WJ, McGovern JP, Duvall EN. Continuous tetanizing (low voltage) currents for relief of spasm. *Arch Phys Med.* 31:766, 1950

64. Bowman B, Bajd T. Influence of electrical stimulation on skeletal muscle spasticity. Proceedings of the International Symposium on External Control of Human Extremities, Belgrade, Yugoslavia, Committee for Electronics and Automation, 1981: 561–576

65. Vodovnik L, Bowman BR, Hufford P. Effects of electrical stimulation on spinal spasticity. *Scand J Rehabil Med.* 16:29, 1984

66. Solomonow M, Shoji H, King A, D'Ambrosia R. Studies toward spasticity suppression with high frequency electrical stimulation. *Orthopedics* 7:1284, 1984

67. Somjen G. *Neurophysiology—The Essentials.* Baltimore, Williams & Wilkins, 1983: 390–393

68. Pierrot-Deseilligny E, Morin C, Katz R, Bussell B. Influence of voluntary movement and posture on recurrent inhibition in human subjects. *Brain Res.* 124:427, 1977

69. Dimitrijevic MR, Faganel J, Gregoric M, et al. Habituation: Effects of regular and stochastic stimulation. *J Neurol Neurosurg Psychiatry.* 35:234, 1972

70. Dimitrijevic MR, Nathan PW. Studies of spasticity in man. 5. Dishabituation of the flexion reflex in spinal man. *Brain.* 94:77, 1971

71. Fuhrer MJ. Interstimulus interval effects on habituation of flexor withdrawal activity mediated by the functionally transected human spinal cord. *Arch Phys Med Rehabil.* 57:577, 1976

72. Cook WA. Effects of low frequency stimulation on the monosynaptic reflex (H reflex) in man. *Neurology.* 18:47, 1968

73. Fuhrer MJ. Dishabituation of flexor withdrawal activity mediated by the functionally transected human spinal cord. *Brain Res.* 63:93, 1973

74. Walker JB. Modulation of spasticity: Prolonged suppression of a spinal reflex by electrical stimulation. *Science.* 216:203, 1982

75. Van Ouwenaller C, Laplace PM, Chantraine A. Painful shoulder in hemiplegia. *Arch Phys Med Rehabil.* 67:23, 1986

76. Basmajian JV. Factors preventing downward dislocation of the adducted shoulder joint. *J Bone Joint Surg.* 41A:1182, 1959

77. Griffin J, Reddin G. Shoulder pain in patients with hemiplegia: A literature review. *Phys Ther.* 61:1041, 1981

78. Teppermann PS, Greyson ND, Hilbert L, et al. Reflex sympathetic dystrophy in hemiplegia. *Arch Phys Med Rehabil.* 65:442, 1984

79. Chino N. Electrophysiological investigation on shoulder subluxation in hemiplegics. *Scand J Rehabil Med.* 13:17, 1981

80. Baker LL, Parker K. Neuromuscular electrical stimulation of the muscles surrounding the shoulder. *Phys Ther.* 66:1930, 1986

81. Van Griethuysen CM, Day GA. Biomechanical analysis of a patient using FES peroneal brace and further developments. *Orthopedics.* 7:1196, 1984

82. Kralj A, Bajd T, Turk R. Electrical stimulation providing functional use of paraplegic patient muscles. *Med Prog Technol.* 7:3, 1980

83. Waters RL, McNeal DR, Clifford B, Falloon W. Functional electrical stimulation of the peroneal nerve for hemiplegia Long-term clinical follow-up. *J Bone Joint Surg.* 67A:792, 1985

84. Stein RB, Charles D, James KB. Providing motor control for the handicapped: A fusion of modern neuroscience, bioengineering and rehabilitation. In: Waxman SG, ed. *Advances in Neurology,* vol 47: *Functional Recovery in Neurological Disease.* New York, NY, Raven Press, 1988: 565–581

85. Brandell BR. Development of a universal control unit for functional electrical stimulation (FES). *Am J Phys Med.* 61:279, 1982

86. Coburn B. Paraplegic ambulation: A systems point of view. *Int Rehabil Med.* 6:19, 1984

87. Crago P. Control of movements by functional neuromuscular stimulation. *Eng Med Biol.* 54:32, 1983

88. Dimitrijevic MR, Gracanin F, Prevec T, Trontelj J. Electronic control of paralysed extremities—Neurolphysiological considerations. *Bio-Med Eng* 3:8, 1968
89. Nathan RH. The development of a computerized upper limb electrical stimulation system. *Orthopedics*. 7:1170, 1984
90. Petrofsky JS, Phillips CA, Stafford DE. Closed loop control for restoration of movement in paralyzed muscle. *Orthopedics*. 7:1289, 1984
91. Solomonow M, King A, Shoji H, D'Ambrosia R. External control of rate, recruitment, synergy and feedback in paralyzed extremities. *Orthopedics*. 7:1161, 1984
92. Altert A, Andre JM. State of the art of functional electrical stimulation in France. *Int Rehabil Med*. 6:13, 1984
93. Bajd T, Kralj A, Sega J, et al. Use of a two-channel functional electrical stimulator to stand paraplegic patients. *Phys Ther*. 61:526, 1981
94. Bajd T, Kralj A, Turk R, et al. The use of a four-channel electrical stimulator as an ambulatory aid for paraplegic patients. *Phys Ther*. 63:1116, 1983
95. Cybulski GR, Penn RD, Jeager RJ. Lower extremity functional neuromuscular stimulation in cases of spinal cord injury. *Neurosurgery*. 15:132, 1984
96. Holle J, Frey M, Gruber H, et al. Functional electrostimulation of paraplegics—Experimental investigations and first clinical experience with an implantable stimulation device. *Orthopedics*. 7:1145, 1984
97. Marsolais EB, Kobetic R. Functional walking in paralyzed patients by means of electrical stimulation. *Clin Ortho Rel Res*. 175:30, 1983
98. Peckham PH, Marsolais, EB, Mortimer JT. Restoration of key grip and release in the tetraplegic patient through functional electrical stimulation. *J Hand Surg*. 5:462, 1980
99. Peckham PH, Mortimer JT, Marsolais EB. Controlled prehension and release in the quadriplegic elicited by functional electrical stimulation of the paralyzed forearm musculature. *Ann Biomed Eng*. 8:369, 1980
100. Hart RL, Thrope GB, Stroh KC, et al. Technology transfer of an upper extremity functional neuromuscular stimulation program. *Proc Rehabil Eng Soc North Am*. 12:389, 1989
101. Keith MW, Peckham PH, Thrope GB, et al. Implantable functional neuromuscular stimulation in the tetraplegic hand: A case report. *J Hand Surg*. 14A:524, 1988
102. Gruner JA, Glaser RM, Feinberg SD, et al. A system for evaluation and exercise-conditioning of paralyzed leg muscles. *J Rehabil R&D*. 20:21, 1983
103. Phillips CA, Petrofsky JS, Hendershot DM, Stafford D. Functional electrical exercise—Comprehensive approach for physical conditioning of the spinal cord injured patient. *Orthopedics*. 7:1112, 1984
104. Ragnarsson KT. Physiologic effects of functional electrical stimulation induced exercises in spinal cord injured individuals. *Clin Ortho Rel Res*. 233:53, 1988
105. Kern H, Bochdansky T, Frey M, et al. Muscle training of paraplegic patients by FES device. *Vienna Int Work Funct Electrostim*. 1:5, 1983
106. Robinson CJ, Jeager RJ, Wurster RD, et al. Restrengthening paralyzed muscle in spinal cord injured patients by electrical stimulation: Predicting restrengthening outcome and measuring therapeutic benefits. *Int Conf Rehabil Eng*. 2:539, 1984
107. Turk R, Kralj A, Bajd T. et al. The alteration of paraplegic patients' muscle properties due to electrical stimulation exercising. *Paraplegia*. 18:386, 1980
108. Glaser RM. Physiological problems with functional neuromuscular stimulation ex-

ercise. In: Engineering Foundation Conference: *Neural Prostheses: Motor Control, Final Report.* Potosi, MO. 1988: 7–8

109. Isakov E, Mizrahi J, Najenson T. Biomechanical and physiological evaluation of FES-activated paraplegic patients. *J Rehabil Res Develop.* 23:9, 1986

110. Isakov E, Mizrahi J, Graupe D. Energy cost and physiological reactions to effort during activation of paraplegics by functional electrical stimulation. *Scand J Rehab Med.* 12 (suppl): 102, 1985

Neuromuscular Stimulation for Improving Muscular Strength and Blood Flow, and Influencing Changes

Dean P. Currier

Progressive-resistance exercise is a traditional physical therapy technique used to increase muscle strength. Neuromuscular electrical stimulation (NMES) has been used therapeutically by physical therapists for several years as a method of facilitating muscle contraction inhibited by pain, preventing denervation atrophy, and decreasing spasticity and spasm.[1-3] A resurgent interest in the use of NMES for increasing the strength of innervated muscle has occurred in the clinical practice of physical therapy. NMES is an effective mechanism for augmenting muscle strength and enhancing local circulation in the contracting muscle.[4-8] The increased popularity of NMES as an alternative approach to traditional progressive-resistance exercise may be attributed to Russian scientist Yadov M. Kots.

Kots's work remained almost unnoticed until members of the Russian Olympic team were observed using NMES as an adjunct to the traditional training regimens at the 1976 Olympics in Montreal.[9] In 1977, Kots visited Concordia University (Montreal) to present his research on the relationship of NMES and increased muscle strength in elite athletes. His lectures sparked renewed interest in the use of NMES. The procedures that he described have frequently been referred to as the *Russian technique*. Kots suggested that the use of NMES may produce a 30- to 40-percent strength improvement in trained athletes over and above that of traditional strength-enhancement methods.

Based in part on these unverified claims of extraordinary gains in muscle strength, a number of North American researchers have investigated the effects of NMES on innervated muscle. Although research findings indicate that electrical current causing excitation of muscles and nerves achieves desired physiological responses, the results of contemporary studies do not appear to verify all of Kots's claims.

The purpose of this chapter is to present a review of research findings about the relationship of NMES to enhancing muscle-strength gains and local blood-flow improvement to contracting muscles. This review should help the reader to apply existing principles of techniques of NMES so as to enhance clinical management of patients and athletes. For the purpose of this chapter, *muscle strength* is defined as the ability to produce external tension against resistance during a muscle contraction, and *neuromuscular electrical stimulation* (NMES) is defined as the use of electricity to produce desired physiological responses through induced facilitation of motor nerves.

THEORY

The tension-developing capacity of muscle during voluntary isometric contraction is a function of both the number of motor units that are recruited and the varying frequency of discharge (firing) of the recruited alpha motoneurons. Tension from weak muscular contractions (up to 50 percent of maximum voluntary contraction, or MVC) is usually graded by the number of active motor units.[10,11] The frequency of discharge of the motoneurons usually remains constant (5 to 15 Hz) during muscle-tension tasks, ranging between 5 and 50 percent of MVC. Although an orderly recruitment of motor units occurs according to size, an overlap of twitch tension is accomplished by asynchronous discharge of motor units at all graded levels of muscle contraction.[12] By the time muscular tension exceeds 50 percent of MVC, all motor units of the activated muscle have been recruited.[13] As muscular tension increases from 50 to 100 percent of MVC, the motor unit discharge frequency similarly increases, affecting the tension. The highest discharge frequencies of the motoneurons range between 40 and 60 Hz (with 100 percent effort).[13] To permit a smooth contraction, the alpha motoneurons of active motor units discharge asynchronously.[14]

The recruitment of motor units through volitional activity does not occur in a random fashion. Motor units are recruited in invariant order, from small to large anterior horn cell size.[15] Slow-twitch (Type I) motor units are morphometrically small and are recruited first in a muscle contraction because these motor units have small anterior horn cells. The slow-twitch motor units have lower tension-developing capacity than do fast-twitch motor units. Slow-twitch motor units have greater endurance than have fast-twitch units. Running a marathon involves muscular contractions of relatively low loads that may be repeated for prolonged periods of time without undue fatigue. Practice and training in physical activities may alter the coordination or timing of muscle response, which is the sequence of muscle activation.[16] Motor unit recruitment patterns may relate to the type of muscular contraction; for example, fast-phasic isometric contraction, as compared with sustained isometric contraction.[13]

Kots' work suggests that the induced form of contraction produced by NMES of muscles and nerves enhances the recruitment of motor units. He theorized that if all motor units were recruited, the muscle would contract maximally, and that with replicated sessions of NMES (training), the muscle would increase its tension-developing capacity (strength). His theory maintains that voluntary contractions cannot reach 100 percent of possible tension because of a force deficit. During volitional effort, not all motor units are recruited, and the motoneuron discharge rate is not maximum (deficit). Kots claims that the amount of force deficit varies from individual to individual because of motivational differences and that individuals only reach 60 to 70 percent of their strength potential through volitional effort. NMES, properly selected (he maintains) can reduce the force deficit in individuals to 10 percent, thereby increasing muscle tension by several percentage points. Some other claims of Kots' NMES regimen (18 training sessions) involved (1) a 40-percent increase in muscular strength; (2) a 10-cm increase in vertical jump; (3) a 10-percent increase in cross-sectional area of the myofibrils of muscle; and (4) a reduction in subcutaneous fat underlying the area of the body being electrically stimulated.[17]

Kots was aware of the physiological facts that human skeletal muscles have different contraction rates and phases and that the induced (electrical) mode of stimulation might not produce contractions similar to those of volitional effort. He found that NMES of a frequency of 100 pps affected the majority of fastest muscle fibers and only a minority of the slowest-contracting fibers. In order to achieve a maximum contraction tension, a NMES frequency of 80 pps was determined to be optimum. Sugai and co-workers reported that the mean maximum muscle force is developed with NMES of 75 pps.[18] Apparently, Kots' assumption was that muscles electrically stimulated at a frequency of 50 pps would behave in the same manner as in voluntary contractions. A volitional motoneuron-discharge frequency of 10 pps produces a smooth contraction with asynchronous activation of motor units, while NMES at a frequency of 19 pps elicits a series of unfused twitches.[19] Various muscles may have varied responses to the frequency of NMES, and the ability to tetanize muscle may require a frequency as fast as 300 pps.[20] Furthermore, the work of Belanger and McComas suggests that during maximum volitional effort, full activation of motor units is achieved easily for the tibialis anterior muscle but with difficulty for plantar flexor muscles.[21]

Kots suggests that the effectiveness of NMES may be attributed to improved recruitment of motoneurons, and that through training an individual might elicit motor units that previously were not activated because of inhibition.[9] Regardless of the acceptance of Kots' theory, much recent work in the area of NMES has been undertaken to either substantiate or refute his claims of augmenting muscle strength.

However, little difference is found in torque produced by a muscle contracting from NMES or from voluntary effort.[4–6] Since the torque-developing capacity of muscle is similar in both traditional active exercise and induced NMES programs, McMikan and associates have stated that the cellular mechanisms of adaptation should be activated during either type of contraction. Changes in muscle, as adaptation mechanisms to stress (exercise), are recognized as structural, physiological, and biochemical alterations. Changes in the central nervous system from volitional exercise have been demonstrated.[7]

EFFECTS OF NMES ON MUSCLE STRENGTH

Although NMES of muscles and nerves was reported as long ago as 1780, it did not appear to receive attention for assisting voluntary movement until 1902, when Bordier noticed its use.[22] Subsequently, NMES of healthy, innervated muscle has enjoyed varied use, and varied success, in physical therapy. Electrical stimulation has been used by physical therapists as a technique preliminary to voluntary muscle contractions and resistance exercise treatment in cases where pain is present.[1,23] Physical therapists have often approached NMES with mixed feelings, possibly because of a lack of understanding that precisely controlled applications may be used successfully in therapeutic interventions.[24] The effectiveness of NMES, compared with that of voluntary exercise was controversial for a long time, because NMES was not perceived as having the same physical value as voluntary exercise. Shriber stated: "In treatment of simple muscle weakness, there can be no argument on the point that voluntary exercise is the most desirable form of action and that no other form of exercise can have the same physical value."[25]

The use of NMES for strengthening healthy muscle has received considerable publicity through recent reports in the literature and is receiving renewed interest among practitioners in the clinic. The literature does support the concept that NMES has the same physical value and response on healthy muscles as does voluntary exercise, but not to the extent claimed by Kots that NMES produces 30 to 40 percent greater isometric strength than voluntary exercise.

Massey and co-workers compared NMES (pulsed square wave, 1000 pps, 10-sec contraction) with both static and dynamic exercise groups and with no exercise (control) groups. Seven muscle groups of the upper extremity were stimulated and exercised over 24 sessions (9 weeks). In comparison with the control group, the electrically stimulated group demonstrated the fewest number of improvements (four of ten measures) among the exercise groups. The dynamic exercise group demonstrated statistical improvement in nine of ten measures, while the static exercise group improved statistically in all ten measures. The investigators concluded that using the current characteristics described, NMES was no more effective (if even as effective) than the conventional types of exercise used in the study. Because NMES did result in modest muscle-strength gains, the investigators thought that under improved procedures and conditions the techniques had promise; however, complaints of muscle fatigue and discomfort from many subjects receiving NMES were made.[26]

In 1979, Currier and co-workers reported that a program of NMES combined with static exercise at MVC was no more effective (21 percent) than a traditional regimen of maximum-effort isometric exercise (19 percent). The NMES consisted of subjects receiving maximally tolerated square-wave stimulation at 25 pps. Six 6-sec contractions, with 10 sec interposed between each group of contractions, were performed in sessions completed on 5 successive days for 2 weeks (ten sessions). The indirect technique of stimulation was used (where one surface electrode was placed over the femoral nerve at the femoral triangle and the other surface electrode was positioned over the distal portion of the quadriceps femoris muscle).[4]

Halbach and Straus examined isokinetic peak torque produced by a volitional exercise group and by an NMES group. Torque was produced by knee extensors at an angular velocity of 120 degrees/sec. Both groups exercised for 3 weeks (15 sessions), after which time it was found that torque had increased in both groups. The isokinetic group increased their torque by 42 percent and the NMES group by 22 percent. The NMES group received a half-wave pulse of 50 pps, with a 10-sec contraction period and a 50-sec rest period between each stimulus. Ten repetitions were given each subject during each session, with the knee positioned in 45 degrees of flexion while exercising with isometric MVC. These investigators reported that pain and a burning sensation were major limiting factors to the subjects' ability to tolerate high-amplitude current.[17]

Eriksson and co-workers reported the effects of NMES with respect to muscle strength performance. The quadriceps femoris muscle was stimulated using square waves of 0.5 msec in pulse duration, at a frequency of 200 pps. They applied NMES for 15 sec, followed by 15 sec of rest between bursts of stimuli, for a total stimulation period of 6 min. Significant gains in peak torque (16 percent) were recorded for the leg receiving NMES, while the contralateral (untrained) leg did not change significantly in performance as a result of NMES of the ipsilateral leg. A control group, that performed dynamic exercise for a similar period of time (5 weeks) showed gains in torque scores of up to 27 percent. The largest torque scores for the NMES group were recorded at or near the knee flexion angle in which the subjects trained, while the dynamic exercise groups revealed a less "position-specific" training effect.[27]

Romero and co-workers stimulated bilateral quadriceps femoris muscle groups of young adult women for ten sessions over a 5-week period. They used a surging (slow ramp-up time) faradic current of 2000 pps with 4 sec of NMES, followed by 4 sec of rest (delay), for a total of 15 min of NMES each session. The training position of the affected legs was 65 degrees of knee flexion. Following treatment produced by isometric MVC, torque increased 31 percent in the nondominant leg and 21 percent in the dominant leg. A control group did not demonstrate a significant difference in mean peak torque between pretest and posttest measurements.[2]

In an effort to evaluate the ability of a specific level of NMES to increase muscle strength, Laughman and co-workers studied three independent groups of subjects: a control group, an isometric exercise group, and a group receiving NMES. The NMES delivered interrupted sine wave pulses at a frequency of 2500 pps, to provide 50 bursts of stimuli each second. Each series of bursts was composed of 10 msec of sinusoidal output, followed by a 10-msec rest period. The sequence of the NMES delivered 15 sec of stimulation followed by a 50-sec rest period. Each series of bursts was ramped on. The experimental subjects exercised for ten repetitions each session, 5 days a week, for 5 weeks (for a total of 25 sessions). Subjects exercised in the sitting position, with their hip and right knee positioned at 60 degrees from full extension. Results revealed that the control group's mean strength increased by 2 percent, the isometric exercise group's by 18 percent, and the NMES group's by 22 percent. The subjects in the NMES group tolerated progressively increasing amounts of current amplitude during the study, ranging from 19 to 88 mA. The investigators concluded that NMES, as used, was an appropriate device for strengthening skeletal muscles without voluntary effort.[6]

McMiken and associates tested the hypothesis that adaptation to ES would be either similar to or less than adaptation to voluntary contraction of the same amplitude. An NMES group and an isometric exercise group trained 4 days per week for 3 weeks. Training by NMES consisted of 10-sec induced muscle contractions with 50-sec rest intervals interposed between the contractions. NMES consisted of a square-wave pulse 0.1 msec in duration and a frequency of 75 pps, with voltage output determined by subject tolerance. Isometric exercise training consisted of ten 10-sec MVCs, with 50-sec rest intervals interposed between the contractions. Both groups demonstrated a marked improvement in strength of the quadriceps femoris muscle on completion of the training. The NMES group increased 22 percent in muscle strength and the isometric exercise group increased 25 percent. No significant difference was found in strength gains achieved by the two groups. No pain was experienced by the subjects in the NMES group during the training. McMiken and co-workers concluded that cutaneous NMES is a viable muscle-strengthening technique.[7]

Currier and Mann added support to the observations made earlier by other investigators.[4,5] Using a method similar to that of Laughman and co-workers, Currier and Mann produced similar findings. The method consisted of 15-sec NMES periods followed by 50-sec rest periods, for ten repetitions each session. A total of 15 sessions was used over a 5-week period (three sessions per week). All subjects trained while seated with their hip and knee flexed at 60 degrees from full extension. The isometric exercise group gained 30 percent in strength from training, the group that received NMES superimposed on isometric exercise gained 25 percent, and the NMES group gained 17 percent. No

significant difference (increase) was found in mean strength measurement between the three groups.[5]

Comparison of four different electrical stimulators and MVC was performed by Walmsley and associates in two experiments. Two stimulators produced currents of 4000 and 4100 Hz (to produce 75 pps) and 2200 Hz
(providing tetanizing currents of 50 pps). The latter unit delivered sinusoidal
current bursts 10 msec in duration, with 10-msec rest periods, a pulse duration
of 0.45 msec, and a maximum current amplitude of 95 mA. Two other stimulators were considered low-frequency units. One low-frequency stimulator delivered a single-spike waveform 0.2 msec in duration at 60 pps, while the fourth
unit produced a biphasic pulse 0.2 msec in duration at 50 pps. Subjects
producing isometric muscle contraction of their quadriceps femoris muscle
during NMES and MVC exercise were seated with their hip angled at 80
degrees flexion and their knee flexed to 60 degrees. Analysis of the peak
torques produced by the subjects revealed that the scores generated by NMES
were significantly less than those produced by MVC. Subjects receiving NMES
superimposed on MVC demonstrated a marked decrease in torque when the
stimulation was added, which suggested that NMES interferes with volitional
activity.[23]

All of these reported studies support the concept that NMES of healthy
muscle will increase strength without requiring volitional effort on the part of
the subject. When NMES is combined with voluntary exercise, the torque
developed from training still remains less than that obtained from voluntary
exercise training alone. To date, research has not confirmed the claims of Kots
that a 30 to 40 percent greater strength increase can be achieved from NMES
techniques than from traditional voluntary exercises.

EFFECTS OF NMES ON ENDURANCE OF HEALTHY MUSCLE

There is little literature available on the effects of NMES on muscle endurance
(the ability of a muscle to sustain activity over extended periods of time) for
muscles that have undergone a training regimen with NMES. Using a regime of
ten stimulus repetitions of 10 sec followed by 50 sec of rest, Kots found that,
during the last few repetitions, the muscle would not produce more than about
80 percent torque of the maximum contraction of the first repetition (due to
fatigue). He claimed that NMES for 7 weeks, with training given 5 days a
week, improved the ability of stimulated muscle for work (work capacity).[9]

The work of Currier and Mann revealed similar observations to those of
Kots, in that NMES resulted in a reduced contraction force between the second
and the tenth (or final) repetition. In their isometric exercise group, the mean
contraction torque on the tenth repetition was 90 percent of the torque recorded on the first repetition (a 10-percent reduction); the group that received
NMES superimposed on isometric exercise showed a 20-percent reduction in
torque, while the mean decrease in the NMES group was 24 percent. These

reductions in torque scores were based on the mean torque of each subject from each repetition over a 5-week training period.[5]

Using an NMES program consisting of 15 sec of stimulation interrupted by 15 sec of rest (200 pps, square-wave current), Eriksson and co-workers reported that levels of isometric endurance at 50 percent of MVC were unchanged from pretest (60 ± 6 sec) to posttest (50 ± 7 sec).[27] Further work needs to be done in order to determine the effects of NMES training on muscle endurance.

EFFECTS OF NMES ON THE ANGULAR VELOCITY OF LIMB MOVEMENT

Eriksson and co-workers reported that a 4-week period of NMES resulted in improved muscle strength; results were similar to those of a corresponding regimen of voluntary dynamic exercises. The results of mean torque of the NMES group appeared less speed-specific than did those of subjects training with slow isokinetic contractions (15 degrees/sec). The effects of NMES appeared to carry over into all speeds of limb movement tested, regardless of whether the rate of training movements was slow or fast. In the case of the subjects undergoing isokinetic training, the largest increments in torque occurred at the speed corresponding to that used in the training (speed-specific). The opposite pattern was reported for subjects training with NMES. Angular velocities tested were 0, 15, 30, 60, 90, and 100 degrees/sec.[27]

In a study by Romero and co-workers, NMES and control groups were measured for knee torque produced at angular velocities of 0, 30, and 60 degrees/sec. The NMES group trained using isometrically produced contractions (0 degrees/sec) while seated with the hip angled at 70 degrees of flexion and the knee at 65 degrees of flexion. Ten sessions of NMES conducted over 5 weeks resulted in a marked improvement of isometric knee extension strength (a 31-percent increase in the nondominant leg and a 21-percent increase in the dominant leg). A significant improvement in isokinetic strength was found in the nondominant leg at 30 degrees/sec. No significant strength improvement was found in either leg at an angular velocity of 60 degrees/sec.[2]

Currier and Mann added support to the observations of Romero and co-workers. Posttest results after 15 training sessions by groups on isometric exercise, NMES combined with isometric exercise, and NMES alone revealed strength improvement over the control group, although no significant differences in torque occurred between the three experimental groups. Each group trained in a seated position, with both the hip and knee joints positioned at 60 degrees of flexion during ten repetitions of passive isometric contraction. No significant changes between pretest and posttest isokinetic torque scores were found for 100, 200, and 300 degrees/sec rates of limb movement. Currier and Mann concluded that the lack of different amounts of torque gains at the various limb velocities following isometric resistance training supports the concept of training specificity.[5]

DOSAGE DETERMINATIONS

In a study designed to establish treatment baselines in an exercise regimen by NMES, Owens and Malone assigned 15 healthy subjects to three groups. Group 1 received NMES to their left knee extensor muscles each day for 10 days; group 2 was given NMES on alternate days of a 10-day period; and group 3 served as controls. Electrical stimulation treatment consisted of 50 sine wave pulses per second, producing ten tetanic muscular contractions for 15 sec each, with an interspaced rest period of 50 sec between bursts of stimuli. Stimulus current was increased as tolerated during the second, fourth, sixth, and eighth contractions in order to maintain torque output of the stimulated muscles. The authors determined that the subjects could tolerate NMES greater than 60 percent of their maximum voluntary isometric knee torque. Knee flexion of 35 degrees was found to be the least-uncomfortable position for receiving the passive style of isometric exercises by NMES. Owens and Malone also reported that current accommodation (subject acceptance) increases during each treatment session, which may indicate that decreasing resistance facilitates increased contraction.[28]

In another study, Selkowitz permitted the amplitude of the stimulating current to increase consistently from contraction to contraction, in order to maintain torque within maximum subject tolerance throughout each training session. He observed that torque increases between the first and seventh contraction with his method.[29]

Liu investigated various numbers of repetitions required by NMES for the augmentation of strength of the quadriceps femoris muscle. Thirty-nine healthy subjects were randomly assigned to one of four groups: a control group that did not receive any treatment, and experimental groups that received six, eight, or ten repetitions of NMES. Experimental subjects received NMES (50 sine wave pulses per second, 15-sec "on" bursts followed by interpulse rest periods of 50 sec) 3 days per week for 5 weeks (for a total of 15 sessions). The results revealed torque gains over time of 5, 21, 35, and 22 percent for the control group and of 6, 8, and 10 percent, respectively, for the repetition groups. A significant difference in strength was reported for women and men. The gains for women were 2, 13, 26, and 35 percent for controls, 6, 8, and 10 percent for the repetition groups, respectively. For men, the strength gains were 5, 16, 19, and 20 percent for controls, 6, 8, and 10 percent, respectively, for the repetition groups. Men in the eight-repetition group and women in the eight- and ten-repetition groups showed significantly greater strength gains after 5 weeks of training with NMES than did control subjects.[30]

Expanding on results revealed by Liu, Soo and co-workers conducted a study to evaluate strength gains when training with a specific NMES dosage. The specific dosages used current amplitudes based on 50 percent of each subject's MVC, eight repetitions of NMES per session, consisting of 15-sec "on" bursts followed by interpulse rest times of 50 sec (2500-Hz carrier sine wave pulse, interrupted 50 times/sec). Subjects trained 2 days a week, using the specific dosage described, for 5 weeks (for a total of ten treatments). Electrical stimulation was applied to the subject's right quadriceps femoris muscle (at the femoral triangle) and midthigh (above the patella). The left leg served as a control. The results showed that torque scores generated by the treated legs were significantly greater than for controls and that the flexor-to-extensor-muscles torque ratio was not altered by the NMES program (R = 52.4 versus 54.9 percent and L = 59.2 versus 50.5 percent pretest and posttest, respectively).[31]

Thus, strength augmentation is possible with the use of electrical stimuli of varied frequencies (33 to 2000 pps), wave shapes, and amplitudes (subject tolerance, 30 to 80 mA and 100 to 400 V). Also, NMES of sufficient amplitude to produce 50 percent of MVC of knee extensor muscles, eight repetitions each session, twice a week (for a total of ten sessions) has been found to be a suitable dosage for augmenting muscular strength in healthy subjects using 50 pps (sine wave).

In summary, examination of the literature reveals certain common characteristics among studies using NMES to augment muscular strength. Investigators have successfully augmented muscular strength while using rates of 33,[32] 50,[5,17] 60,[8] 65,[33] 75,[7] 100,[34,35] 200,[27] 1000,[26] and 2000 pps,[2] and waveforms of trapezoid,[36] rectangular,[32] surging,[5,36] sine,[5,6] and biphasic configurations.[35] The amplitudes of stimuli used have varied considerably. Several investigators reported using current amplitudes within their subjects' tolerance[17,27,33–35]; however, the actual amplitudes were often not cited, or the units of measurement varied from 60 [33] to 90 [5,6] mA and from 100 V[37] to 400 V,[5,6,29] making a common level of current amplitude difficult to identify. Some investigators have established the current amplitude applied to subjects on the basis of an individual's MVC (Table 7–1).[5,29,31] These approaches were attempted to bring about physiologic adaptations of muscle by programs of resistance exercise.

PAIN ASSOCIATED WITH NMES

Subject discomfort may be a limiting factor in many studies and in clinical applications using low-frequency NMES. As current amplitude is increased, the subject's sensory input is also increased, which tends to limit the amount of electrical stimulus amplitude that can be tolerated. According to Kots, a form of electrical current was found that would produce strong tetanic muscular contractions but would also provide an anesthetic effect. The electrical stimulator producing such current characteristics is now available in North America. The so-called "Russian stimulator" produces a carrier frequency of 2500 Hz, which is interrupted so that 50 bursts will produce tetanic contractions.

Halbach and Straus concluded that pain and a burning sensation are the major limiting factors in the current amplitude that can be used in NMES programs.[17] Owens and Malone reported that subjects treated with 50 bursts, per second of NMES found the stimulus somewhat uncomfortable, but that with

TABLE 7–1. CURRENT CHARACTERISTICS USED TO AUGMENT MUSCULAR STRENGTH

Primary Author	Waveform	Pulse Duration (msec)	Frequency (pps)	Amplitude	Repetitions per Sessions	Number of Sessions
Currier[5]	Sine, electrostim 180-2	0.1	2500, modulated at 50	60% MVC[a]	10	15
Eriksson[27]	Square, Grass	0.5	200	Max tolerable 10 mA × 30–60 V	15 sec on, 15 sec off × 6	4–5 times per week for 5 weeks
Godfrey[8]	Medcosonlator Dublett	—	60	Max tolerable	10 sec on, 50 sec off × 10	12
Halbach[17]	Half sine, Jono-Modulator	—	50	Max tolerable	10 sec on	15 (3 weeks)
Johnson[33]	Triangular, then rectangular, Siemens neuroton	—	65	Max tolerable 60 mA × 110 V	10 sec on, 50 sec off × 10	19 (95% patients)
Kramer[35]	Biphasic rectangular, Teca SPS/T	—	100	Max tolerable, 34.1 mA	10 sec on, 10 sec off	10–12 (4–5 weeks)
Lainey[34]	Interferential Medelco, Nemectrodyn	—	100 (4000, 4100)	Max tolerable	10 sec on, 50 sec off	17 (5–6 weeks)
Laughmann[6]	Sine, Electrostim 180-2	0.1	2500, modulated at 50	Max tolerable 90 mA	15 sec on, 50 sec off × 10	25
Massey[26]	Square, Isotron	—	1000	Max tolerable 5 W	10–15 sec on × 10	9 weeks
McMiken[7]	Faradic, Stewart Faradic GF01	0.1	75	Up to 80% MVC,[a] 10 V	10 (1:5 ratio)	4 times per week (3 weeks)

(continued)

181

TABLE 7-1. Continued

Primary Author	Waveform	Pulse Duration (msec)	Frequency (pps)	Amplitude	Repetitions per Sessions	Number of Sessions
Munsat[32]	Rectangular	0.2	33	50% MVC[a]	5 sec on, 25 sec off × 1 hour	Daily for 1–2 weeks
Romero[2]	Biphasic, Teca SP5	—	2000	Max tolerable 8–15 V	4 sec on, 4 sec off × 15 min	10 (5 weeks)
Williams[36]	Trapezoid, Multitone	—	—	—	10 × 20 min (2:3 ratio)	8–22 treatments, $\overline{x} = 13.1$

[a]Maximum voluntary contraction.

repeated use these same individuals adjusted to the discomfort and accepted increasing amplitudes over time. Their subjects were able to tolerate electrical current amplitudes that artificially produced greater than 60 percent of their maximum levels of contraction.[28]

In a more detailed study than others have reported, Currier and Mann assessed the pain experiences of 17 healthy subjects who complained of discomfort while completing 5 weeks of training with isometric exercise, NMES, or a combination of both. The McGill Pain Questionnaire was administered to all of the subjects experiencing pain. Results of the questionnaire revealed that the healthy subjects who received the NMES mode of training experienced similar torque gains but less muscle soreness than did those who performed conventional exercises. Most of the subjects in the exercise and NMES groups experienced pain at the medial aspect of their exercised knee. Pain felt by those receiving NMES (n = 12) was predominantly expressed as being of a sensory (spatial, temporal, and tactile) rather than an affective (pressure and autonomic) or an evaluative (overall pain) quality. The authors concluded that NMES does not appear to increase the risk of discomfort more than does conventional resistance exercise designed to achieve similar torque-developing capacities of muscles in healthy subjects.[38]

Franklin and associates found that individuals who receive a commonly used NMES protocol of 10 contractions over a 15-sec period develop significant increases in delayed onset muscle soreness. Muscle soreness and damage may result from a single session of NMES with peak amplitudes sufficient to produce torques equivalent to 30 percent of an individual's MVC. Their subjects' blood CK levels were still increasing at 72 hours poststimulation.[39]

FATIGUE WITH NMES

Torque produced by contracting muscle declines with time and numbers of contractions. This decrement of torque produced by contracting muscle(s) is referred to as *fatigue*. Muscle contractions induced by NMES fatigue more rapidly than those of equal force produced by volitional effort. Currier and Mann applied NMES that generated a 2500-Hz carrier frequency of sine wave current that was modulated to produce bursts for 15 sec; there were 750 individual pulses in each burst. Stimulated subjects' torque, developed during each burst, was recorded for each set of the ten repetitions or bursts per session during the 15 sessions. The torque decrement (fatigue curves of the knee extensors) over a continuum of repetitions amounted to 24 percent for the subjects receiving only NMES, 10 percent for subjects performing isometric exercises of equal contraction force, and 20 percent for individuals undergoing a concurrent combination of both.[5] When muscle contractions are induced by NMES, the same participating motor units are being continuously activated to produce torque, whereas with volitional effort the torque production is divided among different motor units of the muscle, which results in less fatigue. Additionally, Cabric and co-workers postulate that electically stimulated muscle contractions show greater fatigue when compared with volitional efforts because NMES has a more pronounced affect on Type II muscle fibers than on Type I fibers.[40]

Hosking and co-workers showed that the decrement in muscle force was dependent on the frequency of the stimulation. Prolonged NMES (18 sec) of the quadriceps femoris muscle at 30 and 100 pps produced patterns of force decrement. This force decrement was characteristic when the muscle was stimulated indirectly by its nerve or by electrodes placed over the muscle group. A 10-percent force decrement was recorded for the 30-pps frequency and a 59.6-percent decrement was recorded for the maximum force produced by 100 pps.[41]

In a study designed to determine the lowest number of stimulus repetitions needed to augment muscle strength, Liu found a mean decrease of torque with successive repetitions during training for three experimental groups. The mean torque decrement, from first to last contraction, for men in a ten-repetition group was 20 percent. The eight-repetition group showed a 19-percent decrease, and the six-repetition group showed a 17-percent decrease, in torque from the first to the last muscle contraction (repetition) in the session. For women, the decrease in torque between the first and last repetition by NMES was 20, 18, and 16 percent, respectively, for the ten-, eight-, and six-repetition groups.[30]

Rooney showed clinically that after every two muscle contractions induced by NMES the torque decrement could be prevented or reduced by manually increasing the current amplitude of the NMES. By increasing the current amplitude, additional motor units are activated to help reduce the torque decrement with continued NMES. Using a random selection of combination of various bursts with various carrier frequencies (50, 70, and 90 bps with 2500, 5000, and 10,000 Hz carrier frequencies) to stimulate the quadriceps femoris muscle of 27 subjects, Rooney found a trend for greater current amplitude requirements to maintain the target 50 percent of MVC as the combination of frequencies increased. That is, the combination of 50/2500 Hz required less amperage than 90/5000 Hz frequencies to obtain equal torque and thus reduce torque decrement of the contracted muscle. The mean torque decrement (fatigue) in his study was 30.3 percent between the first and tenth muscle contractions.[42]

When using NMES with burst modes, the relationship between "on" time and "off" time of the current stimulus is important to minimize fatigue. In NMES the "on" time to "off" time of the stimulus may be expressed as a ratio. Fatigue occurs more rapidly at a 1:1 ratio (on:off time) than at ratios of 1:2, 1:3, and 1:5.[43,44]

Peripheral fatigue results from failure of the muscle contractile apparatus and yields a decreased force generating capacity in the individual muscle fibers.[45] When muscles are electrically stimulated the larger fibers respond before the smaller-sized fibers. The larger, more powerful Type II fibers are elicited before Type I fibers during NMES, and the Type II fibers are more fatigable. Type II muscle fibers produce more lactic acid than Type I fibers and lactic acid contributes to peripheral fatigue.[46]

CLINICAL NMES

Clinical NMES is used in the rehabilitation of patients having abnormal physical conditions. Williams and Street reported on an electrical re-education technique that was successfully used with patients unable to produce voluntary contractions of the quadriceps femoris muscle. They used a trapezoid waveform of current followed by rest periods of 3 to 4 sec. The total treatment time was 20 min. NMES was reported to have disappointing results when not combined with active exercise. No strength scores were reported, but a mean thigh girth increase of 1 cm was observed after about 12 treatments.[36]

In 1977, Johnson and co-workers reported on the successful use of NMES in reducing pain and in increasing the strength and size of the quadriceps femoris muscle in 50 patients with chondromalacia patellae. Their results differed with variations in the number of treatment periods, the amplitudes of NMES used, and the degree of muscle atrophy present in each patient.[33]

Muscle atrophy and weakness often follow the first 6 weeks of reconstructive surgery of the anterior cruciate ligament. Eriksson and Haggmark divided two groups of patients, recovering from major knee ligament surgery and wearing casts, into an isometric exercise group and a group receiving both NMES and isometric exercise. This latter group received NMES with a frequency of 200 pps, producing intermittent muscle contractions for 5 to 6 sec, followed by a rest period of 5 sec. The NMES was administered by placing the first electrode through a hole cut in the cast proximal to the knee and by placing the second electrode over the femoral nerve in the groin. All patients exercised for 1 hour each day, 5 days a week, for 4 weeks. All patients were examined clinically, and muscle biopsies were taken prior to surgery and at 1 and 5 weeks after surgery. The group receiving the NMES had less atrophy and better muscle function, and their muscles contracted earlier after surgical procedures than did those in the control group performing isometric exercises. Eriksson and Haggmark concluded that NMES might prevent a fall in oxidative enzyme activity; thus, NMES may be a possible means of preventing muscle atrophy after major knee ligament surgery.[37]Delitto and co-workers showed that anterior cruciate ligament (ACL) surgery patients receiving a 3-week regimen of NMES had higher percentages of both extension and flexion torque when compared with patients performing voluntary exercises. Each group of patients received five treatments a week for 3 weeks. Treatments consisted of 15 co-contractions of the quadriceps femoris and hamstring muscles using a 15-sec duration and a 50-sec rest period between contractions. Both NMES and voluntary efforts were at the patients' tolerance.[47] Patients receiving NMES at the University of Kentucky, in addition to gaining more strength than those performing equal loads with conventional exercises, also do not incur muscle atrophy postsurgically while on the NMES regimen. The NMES regimen consists of NMES equivalent to 50 percent of the patients' presurgically measured torque, co-contractions, 10 contractions each of 3 days a week for the 6-week period after surgery.

Godfrey and co-workers compared patients postsurgically who had received NMES with patients undergoing a voluntary exercise program. After 12 treatments, the dynamic torque gains (measured at angular velocities of 3, 10, and 25 repetitions per min) were found to be significantly greater for patients using NMES than for those exercising isometrically.[8]

Standish and associates examined the use of NMES of muscle in the prevention of atrophy in immobilized limbs. Six patients were assigned to each of two groups following knee surgery. Each group of patients had their affected knees immobilized for a period of 6 weeks. One group, after 10 days of immobilization, received NMES of 2500 Hz, modulated to produce tetanic muscular contractions (50 pps) lasting 15 sec. Each treatment session consisted of ten repetitions of NMES applied to the affected knee extensor muscles, producing passive isometric exercise to patients' tolerance. Following cast removal, both groups of patients received similar rehabilitation programs. Biopsies of the vastus lateralis muscle, taken from subjects of both groups at the end of the period of NMES, revealed that the ATPase levels of the stimulated patients increased, while the ATPase levels in the immobilized control group decreased.[48]

Using an interferential current generator (two circuits carrying currents with frequencies of 4000 and 4100 Hz, respectively), Lainey and co-workers sequentially assigned eight patients to two groups. A double-crossover design was used to permit group 1 patients to engage in a pattern of volitional isometric exercise for 1 week, exercises combined with NMES for 1 week, exercises alone for 2 weeks, and exercise and NMES for the final 2 weeks. Group 2 patients reversed the regimen of group 1 for the 6-week experimental program. Results revealed that during the first 2 weeks of training patients receiving only isometric exercise tended to show greater increases in strength than those receiving the combination of exercise and NMES. However, in contrast, during the last 4 weeks of the training regimen, patients who received the combination of exercise and NMES recorded greater strength gains (39.5 percent) than did the exercise-only patients (7.4 percent). The authors concluded that NMES may be a worthy adjunct to exercise in the rehabilitation of patients that have undergone recent knee surgery.[34]

In summary, the literature indicates that NMES using surface electrodes is useful, by itself or in combination with isometric exercise, for restoring muscle size, enzymes, and torque output in patients with muscle atrophy and dysfunction following injury or major knee surgery. Furthermore, the best results of the therapy seem to occur among patients having the most severely atrophied muscles. Electrical stimulation appears to be helpful in the management of pain among patients where joint function is impaired as a result of inflammation, injury, and surgery.

EFFECT OF NMES ON GIRTH

Millard used NMES (square-wave pulse, 50 pps, 0.1 msec in duration) for 10-min periods in order to determine its value in the restoration of knee extensor strength, thigh girth, and knee effusion. The stimulus amplitude produced a contraction force sufficient to raise the subject's heel off the resting surface. Results of treatment revealed a slightly greater thigh girth in subjects receiving NMES than in the voluntary exercise group. No differences in muscle strength or joint effusion were observed between the two groups following 21 days of treatment.[49]

In another study of strength gain, measurements of both right and left upper and lower arm girths were made by Massey and co-workers of subjects involved in an NMES program 9 weeks (24 sessions) in duration. Using a steel anthropometric tape, they measured the largest portion of the arm twice at each site. The average of the two measurements was used for the accepted girth measure. The investigators reported statistically significant increases in right upper arm and lower left arm girths over those of a control group of subjects.[26]

Johnson and associates reported increased thigh girth in 50 patients having chondromalacia patellae who were treated with NMES. The stimulator produced rectangular pulses (65 Hz) and was used to provide a 10-sec maximum tetanic contraction within the patient's tolerance. The timing sequence of the stimulator provided a 50-sec rest period after each 10-sec contraction, and this timing sequence was repeated for ten repetitions during each of the 20 treatments. Thigh girth was measured at 7 and 15 cm proximal to the patella. Patients having mild chondromalacia patellae were found to have an increased thigh girth of 4.3 percent following 20 treatments of the vastus medialis muscle and femoral nerve. The patients with severe patellar problems improved 6.8 percent in girth, which the authors reported as probably reflecting improvement relating to the initial degree of atrophy. That is, the greater the initial muscular atrophy, the greater the improvement noted from treatment using NMES.[33]

Godfrey and co-workers treated a group of patients, referred for rehabilitation following surgery or injury, with tetanizing NMES in a double-blind study. The NMES (60 pps) was applied to the vastus medialis muscle and to the middle third of the thigh for 10 sec, followed by a rest period of 50 sec. Each patient received ten repetitions of the 10-sec stimuli at maximum tolerable current amplitude on a daily basis (for a total of 12 treatments). The circumferences of the patients' thighs were measured at 10 and 20 cm superior to the adductor tubercle, on a line drawn from the tubercle to the anterior superioriliac spine. The measured thigh girths were not found to be greater for electrically stimulated patients than for those receiving isometric exercise.[8]

A clinical study of three subjects receiving 15 NMES treatments (half-wave, 50-pps, timing sequence of 10-sec contractions followed by 50-sec rest periods between contractions) to the thigh was reported by Halbach and

Straus. Each treatment consisted of ten repetitions. No definitive change in thigh girth (measured 20 cm superior to the knee joint) was reported, although the torque scores improved 22 percent from the isometric exercise training.[17]

Romero and co-workers, studying the effects of NMES on control and experimental groups composed of nine women each, reported no differences in thigh girth between the groups. Surging intermittent faradic stimulation (2000 pps, 4-sec on and 4-sec off timing sequence for 15 min, average amplitude of 10.8 V or about 50 mA) was administered in twice-weekly sessions for a total of 5 weeks (ten treatment sessions). The quadriceps femoris muscles of both legs of each subject were exercised electrically and tested. Torque scores improved significantly compared with those of the control group, but no differences between the groups were reported for girth measurements.[2]

The work of Currier and Mann revealed similar findings to those of Romero and co-workers. Although torque was increased through training with isometric exercise, NMES, and a concurrent combination of both, when compared with control subjects no statistically significant differences in the posttest girths were found.[5]

The effectiveness of NMES for increasing girth measurements of the thighs remains unresolved. The literature reveals that muscle mass of animals is definitely increased as a result of short-term (less than 6 weeks) and long-term (more than 6 weeks) NMES treatments. The literature pertaining to studies of humans is mixed regarding the effectiveness of NMES for increasing girth measurement. Some studies are positive on its effectiveness, while an equal number have not confirmed that NMES increases muscle mass, particularly when a training routine involves isometric muscle contractions.

EFFECTS OF NMES ON BLOOD FLOW

Long- and short-term NMES of muscle results in an increased vascular supply, with a concomitant increase in the number of capillaries within the muscle. Over 4-, 14-, and 28-day periods of intermittent NMES (10-pps frequency), Myrhage and Hudlicka reported a 20-, 50-, and 100-percent increase in capillary density to the stimulated tissue, respectively.[50] Applying both direct and percutaneous NMES to the nerve of a particular leg muscle in dogs on different trials, Wakin found that maximum blood flow to the muscle resulted with stimuli of 8 to 32 pps.[51] Randall and co-workers reported a greater hyperemia following NMES than that occurring during contraction of the stimulated muscle in dogs.[52] Folkow and Halicka found a progressive increase in blood flow to the gastrocnemius muscle of cats when using NMES at rates of 1, 2, and 4 pps, but blood flow increased proportionally less as the stimulus frequency increased to 8, 16, 20, 30, and 60 pps, respectively.[53] Using various stimulus frequencies and various levels of muscular contractile forces on cat muscles, Petrofsky and associates found that blood flow increased during most levels of contractions but that it increased to a greater extent immediately following contraction regardless of the level of contractile force used. Using computer assistance, they administered NMES that corresponded to the asynchronous recruitment of motor units, as occurs in voluntary muscle contractions. Other investigators administered NMES so that the muscle responded in a synchronous manner. Although the synchronous mode differs substantially from the voluntary asynchronous mode of motor-unit recruitment, the effects on blood flow appear to be similar.[54]

In a study designed to determine the effect of 2500-Hz carrier frequency modulated at 50 bursts per sec on microvascular perfusion, Clemente found that NMES can increase the degree of microvascular perfusion in skeletal muscle. He also noted that muscle contraction is essential for increasing the degree of perfusion and that mechanisms other than sympathetic outflow effect the changes in microvascular perfusion.[55]

Currier and co-workers investigated the effect on vascular dynamics of NMES and graduated muscular responses produced by the stimulator. (The electrical stimulator used has a 2500 Hz carrier frequency modulated at 50 bursts per second. The effects of these new stimulators on blood flow dynamics have not been established by controlled study.) In this particular study, healthy volunteers were randomly assigned to an experimental group (N = 14) receiving tetanic NMES to the gastrocnemius muscle or to a control group (N = 14) receiving no treatment. Using a Doppler device, the results revealed a mean 25- and 27-percent increase in pulsatility index scores (peak-to-peak pulse divided by mean distance of cardiac cycles) following 10 min of electrical stimuli bursts, producing torques at 10 and 30 percent of maximum voluntary contraction torques. No significant change in blood flow dynamics was found for the untreated control subjects. The blood flow dynamics in the experimental subjects increased significantly during the first minute of NMES and remained elevated at a steady-state level throughout the stimulation period and for 10 min following the termination of treatment. The results demonstrated that NMES (2500 Hz interrupted for 50 bps) applied with a stimulus sequence of 15 sec on and 50 sec off, can alter the vascular dynamics affecting local muscle blood flow.[56]

In a related study investigating whether finger blood flow is altered by NMES of the gastrocnemius muscle at intensities of 15 and 30 percent of prestimulation maximum voluntary contraction torques, Liu and associates found that a significant difference in finger blood circulation occurred between levels of contraction torques and between individuals receiving NMES and control subjects not receiving NMES. Twenty-six healthy subjects participated in this study and were assigned randomly to either an experimental group (N = 13) receiving 10 min of NMES (with bursts of 15 sec followed by 50-sec rest periods) or to a control group (N = 13) receiving no treatment. The significant finding of decreased blood flow dynamics in the fingers of the NMES subjects demonstrates that NMES of 50 bps frequency does influence circulation systematically. Electrical stimulation of these specific current output characteristics brings about alterations in circulation because of metabolic changes in muscles undergoing the exercise produced by the stimulation.[57]

Most recent studies involving short-term NMES have used isometric muscular contractions. This type of exercise by NMES has not been examined to determine whether there is an increase in capillaries of the muscles being stimulated.[58] Further research is indicated to clarify the effects of short-term NMES of various frequencies on the density of capillaries in stimulated muscles.

Tracy and associates measured the effects of selected frequencies from two different pulsed electrical stimulators on blood flow, blood pressure, and heart rate. All subjects received NMES at an amplitude sufficient to produce torque equal to 15 percent of prestimulation MVC of the quadriceps femoris muscle. Blood flow was found to be dependent on pulse frequency but independent of stimulator type. Pulsed frequencies of 10, 20, and 50 pps were found effective for clinical use of NMES for promoting arterial blood flow to muscle. Inconsistent changes in blood pressure and heart rate from NMES were reported.[59]

Not all types of NMES affect the blood flow dynamics of the muscle receiving the stimuli. To date, there is a dearth of literature to support the claim that so-called high-voltage stimulation (HVS) increases blood flow to muscle in a clinical situation. In an abstract, Alon and associates reported no significant changes in posterior tibial artery blood flow in 20 subjects receiving HVS of an amplitude up to, but below, muscle contraction threshold.[60] In an unpublished pilot study at the University of Kentucky in 1981, Loze was unable to find an increase in localized blood flow in the femoral artery of five healthy subjects after stimulating their right gastrocnemius muscles with a frequency of 4 and 80 pps and a switching rate (activation time between the two small electrodes) of 2.5 sec. Current amplitude was set to subjects' level of tolerance and was maintained for 2 min of muscular contractions.[61] In 1982, Fields stimulated the gastrocnemius muscle of 14 healthy subjects using HVS amplitude to levels of tolerance and frequencies of 15 and 30 pps. The switching rate between electrodes was 2.5 sec. Again, no increased blood flow was found in the popliteal artery after 10 min of HVS.[62]

As a culmination of the previous studies on blood flow and HVS on healthy individuals, Walker and associates investigated different NMES locations and amplitudes. They randomly assigned healthy subjects to one of three groups: NMES (n = 16), isometric exercises (N = 18), and control (N = 8). The HVS was set for 10 pps, a 2.5-sec switching rate between electrodes, and voltage amplitudes designed to produce contraction of the plantar flexors so as to simulate 10 and 30 percent of the prestimulation MVC torque scores and back extensors of 10 percent of MVC. The voltage amplitudes ($\bar{x}$ = 271 V, range 150 to 350 V, for 10 percent of MVC of plantar flexors; $\bar{x}$ = 271 V, range 190 to 415 V, for 30 percent of MVC of plantar flexors; and $\bar{x}$ = 445 V, range 420 to 450 V, for 10 percent of MVC of back extensors) were then used to produce rhythmic muscular contractions during the experimental procedure. Thirty percent of MVC by NMES for back extensors could not be obtained by the HVS unit because of subject tolerance and insufficient pulse change. A Doppler device was used to measure vascular dynamics of the popliteal artery. There were no significant changes in blood flow dynamics in the popliteal artery from HVS applied with the intensities of 10 and 30 percent of MVC to the plantar flexors and back extensors, respectively.[63] The results are difficult to explain because isometric muscle contractions were obtained in all subjects by HVS. The pulse durations of the stimuli are extremely short (range 0.050 to 0.075 msec), and the total pulse charge is small. This small current charge coupled with a small total current (≤ 2.0 mA) may account for the very small effect on the metabolism of the contracted muscle.[60–63] Whatever the reason, no change in blood flow dynamics has been demonstrated in healthy subjects by high-voltage stimulation when used clinically.

METABOLIC AND ULTRASTRUCTURAL ALTERATIONS

The muscle fiber cells of mammalian skeletal motor units have remarkable adaptive potential and are perhaps the most adaptable tissue in the body (in response to a wide variety of stimuli, including NMES).[64] Muscle adapts to changes in demand and acquires biochemical and ultrastructural characteristics that are probably better suited to its new functional needs.[65] The metabolic demand on muscle decreases as a result of disuse (joint immobilization, various diseases, aging, and bed rest), while increased metabolic demand occurs with both exercise and NMES.[40,66] This section concentrates on the effect of increased demand from exercise, both volitional and passive, by NMES.

Long-term NMES (greater than 6 weeks) of peripheral nerves and muscles by means of implanted electrodes has been used to correct "drop foot" and hip-extensor weakness of stroke patients and as an orthotic substitute.[32,67] This approach has provided much of the data about NMES effects on the ultrastructure of muscle.

Eriksson and Haggmark studied the acute effects of NMES on the quadriceps femoris muscles of 23 healthy subjects. Muscle biopsies were taken from the stimulated leg prior to the daily training phase and within 2 days after the training period (4 to 5 weeks). Metabolic changes were observed: a depletion of ATP and CP stores, a decrease of enzymes (ATPase, MK, CPK, phosphorylase, lactic dehydrogenase, and succinic dehydrogenase), and an increase of lactate resulted from 6 min of continuous NMES, These changes in enzymes from NMES have also been reported following intense muscular exercise. However, when the NMES was intermittently applied 4 or 5 days a week, no significant enzyme, muscle fiber characteristics, or mitochondrial changes occurred.[37]

The effects of 5 to 6 weeks of immobilization on myofibrillar ATPase and muscle glycogen concentration following major surgical repair of the knee ligaments of nine patients were studied by Standish and co-workers. A control group ($n = 3$) and an experimental group ($n = 6$) engaged in conventional physical therapy following cast removal, but the experimental group also received NMES beginning 10 days after surgery and continuing until 4 weeks after cast removal. Results revealed that ATPase actively diminished in the control group but remained essentially the same in the experimental group receiving NMES. Between biopsies, the glycogen concentrations remained unchanged in both groups following rehabilitation exercise. This study indicated that myofibrillar ATPase levels of muscle can be maintained by NMES applied while the knee joint is immobilized.[48]

The effects of short-term NMES of two different frequencies on the metabolism of the vastus lateralis muscle in ten healthy subjects were studied by Houston and co-workers. The vastus lateralis muscle of one leg was stimulated for 60 min (with continuous stimuli pulses 0.6 msec in duration at 10 pps), while the other leg was stimulated intermittently at a frequency of 50 Hz (12-sec bursts followed by 48-sec interpulse rest periods). Biochemical analyses revealed increases in muscle lactate and citrate concentrations; no significant changes in ATP, CP, and metabolite concentration; and reductions in glycogen for both stimulation conditions. Fast-twitch muscle fibers had lower glycogen contents than did slow-twitch fibers after 10-pps stimulation, whereas 50-pps stimulation only affected glycogen reduction in 50 percent of the fibers. Reported changes from biochemical analyses were less than have been noted following traditional exercise programs. The authors conjectured that NMES similar to that used in their experiment is indicated for certain clinical conditions.[68]

In-vivo NMES of frog muscles showed that glycogen concentration decreases consistently with increasing voltage and pulse frequency. Total protein content did not change with various pulse frequencies. The extent of depletion of total carbohydrates decreased with increasing days of stimulation. These results led the investigators to advocate NMES as a method of preventing muscle waste in atrophic conditions of muscles.[69]

Concurrent with the physiological (strength) and biochemical (metabolic) changes are transformations in the muscle ultrastructure following periods of NMES. Skeletal-muscle cells can be classed into slow-twitch (Type I) and fast-twitch (Type II) categories by ultrastructural studies conducted by electron microscopy. The classification may be made by quantitative analyses of the sarcoplasmic reticulum, T-tubular system, the number of mitochondria and glycogen particles, the width of the Z line, and the presence of M-band proteins.

Contractile characteristics of mammalian skeletal muscle are altered by changing the pattern of activity imposed upon the muscles.[70] Using NMES of 200 rectangular pulses 0.05 msec in duration, amplitude of twice threshold, and a very slow frequency of 1 pps, Eisenberg and Gilai found no gross structural alterations but reported the occurrence of subtle changes. The mitochondria contained granules of normal size and number, but the matrix width of the inner crista was increased by NMES. The width of the inner crista was unchanged. The myofibrils were also unchanged, except for a slight swelling in the myosin lattice. The transverse T system and sarcoplasmic reticulum were essentially unchanged, except that the minor diameter of the transverse tubule was increased. The stimulated muscle fibers had a marked increase in the electron-dense content of the terminal cisternae.[71]

Other researchers have reported more dramatic ultrastructural changes in skeletal muscle following a more prolonged period of NMES than that reported by Eisenberg and Gilai. With NMES, fast-twitch muscle fibers seem to adapt a wider Z disc, which is characteristic of slow-twitch fibers.[72] Increased numbers of mitochondria have also been reported following prolonged NMES. The number of T tubules and elements of the sarcoplasmic reticulum decrease after a few days of stimulation.[65]

During the transformation from fast- to slow-twitch fiber characteristics as a result of NMES, the contractile speed and activity of myosin ATPase, and the calcium uptake by the altered sarcoplasmic reticulum, change to traits that are slower than usual for a typical slow muscle (eg, the soleus).[65] Prolonged stimulation does not seem to affect the number of muscle fibers. Stimulated fibers acquire diameters typical of slow-twitch fibers; this finding parallels the reported reductions in wet weight and in cross-sectional area.[73] To date, all of the ultrastructural changes reported as an adaptation response to NMES are reversible within 6 weeks of discontinuing the stimulation.[65]

All studies conducted so far on ultrastructural changes of skeletal muscle by NMES have been based on prolonged periods (6 weeks) of stimulation. Greathouse and co-workers studied the short-term (4 weeks) effects of NMES on rat hind-limb skeletal muscles. The rats were assigned to one of three groups: group 1 was treated daily, group 2 every other day, and group 3 received no stimulation. Electrical stimulation (2500-Hz carrier sine wave, interrupted for 50 bps, to produce fused tetanic contractions) was directed to the knee extensor and flexor muscles of the rats for 15-min sessions over a period of 22 days. Electron micrographs of the excised muscles revealed that the A-bands, I-bands, Z-disc, and actin and myosin filaments were not changed by NMES. The number and volume density of mitochondria increased significantly in both extensor and flexor muscles. The number of T-tubular systems was reduced in both muscle groups. These observed ultrastructural alterations appear similar to those reported for prolonged stimulation of muscle and to reports that fast-twitch fibers change to slow-twitch fibers within 4 weeks of stimulation.[74]

OTHER INFLUENCES OF NMES ON MUSCLE*

Histochemical-Enzyme Changes

NMES of low-frequency applied to the fast muscles of rabbit for several weeks will cause them to acquire the biochemical and physiologic characteristics of slow muscles.[65] Changes in both heavy- and light-chain components of myosin

---

* Adapted from: Cummings J: Electrical stimulation of healthy muscle. In: Nelson RM, Currier DP (eds). *Clinical Electrotherapy.* 1st ed. Norwalk, Appleton & Lange, 1987.

are involved in this orderly transformation as revealed by gel electrophoresis, myosin paracrystal formation, and immunocytochemistry.[73,75–77]

In addition to influences on myosin, other myofibular changes may follow chronic NMES. After 3 weeks of NMES, Roy and associates showed that the ratio of alpha to beta forms of tropomyosin changes to that ratio characteristic of slow muscles.[78]

Chronic, low-frequency NMES of fast muscles can also cause some contractile properties of fast muscles to resemble those of slow muscles, regardless of the frequency of stimulation, provided that the total number of stimuli is comparable, that the duration of the stimuli is sufficient (a minimum of 2 weeks), and that all motor units are elicited.[79] These findings indicate that NMES influences enzymatic plasticity in healthy mammalian muscles.

Membrane Changes

Maintenance of the membrane properties of muscles are greatly influenced by the muscle impulse activity.[80,81] Jansen and associates have shown that chronic NMES can prevent the spread of acetylcholine sensitivity that follows denervation, and that reinnervation may be prevented by NMES.[82] Lomo and coworkers showed that chronic NMES of denervated muscle can slow the speed of muscle contraction and can actually convert a muscle with predominantly slow-twitch fibers into one dominated by fast-twitch fibers.[83] Other researchers have similarly demonstrated that fast-twitch muscle fibers can be transformed into slow-twitch fibers through chronic NMES.[70,84,85] Although the issue of whether or not nerve-generated activity is the only factor responsible for the maintenance of healthy muscle remains clouded, studies have demonstrated that impulse frequency does have profound effect on the membrane properties of muscle and, therefore, on the contractility of mammalian muscle.

SUMMARY

NMES designed to artificially produce muscle contraction is similar, in some respects, to volitional efforts. NMES of specific current characteristics elicits enough motor units to produce torque similar to that produced by the voluntary efforts of subjects.

A considerable number of studies supports the concept that NMES of healthy muscle increases strength without requiring voluntary effort by the subject. These increases have been clearly demonstrated for patients having chondromalacia patellae or recovering from major knee surgery, as well as for subjects having no physical malady. NMES has also been successfully used to prevent atrophy during joint immobilization.

Although various dosages have been reported that produce strength gains in muscle, specific current characteristics have been shown to be successful. Since several types of NMES have been used successfully, waveform is probably not as important to augmenting muscle performance with training as are amplitude, frequency, and pulse duration. Electrical-stimulation amplitude sufficient to produce 50- to 60-percent maximum voluntary contraction during each of eight to ten repetitions per session, along with a frequency capable of producing a fused tetanic muscle contraction (50 to 90 pps), are apparently essential ingredients to improving the torque output of muscle tissue.

Subject tolerance to different electrical stimulators varies considerably, so that no single waveform or device is more comfortable than another. Limiting the duration of pulses seems to contribute to subject comfort, and a range of 0.05 to 0.50 msec appears to be very tolerable to most subjects.

Although most electrical stimulators may improve or increase the circulatory dynamics of muscles being stimulated, those with a frequency of 10 to 50 pps seem to be better than those with faster frequencies. Stimulators must be capable of increasing the metabolism of the contracting muscle, in order to improve the blood flow to the working muscle. To improve blood circulation, short interpulse intervals (1:1 to 1:2) may be better than long interpulse intervals. To improve muscle performance, such as torque, the interpulse interval should be set at a 1:3 to 1:5 ratio, in order to avoid excessive fatigue.

NMES of short-term duration (less than 6 weeks), as well as that of long-term duration (greater than 6 weeks), influences the biochemical and structural components of muscle. Evidence obtained thus far supports the conversion of Type II to Type I fibers through altered composition and organelles of the muscle and muscle cell, respectively. Alterations in muscles obtained by NMES seem to be reversible with discontinuation of the program. The amount of time necessary for reversing the altered features of muscles upon termination of NMES has been reported as being 6 weeks.

REFERENCES

1. Kramer JF, Mendryk SW. Electrical stimulation as a strength improvement technique: A review. *J Orthop Sports Phys Ther.* 4:91, 1982
2. Romero JA, Sanford TL, Schroeder RV, et al. The effects of electrical stimulation of normal quadriceps on strength and girth. *Med Sci Sports Exerc.* 14:194, 1982
3. Chase J. Elicitation of periods of inhibition in human muscle by stimulation of cutaneous nerves. *J Bone Joint Surg (Am).* 54:1737, 1972
4. Currier DP, Lehman J, Lightfoot P. Electrical stimulation in exercise of the quadriceps femoris muscle. *Phys Ther.* 59:1508, 1979
5. Currier DP, Mann R. Muscular strength development by electrical stimulation in healthy individuals. *Phys Ther.* 63:915, 1983
6. Laughman RK, Youdas JW, Garrett TF, et al. Strength changes in the normal quadriceps femoris muscle as a result of electrical stimulation. *Phys Ther.* 63:494, 1983
7. McMiken DF, Todd-Smith M, Thompson C. Strengthening of human quadriceps muscles by cutaneous electrical stimulation. *Scand J Rehab Med.* 15:25, 1983
8. Godfrey CM, Jayawardena H, Quance TA, et al. Comparison of electro-stimulation and isometric exercise in strengthening the quadriceps muscle. *Physiother Can.* 31:265, 1979

9. Babkin D, Timtsenko N, eds. Notes from Dr Kots' (USSR) lectures and laboratory periods. Canadian–Soviet exchange symposium on electrostimulation of skeletal muscles. Concordia University, Montreal, December 6–15, 1977

10. Bigland B, Lippold OCJ. The relation between force, velocity, and integrated electrical activity in human muscles. *J Physiol.* 123:214, 1954

11. Clamann PH. Activity of single motor units during isometric tension. *Neurology.* 20:254, 1970

12. Milner-Brown HS, Stein RB. The relation between the surface electro-myogram and muscular force. *J Physiol.* 246:549, 1975

13. Petrofsky JS. *Isometric Exercise and Its Clinical Implications.* Springfield, IL, Charles C. Thomas, 1982

14. Rack PMH, Westbury DR. The effects of length and stimulus rate on tension in the isometric cat soleus muscle. *J Physiol.* 204:443, 1969

15. Olson CB, Carpenter DO, Henneman E. Orderly recruitment of muscle action potentials. *Arch Neurol.* 19:591, 1968

16. Normand MC, Lagase-PP, Rovillard CA, et al. Modifications occurring in motor programs during learning of a complex task in man. *Brain Res.* 241:87, 1982

17. Halbach JW, Straus D. Comparison of electromyostimulation to isokinetic training in increasing power of the knee extensor mechanism. *J Orthop Sports Phys Ther.* 2:20, 1980

18. Sugai N, Worsley R, Payne JP. Tetanic force development of adductor pollicis muscle in anesthetical man. *J Appl Physiol.* 39:714, 1975

19. Buller AJ, Lewis DM. Further observations on the differentiation of skeletal muscles in the kitten hind limb. *J Physiol.* 176:355, 1965

20. Brown GL, Burns BD. Fatigue and neuromuscular block in mammalian skeletal muscle. *Proc R Soc Lond (Biol).* 136:182, 1949

21. Belanger AV, McComas AJ. Extent of motor unit activation during effort. *J Appl Physiol.* 51:1131, 1981

22. Licht S. History of electrotherapy. In Stillwell GK, ed. *Therapeutic Electricity and Ultraviolet Radiation*, 3rd ed. Baltimore, Williams & Wilkins, 1983

23. Walmsley RP, Letts G, Vooys J. A comparison of torque generated by knee extension with a maximal voluntary muscle contraction vis-a-vis electrical stimulation. *J Orthop Sports Phys Ther.* 6:10, 1984

24. Wolf SL, ed. *Electrotherapy.* New York, Churchill Livingstone, 1981: vii–viii

25. Shriber WJ. *A Manual of Electrotherapy*, 4th ed. Philadelphia, Lea & Febiger, 1975

26. Massey BH, Nelson RC, Sharkey BC, et al. Effects of high frequency electrical stimulation on the size and strength of skeletal muscle. *J Sports Med Phys Fit.* 5:136, 1965

27. Eriksson E, Haggmark T, Kiessling KH, et al. Effect of electrical stimulation on human skeletal muscle. *Int J Sports Med.* 2.18, 1981

28. Owens J, Malone T. Treatment parameters of high frequency electrical stimulation as established on the electro-stim 180. *J Orthop Sports Phys Ther.* 4:162, 1983

29. Selkowitz DM. Improvement in isometric strength of the quadriceps femoris muscle after training with electrical stimulation. *Phys Ther.* 65:186, 1985

30. Liu HI. *Optimum Repetitions for the Development of Strength and Muscle Hypertrophy by Electrical Stimulation.* Master's thesis, University of Kentucky, Lexington, 1984

31. Soo CL, Currier DP, Threlkeld AJ. Exercise dosage of electrical stimulation for improving performance of healthy muscle. *Phys Ther.* 68:333, 1988

32. Munsat TL, McNeal D, Waters R. Effects of nerve stimulation on human muscle. *Arch Neurol.* 33:608, 1976
33. Johnson DH, Thurston P, Ashcroft PJ. The Russian technique of faradism in the treatment of chrondromalacia patellae. *Physiother Can.* 29:1, 1977
34. Lainey CG, Walmsley RP, Andrew GM. Effectiveness of exercise alone versus exercise plus electrical stimulation in strengthening the quadriceps muscle. *Physiother Can.* 35:5, 1983
35. Kramer JF, Semple JE. Comparison of selected strengthening techniques for normal quadriceps. *Physiother Can.* 35:300, 1983
36. Williams JGP, Street M. Sequential faradism in quadriceps rehabilitation. *Physiotherapy.* 62:252, 1976
37. Eriksson E, Haggmark T. Comparison of isometric muscle training and electrical stimulation supplementing isometric muscle training in the recovery after major knee ligament surgery. *Am J Sports Med.* 7:169, 1979
38. Currier DP, Mann R. Pain complaint: Comparison of electrical stimulation with conventional isometric exercise. *J Orthop Sports Phys Ther.* 5:318, 1984
39. Franklin ME, Currier DP, Smith S, et al. Effect of varying the electrical stimulation of muscle contraction to rest time ratio on muscle damage and soreness. Submitted for publication
40. Cabric M, Appell HJ, Resic A. Fine structural changes in electrostimulated human skeletal muscle. *Eur J Appl Physiol.* 57:1, 1988
41. Hosking GP, Young A, Dubowitz V, et al. Tests of skeletal muscle function in children. *Arch Dis Child.* 53:224, 1978
42. Rooney JG. *Effect of Variation in the Burst Mode and Carrier Frequency of High Amplitude Electrical Stimulation on Muscle Fatigue and Pain Perception of Healthy Subjects.* Doctoral dissertation, University of Kentucky, Lexington, 1988
43. Benton LA, Baker LL, Bowman BR, et al. *Functional Electrical Stimulation: A Practical Clinical Guide*, 2nd ed. Downey, CA, Randho Los Amigos Rehabilitation Engineering Center, 1981
44. Packman-Braun R. Raltionship between functional electrical stimulation duty cycle and fatigue in wrist extensor muscles of patients with hemiparesis. *Phys Ther.* 68:51, 1988
45. Bigland-Ritchie B, Furbush F, Woods JJ. Fatigue of intermittent submaximal voluntary contractions: Central and peripheral factors. *J Appl Physiol.* 61:421, 1986
46. Appell HJ. Skeletal muscle atrophy during immobilization. *Int J Sports Med.* 7:1, 1986
47. Delitto A, Rose SJ, McKowen JM, et al. Electrical stimulation versus voluntary exercise in strengthening thigh musculature after anterior cruciate ligament surgery. *Phys Ther.* 68:660, 1988
48. Standish WD, Valiant GA, Bonen A, et al. The effects of immobilization and of electrical stimulation on muscle glycogen and myofibrillar ATPase. *Can J Appl Sports Sci.* 7:267, 1982
49. Millard JB. The use of electrical stimulation in the rehabilitation of knee injuries. *Proc Int Congr Phys Med (Lond).* 317, 1952
50. Myrhage R, Hudlicka O. Capillary growth in chronically stimulated adult skeletal muscle as studied by intravital microscopy and histological methods in rabbits and rats. *Microvasc Res.* 16:73, 1978
51. Wakin KG. Influence of frequency of muscle stimulation on circulation in the stimulated extremity. *Arch Phys Med Rehabil.* 34:291, 1953

52. Randall BF, Imig CJ, Hines HM. Effect of electrical stimulation upon blood flow and temperature of skeletal muscle. *Am J Phys Med.* 32:22, 1953

53. Folkow B, Halicka HO. A comparison between "red" and "white" muscle with respect to blood supply, capillary surface area and oxygen uptake during rest and exercise. *Microvasc Res.* 1:1, 1968

54. Petrofsky JS, Phillips CA, Sawka MN, et al. Blood flow and metabolism during isometric contractions in cat skeletal muscle. *J Appl Physiol.* 50:493, 1981

55. Clemente FR. *The Effects of 2500 Hz Frequency Transcutaneous Electrical Stimulation on the Degree of Microvascular Perfusion of Rat Skeletal Muscle.* Doctoral dissertation, University of Kentucky, Lexington, 1989

56. Currier DP, Petrilli CR, Threlkeld AJ. Effect of medium frequency electrical stimulation on local blood circulation to healthy muscle. *Phys Ther.* 66:937, 1986

57. Liu HI, Currier DP, Threlkeld AJ. Circulatory response of unexercised body part to electrical stimulation of calf muscle in healthy subjects. *Phys Ther.* 68:340, 1988

58. Brown M D, Cotter MA, Hudlicka O, et al. The effects of different patterns of muscle activity on capillary demity, mechanical properties and structure of slow and fast rabbit muscles. *Pflugers Arch.* 362:241, 1976

59. Tracy JE, Currier DP, Threlkeld AJ. Comparison of selected pulse frequencies from two different electrical stimulators on blood flow in healthy subjects. *Phys Ther.* 68:1526, 1988

60. Alon G, Bainbridge J, Croson G, et al. High-voltage pulsed direct current effects on peripheral blood flow. *Phys Ther.* 61:678, 1981

61. Loze G. Pulsed, high voltage Galvanic stimulation. Effect on localized blood flow. Unpublished study, University of Kentucky, Lexington, 1981

62. Fields SA. High voltage Galvanic stimulation: Effect on peripheral blood flow. Unpublished study, University of Kentucky, Lexington, 1982

63. Walker DC, Currier DP, Threlkeld AJ. Effects of high voltage pulsed electrical stimulation on blood flow. *Phys Ther.* 68:481, 1988

64. Rose SJ, Rothstein JM. Muscle mutability: Part 1. General concepts and adaptations to altered patterns of use. *Phys Ther.* 62:1773, 1982

65. Salmons S, Heriksson J. The adaptive response of skeletal muscle to increased use. *Musc Nerve.* 4:94, 1981

66. Rothstein JM, Rose SJ. Muscle mutability: Part 2. Adaptation to drugs, metabolic factors, and aging. *Phys Ther.* 62:1788, 1982

67. Gracanin F, Vrabic M, Vrabic G. Six years experience with FNMES method applied to children. *Eur Medicophys.* 12:61, 1976

68. Houston ME, Farrance BW, Wight RI. Metabolic effects of two frequencies of short-term surface electrical stimulation on human muscle. *Can J Physiol Pharmacol.* 60:727, 1982

69. Reddana P, Moortly CV, Govidappa S. Pattern of skeletal muscle chemical composition during in vivo electrical stimulations. *Ind J Physiol Pharmacol.* 25:33, 1981

70. Salmons B, Vrbova G. The influence of activity on some contractile characteristics of mammalian fast and slow muscles. *J Physiol.* 201:535, 1969

71. Eisenberg BR, Gilai A. Structural changes in single muscle fibers after stimulation at a low frequency. *J Gen Physiol.* 74:1, 1979

72. Salmons S. Functional adaptation in skeletal muscle. *Neuroscience.* 3:134, 1980

73. Pette D, Muller W, Leisner E, et al. Time dependent effects on contractile properties, fibre population, myosin light chains and enzymes of energy metabolism in

intermittently and continuously stimulated fast twitch muscle of the rabbit. *Pfluegers Arch.* 364:103, 1976

74. Greathouse DG, Nitz AJ, Matulionis D, et al. Effects of electrical stimulation on ultrastructure of rat skeletal muscles. *Phys Ther.* 64:755, 1984

75. Sreter FA, Pinter K, Jolesz F, et al. Fast to slow transformation of fast muscles in response to long-term phasic stimulation. *Exp Neurol.* 75:95, 1982

76. Sreter FA, Romanul FCA, Salmons S, et al. The effect of a changed pattern of activity on some biochemical characteristics of muscle. In: Milhorat AT, ed. *Exploratory Concepts in Muscular Dystrophy, Vol. II.* Amsterdam, Excerpta, 1974: 338–343

77. Rubinstein NA, Kelly AM. Myogenic and neurogenic contributions to the development of fast and slow twitch muscles in rat. *Dev Biol.* 62:473, 1978

78. Roy RK, Mabuchi K, Sarkar S, et al. Changes in tropomyosin submit pattern in chronic electrical stimulated rabbit fast muscles. *Biochem Biophys Res.* 89:181, 1979

79. Hudlicka O, Tyler KR, Srihari T, et al. The effect of different patterns of long-term stimulation on contractile properties and myosin light chains in rabbit fast muscles. *Pfluegers Arch.* 393:164, 1982

80. Gutmann E. Considerations on neurotrophic relations in central and peripheral nervous system. *Acta Neurobiol Exp (Warsaw).* 35:841, 1975

81. McComas AJ, Discussion. In: Korr IM, ed. *Neurological Mechanisms in Manipulation Therapy.* New York, Plenum Press, 1977: 369–370

82. Jansen JKS, Lomo T, Micolaysen K, et al. Hyperinnervation of skeletal muscle fibers: Dependence on muscle activity. *Science.* 181:559, 1973

83. Lomo T, Westgaard RH, Dahl HA. Contractile properties of muscle: Control of pattern of muscle activity in rat. *Proc R Soc Lond (Biol).* 187:99, 1974

84. Pette D, Smith ME, Staudte HW, et al. Effects of long-term electrical stimulation on some contractile and metabolic characteristics of fast rabbit muscles. *Pfluegers Arch.* 338:257, 1973

85. Salmons S, Sreter FA. Significance of impulse activity in the transformation of skeletal muscle type. *Nature.* 263:30, 1976

CHAPTER 8

High-Voltage Pulsed Current: Theoretical Bases and Clinical Applications

Roberta Newton

High-voltage pulsed current (HVPC) gained widespread use in the United States in the 1970s. Because of its unique waveform characteristics and expanded clinical application, HVPC is associated with a separate class of electrotherapeutic devices.[1] Devices in this class have a "twin-peak monophasic wave form with a fixed duration in the microsecond range (up to 200 μsec) and a voltage greater than 100 volts" (Fig. 8–1).[2] Classes of electrical stimulators are compared in relation to the physiological and electrophysical effects of their waveform characteristics. The key to successful treatment with HVPC is flexibility in selecting appropriate waveform parameters to promote recovery from injury, re-educate muscles, or modulate pain.

The purposes of this chapter are to (1) describe the waveform characteristics of HVPC; (2) discuss the theoretical physiological and electrophysical bases of HVPC; (3) present clinical applications, including known or postulated rationales, for using HVPC; and (4) provide the practitioner with ideas for clinical research. Without clinical research to determine the efficacy of HVPC, a decline in its use as an effective modality will occur.

HISTORICAL BACKGROUND

In 1945, Haislip and colleagues from Bell Telephone Laboratories developed the first high-voltage stimulator. By decreasing the pulse duration and increasing the voltage, stimulation of deeper tissues occurred without tissue damage. The unit is the DynaWave Neuromuscular Stimulator.[3] Anecdotal evidence

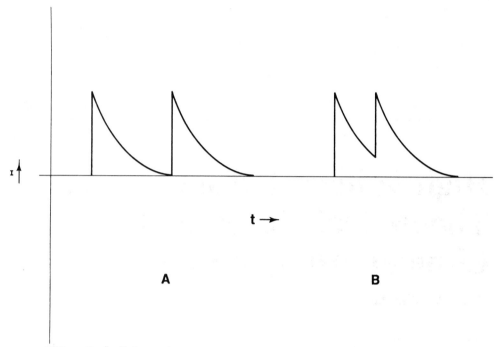

I

t →

A   B

Figure 8—1. Schematic representation of a high-voltage pulsed waveform.

described DynaWave treatment for decubiti, burns, acute sprains, strains, lower back pain, and phantom limb pain.[3,4]

The first published report using this modality appeared in 1966. The purpose of the study was to examine the effectiveness of electrotherapy in promoting wound healing. Eight dogs (litter mates) were divided into two groups, experimental and control. Each dog had a tourniquet applied to the left lower extremity for 12 hours. Twenty-four hours after removal of the tourniquet, the experimental group received electrotherapy consisting of a 4-μsec dual pulse at 150 V (polarity not stated). Stimulation occurred at different sites for 10 sec each until the entire limb was treated. Total time of electrical stimulation was 5 min. Twenty-four hours following stimulation, a marked difference in edema between the control feet and the treated feet occurred. By day 6, all of the untreated limbs were gangrenous. By day 11, healing was complete in the treated group and severe gangrene was still present in all of the untreated limbs. The rationale for healing proposed by the authors was that muscle contraction elicited by neuromuscular electrical stimulation (NMES) increased circulation to the injured area.[5]

A case report published in 1971 described the use of DynaWave for the treatment of an abscess on the foot of a diabetic patient. A 20-min electrotherapeutic treatment followed whirlpool. The only stimulus parameter reported was a frequency of 5 pps. After 3 days of treatment, an increase in circulation to the area and retardation of the infection occurred. The patient received electrotherapy twice a day for 4 weeks until discharge. Rationale for the treatment was to "stimulate muscular contraction around the infected area to increase blood flow to the part to promote healing."[6]

The upsurge in HVPC began in 1974, when Lehmann (Electro-Med Health Industries) began nationally advertising the High-Voltage Electro Galvanic Stimulator (EGS).[7] Since then there has been a significant increase in the clinical use of HVPC, as well as in educational programs on its physics, physiology, and clinical operation. To keep pace with clinical demands, manufacturers developed newer (improved) units.

WAVEFORM CHARACTERISTICS

The name of this particular electrical stimulator varies: high-volt, high-voltage galvanic, high-voltage pulsed galvanic, and high-voltage pulsed current. The term "pulsed" prevents the therapist from thinking the unit produces continuous direct current (DC), (ie, galvanic). Some descriptors include the term "galvanic," but the shape of the waveform is not similar to the traditional low-voltage interrupted galvanic waveforms (Fig. 8–2). A more complete description of this device is as follows:

> HVPC stimulator is a unit that has a twin peak monophasic waveform with a fixed duration. Duration is expressed in the microsecond range (up to 200 μsec). A (therapeutic) voltage is larger than 100 volts. The units are constant voltage units. Frequency is independently controlled. Depending on the unit, the on/off cycle is either fixed or controlled independently.[2]

"High-voltage" is a term applied to a class of electrical stimulation devices capable of delivering amplitudes greater than 100 volts. A therapist treating with less than 100 volts on a HVPC unit is still using a class of HVPC units. Waveform characteristics are described as follows (Fig. 8–1).

Wave Shape. The pulse is a monopolar twin peak with an instantaneous rate of rise and a slope on the downside of each peak. The pulse is dual peaked because a single peak of ultrashort duration cannot stimulate nerve axons. The wave shape is fixed and cannot be changed by the clinician.

Duration. Duration is the period that current flows during one waveform (pulse). Measurement of duration varies. For example, duration of the first phase serves as the pulse duration; or, pulse duration is measured at one-half the pulse height (for example, 28 μsec and 17 μsec).[8] Duration is a fixed value and cannot be changed.

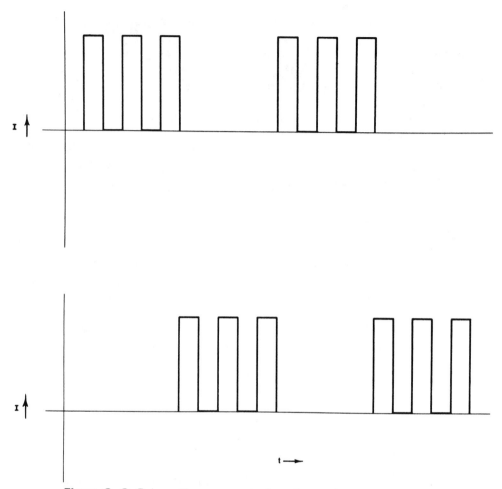

Figure 8–2. Schematic representation of a reciprocate mode.

Current Density. Since HVPC units have a high peak and a low effective value of current flow, current density is the parameter to consider. Current density is examined by comparing waveforms. Compare the waveform that has the downslope of the first pulse reaching the isoelectric line (where no electrons flow) with the waveform that has a downslope of the first pulse not reaching the isoelectric line (Fig. 8–2). Note that the second waveform will have more current density; that is, more electrons will flow per unit time.

Current density per unit time is changed by several methods. One is by adjustment of the *microspace pulse* (or *intrapulse interval*). This interval is the period between the end of the first phase and the start of the second phase of the waveform. Only a few HVPC units have this feature. The shorter the intra pulse interval (ie, microspace) the larger the number of electrons flowing per unit time. To date, clinical researchers have not determined the physiological value of microspacing the dual pulse.

A second method used to increase current density is to increase frequency. This permits more waveforms per unit time, thereby increasing electron flow per unit time.

Frequency. Frequency is the number of waveforms per second. The unit of measurement is pulses per second (pps). Do not become confused because the wave shape has a dual peak. A frequency of 2 pps is a rate of two complete waveforms per second: however, the number of peaks seen on an oscilloscope is four.

Train. The term *train* refers to the pattern of pulses generated. The three most common modes on HVPC machines are continuous, reciprocate, and surge.

1. *Continuous train* refers to the repetitive sequence of pulses used for the entire duration of treatment (refer to Fig. 10–8). The term refers to a series of pulses and does not mean galvanic (direct or continuous) current. The amplitude of each pulse is at the same preselected height.
2. *Reciprocate* refers to alternate on-and-off current flow of one active pad (electrode) in relation to the other (Fig. 8–2). *Active pad* refers to the pad used to deliver treatment. The *dispersive pad* completes the patient circuit. Thus, when current is flowing from one active pad for 2.5 sec, no current is flowing from the other active pad, and vice versa. Reciprocate modes are fixed at 2.5, 5, and 10 sec "on" and 2.5, 5, and 10 sec "off". Each setting then gives an on/off cycle for each active pad of a 1:1 (on:off) ratio. The amplitude of each pulse in the pulse train is at the same preselected height.
3. *Surge* (or ramp) is a series of waveforms whereby each successive waveform increases in amplitude until reaching the preselected maximal amplitude. An advantage of this mode is that because the amplitude builds up over time, the patient does not experience the maximum preset voltage at the onset of stimulation. Many surge trains have a 2.5, 5, and 10 sec on/off cycle, producing a 1:1 on/off ratio. Some units have independently controlled on/off switches.

The advantages of the surged mode are that (1) the stimulus amplitude will not surprise the patient; that is, amplitude builds up gradually rather than stimulating the patient with the preselected maximum on the first pulse; and (2) the gradual buildup in amplitude prevents a stretch reflex in a spastic muscle when stimulating the antagonistic muscle. HVPC is the unit of choice when using NMES for neurologic patients.

Importance of Waveform Characteristics

Each waveform characteristic, alone or in combination with other waveform characteristics, produces a variety of physiological and electrophysical responses. To select proper parameters for treatment, therapists need knowledge of their effects on normal tissue.

When current passes through a circuit containing resistors, voltage drops occur, thereby losing energy. Skin offers impedance (a form of resistance) to the flow of electrical current. Impedance of skin may be as high as 100,000 Ω. This phenomenon occurs in some treatment applications with traditional low-voltage units. A high-voltage device produces a spontaneous breakdown in skin impedance. Little if any voltage drop occurs as current flows through the skin.

Procacci and colleagues developed an electrical circuit composed of resistors and capacitors designed to mimic the skin's electrical circuit.[9] When a high-voltage stimulus (100 V) passes through a circuit, current flows toward the path of the capacitor. Since crossing a capacitor wastes little energy compared to crossing a resistor, the benefits are twofold: (1) more current density beneath the skin to reach target tissues; and (2) negligible, if any, cutaneous vasodilation. Lost energy due to tissue impedance, is converted to heat. This in turn produces direct vasodilation of cutaneous blood vessels. Since a minimal amount of the high voltage current passes across the resistor side of the circuit, energy loss is minimal. This lessens the occurrence of vasodilation.

A second important factor to consider for NMES treatment is that HVPC produces negligible, if any, chemical buildup under the electrode pads. Newton and Karselis measured skin pH for 3 consecutive days before stimulation of 40 subjects. On the treatment day, the active electrode placed on the ventral forearm delivered a 100-V, 80-pps cathodal stimulation for 30 min. Skin pH measurement followed the treatment. No significant acid or base buildup under the pads, as measured by skin pH, occurred.[1]

In summary, HVPC passes through the skin with negligible thermal and electrochemical effects. Increased current density is available to target tissues, because of the route undertaken by the current through the skin.

Nerves and muscles are the target tissues treated by most practitioners. Since the HVPC unit has an ultrashort duration, the unit does not stimulate denervated muscle. A denervated muscle requires a pulse duration (chronaxie value) of at least 1 msec. HVPC treatment of partially denervated muscle activates only neurally intact motoneurons.

The advantage of the ultrashort pulse duration relates to stimulation of sensory nerve fibers. Li and Bak noted that chronaxie values for A-beta (touch), A-delta (pain and temperature), and C (pain) sensory axons were 0.20, 0.45, and 1.50 msec, respectively.[10] Since the pulse durations of HVPC units range up to 200 μsec, the chance for stimulating A-delta and C sensory axons decreases, thus increasing patient comfort. Current density also affects patient comfort by influencing sensation arising from electrical stimulation. The section on clinical applications includes a more detailed outline of the effects of HVPC on the various target tissues.

HVPC DEVICES

The more waveform characteristics controlled by the practitioner, the greater the flexibility in selecting the proper combination of waveform parameters. Various accessories also increase the capabilities of the unit. Since variations exist, this section presents only the most common parts of HVPC units. The reader should refer to the technical manual for specifics of each unit.

Wave Shape and Pulse Duration. The fixed shape (twin peak) and pulse duration cannot be changed by the practitioner. To classify a device as a HVPC unit, the unit has a dual-peak monophasic waveform.

On/Off Timer Control. This switch turns the power on and sets the length of the treatment. When the switch is in the "off" position, no current flows through the patient circuit.

Polarity Switch. The polarity switch sets the polarity of the active electrode in relation to the dispersive electrode. The active pad (electrode) is the pad that delivers the treatment current. The dispersive (inactive) pad completes the patient circuit.

Amplitude Control. The (amplitude) control sets the output voltage of the active electrode within a range from 0 to 500 V. Most units have a reset, safety feature. Turning the unit off without returning the voltage output to zero activates the reset feature. Current will not flow until the unit is reset, by resetting the amplitude control dial. This safety feature prevents the patient from receiving an unnecessary shock.

Pad Balance. This switch permits independent amplitude control over the two active pads (electrodes). It permits an increase in amplitude of one pad in relation to the other. The advantage of this feature occurs when using HVPC for modulation of pain. A patient tolerates less NMES when an active electrode delivers current directly over the painful site. Therefore, two active pads delivering current at different amplitudes provide a maximal amplitude in each pad. The electrode directly over the painful site should deliver *less* current than the pad in proximity of the painful site.

Pad/Probe Mode Switch. This switch regulates the pattern of stimulation; that is, continuous or reciprocate. *Continuous* means a continuous flow of pulses through the active pads. The positions 2.5, 5, and 10 sec *reciprocate* indicate current alternates by flowing from one then the other active pad. Depending upon the unit, reciprocate position may be either interrupted (all pulses at the same predetermined amplitude) or surged (amplitude increasing with each pulse until reaching the predetermined amplitude).

Surged Train. Several units contain both the reciprocate dial (with interrupted mode) and a separate surge train. When the surged train is separate, the therapist independently controls the on/off cycle. This control permits alteration of the ratio of the on/off cycle up to a 1:5 ratio.

Output Meter. A meter (needle deflection) or a digital readout records output from the unit, which may be units of measurement in voltage, peak current, or both.

Microspace Switch. Some units have this function, which enables manual regulation of the distance between the two peaks of a waveform (intrapulse interval).

Indicator Lights. These lights provide the practitioner with a visual acknowledgment that a particular function is in operation.

Output Jacks. Receptacles for the electrode heads are available for the active pads, handle (probe) electrode, and dispersive pad.

Electrodes. The active electrode may be either a pad electrode or a handle (probe) electrode. The number of active pads may vary from one to four. The size of each active pad may range from 5.7 to 7.56 cm. The dispensive pad may be 2.16 by 25.4 cm. The composition of the active pad varies. Some pads consist of a metal plate encased in a rubber housing with a sponge placed between the metal plate and the patient. Other pads are flexible and contain an impregnated conductive medium. The flexible pad has the advantage of conforming to the body part better than the pad with the metal plate.

A major treatment consideration for both active and dispersive pads is the accumulation of dirt and oils on the pad surface. This accumulation increases resistance to current flow and therefore decreases the electrical efficiency of the unit. Frequent changes of the sponge, a disposable covering, or frequent cleansing of the electrodes will prolong the pads' effectiveness.

Accessories for the handle electrode increase the clinical usefulness of the electrical stimulator. In some first-generation HVPC units, the handle electrode had a fixed applicator. External applicators include spot (disk) electrode, rectangular electrode, point stimulator (acuspot), and roller. Internal probes include intraoral, vaginal, and rectal electrodes. The intraoral electrode has an insulated shaft that permits stimulation only at the tip. All externally applied electrodes use a conductive medium or a wet-sponge cover. Manufacturers have the capability of manufacturing special electrodes for specific applications.

CLINICAL APPLICATION

To increase the effectiveness of HVPC treatment, the practitioner should take a problem-solving approach. First, the practitioner needs to identify all of the patient problems that can benefit from NMES. More than one problem is treatable with a single treatment. For example, with a painful ankle sprain, both edema and pain are treated. Second, the practitioner should state the known and postulated rationales for the use of HVPC. Third, the practitioner must identify the intervening tissues through which the current passes before reaching the target tissue; this aids the therapist in determining the effect that each tissue has upon current flow.

Fourth, the clinician visualizes current flow from the active electrode to the dispersive electrode. The dispersive electrode is an integral part of the patient circuit and should not be placed improperly, because current needs to flow through the target tissue. Misplacement of the dispersive electrode decreases current flow through the target tissue and diminishes the effects of treatment. For the fifth and final step in the problem-solving approach, proper documentation procedures are essential to measure the effectiveness of the treatment and substantiate its efficacy. The tissues of the body have "fail-safe" mechanisms; that is, they respond to more than one combination of stimuli to maintain viability. Therefore, more than one set of waveform parameters could and would (no doubt) be effective. The practitioner should be careful to avoid set protocols for patients with similar problems.

In summary, the therapist conducts a thorough assessment for the use of HVPC for treatment. Factors to consider include (1) its electrophysical and physiological effects upon various tissues; (2) optimal stimulus parameters and electrode placement, based upon scientific and clinical literature; and (3) duration of treatment. The standard treatment time of 20 min may not be correct, so the therapist adjusts treatment times accordingly. Documentation of current permanent and patient response is suggested.

Wound Healing

Rationale. NMES for wound healing includes the effect of an electrical stimulus on microorganisms, the type of injury, and the tissue repair process. Studies using low amplitudes of direct current provide most of the bases for HVPC in promoting wound healing.

A cathodal current of 6 μA to 1.4 mA DC affects microorganism growth in both in-vivo and in-vitro models. Rowley noted a decrease in *Escherichia coli* B growth rate in an in-vitro study.[11] Rabbit skin wounds infected with *Pseudo-*

monas aeruginosa showed similar results.[12] A 72-hour stimulation period with a 1-mA DC cathodal current either decreased or inhibited growth rate of the microorganisms. A 6 μA negative DC stimulus on rat and rabbit femurs infected with *Staphylococcus aureus* caused a decrease in growth rate after 1 hr of NMES.[13]

Wheeler and co-workers proposed two mechanisms for the decrease in the growth rate of the microorganisms. Continued electrical stimulation of the single-celled organism disrupts its homeostatic mechanism to the point of death. The second hypothesis they proposed was a disruption of intracellular activity. This disruption occurs either by irreversible disruption of enzyme processes or regulatory mechanisms involved in transport across the cell membrane.[14] Disruption or alteration of the enzymatic processes of the microorganism is also proposed by Pilla.[15] Thus, research studies support the use of negative DC current for retarding the growth rate of microorganisms.

Many researchers applied electrical current to facilitate recovery. Tissue damage causes disruption of cell membranes and alteration of cellular constituents. This produces an electrical potential difference between injured and intact tissues, termed *injury potential*. Burr and co-workers noted that as the wound healed, the injury potential varied until recovery occurred. At the onset, the potential was positive, peaking at 48 hrs postinjury. This peak gradually declined and the potential became negative 8 to 9 days postinjury. Smaller fluctuations occurred until recovery was complete.[16,17] These fluctuations in the electrical potential of the wound need to be correlated with the repair process.

Carey and Lepley were the first researchers to examine blood cell migration in wounds. They applied a 0.2 to 0.3-mA DC to rabbit skin wounds for 2 to 5 days. A clumping of leukocytes and a thrombosing in small vessels occurred near the positive pole with no such activity at the negative pole.[18] Harrington and colleagues examined dermal cell movement in rat skin wounds. After a 24-hr application of 200 to 800 μA, they noted migration of epithelial cells and larger numbers of dermal cells under the anode than under the cathode. They concluded that using the anode as the active pole had a "beneficial influence" upon the early phase of wound healing.[19] These studies show that the anodal current can facilitate cell movement in a wound.

More recently, Bourguignon and colleagues examined HVPC influence on cellular constituents.[20,21] They electrically stimulated human fibroblast cell cultures for 20 min. Specific combinations of HVPC frequency and voltage significantly increased the rate of protein and DNA synthesis. Frequencies of 100 pps and voltages of 50 and 100 V produced the greatest rate of synthesis. Voltages greater than 250 V inhibited the synthesis rate of protein and DNA. This study represents the first research examining HVPC on cellular biosynthesis.

To date, studies of HVPC for wound healing are limited. Reports of anecdotal evidence, treatment protocols, and pilot studies on the effects of HVPC (alone or in combination) are found in the literature. Akers and Gabreilson conducted a descriptive study on 14 patients with pressure sores.[22] The patients were divided into three treatment groups: (1) HVPC; (2) HVPC and whirlpool; and (3) whirlpool. NMES was given twice a day and whirlpool once a day. Stimulation parameters and electrode placement were not stated. Wound size, measured weekly, was used in a correlation analysis. They reported the largest rate of change in wound size with HVPC only and the least amount of change in the group receiving whirlpool only. Because of the lack of detailed methodology, these results are interpreted with caution. In a study by Alon and associates, patients received hydrotherapy, debridement, and HVPC; no parameters were stated.[23] Twelve of 15 diabetic ulcers completely healed in an average of 2.5 months. Feedar and Kloth found similar results in a group of patients with decubitus ulcers.[24]

Ross and Segal described the use of HVPC for wound healing following podiatric surgery. Negative polarity was used to move fluid from the area to increase blood flow, and to facilitate the wound healing process. A positive polarity was utilized for its germicidal effect and for its "sedative effect on the nerve."[25]

In summary, studies show that polarity is the predominant current characteristic to consider in wound healing. The negative pole retards microorganism growth. The positive pole facilitates cellular migration, particularly in the proliferation phase of wound healing. Current density is also an important consideration because most of the studies reviewed use a continuous direct current. To increase the amount of current flow per unit time when using pulsed current amplitude and frequency are increased. Both basic science and clinical research have to examine the influence of electrical current on all phases of wound healing.

Treatment Methods. The protocol described below was developed for the treatment of decubiti.[2] The protocol is adapted to treat other types of wounds and burns (discussed below).

I. Documentation: should include, but not be limited to, the following:
   A. Measurement of the wound: a set of concentric circles, or tracing the wound on sterile transparent paper are used to measure the wound.
   B. Measurement of the depth: measure at the approximate center.
   C. Description of undermining of the wound.
   D. Statement of the type of microorganism(s) present.
   E. Description of the general characteristics of the wound.
   F. Record of the medications and dressings.
   G. Photography: a weekly photograph, taken at a standard distance from the wound, is a valuable documentation procedure.
II. Procedure
   A. Treatment out of water
      1. Remove housing and sponges, and wrap the active electrode(s) in sterile gauze. Soak them in sterile saline.
      2. Attach one or more active electrodes directly over the wound, or

attach one active electrode over the wound and a second active electrode distal to the first.

   3. Attach the dispersive pad proximally. Visualize the current path to be sure that current flows through the wound and does not circumvent it.

  B. Treatment in water

    1. Use either a plastic container or a whirlpool with a recent electrical safety check. The whirlpool and electrical stimulator are plugged into a ground fault interruption receptacle.

    2. Remove housing and sponge from the active electrode(s) and wrap them in gauze.

    3. Attach the active electrode(s) distal to the wound. To increase the effectiveness of the treatment, the active electrode(s) must be attached to the body.

    4. Attach the dispersive electrode OUT of the water and proximal to the wound. Visualize the path of current flow so current flows through the wound.

III. Treatment parameters

  A. Frequency: high.

  B. Amplitude: subthreshold to muscle contraction. Amplitude is increased as accommodation occurs.

  C. Polarity

    1. Negative polarity is used if microorganisms are present. Continue to use negative polarity until the wound is culture-free for 3 days.

    2. Positive polarity is used if the wound is culture-free or is used after the wound is culture-free for 3 days.

  D. Duration and frequency of treatment: Since most of the studies on the use of electrical stimulation for wound healing used direct current, the length and frequency for treatment is adjusted to permit the greatest amount of current flow per unit time.

  E. Rate of healing: a healing rate of 1 mm per week has been documented.[14] If the wound healing slows, polarity is changed for ONE treatment only. Switching polarity is hypothesized to reactivate the wound healing process.

IV. Assessment: Assess the wound after each treatment and perform a complete assessment weekly.

 V. Sterilization of the electrodes: Appropriate sterilization procedures, particularly for the flexible electrodes, are provided by manufacturers.

Clinical Application. The following section describes three conditions treated with HVPC. Guidelines for documentation and treatment are adapted from those procedures described in the protocol for healing of decubiti.

Burns. HVPC treatment before debridement affects pain modulation (see "Modulation of Pain" later in the chapter) and aids healing. HVPC (negative polarity) applied over scar tissue facilitates movement of the injured part. Although the mechanism for this clinical observation is unknown, pain reduction may be a key element.

Postsurgical Wounds. The active and dispersive electrodes are placed on either side of the wound (similar to TENS). Both pain modulation and wound recovery can benefit from HVPC treatment.

Hand Injuries, Traumatic and Postsurgical. HVPC is used for pain modulation, wound healing, and edema reduction. When treating in a pan of water with amplitude of stimulus subthreshold to muscle contraction, the patient can voluntarily exercise the hand muscles. This voluntary exercise will also reduce edema via muscle pump action.

NMES producing muscle pump action can also be used.[26] The active electrode is placed over the area of edema or of distal nerve distribution and the dispersive electrode placed proximally. Treat with 2 to 8 pps for about 30 min. A decrease in edema, as measured by circumferential measurements and an increase in total active motion (TAM), documents treatment outcome.

Edema Reduction

Rationale. Edema due to physical disruption of blood vessels may be alleviated with HVPC. The electrical stimulus parameter, polarity, is used to induce muscle pump action and to shift fluid from the area. Muscle pump action is voluntary or elicited by NMES. Polarity repels fluid from the area. All blood cells and plasma proteins are negatively charged at normal blood pH of 7.4.[27] Williams and Carey proved that stimulation of the dog's jugular vein with positive polarity produced clumping of blood cells. Application of a negative current reversed this clumping.[28] Whenever electric current shifts blood components, the fluid medium also shifts. Albumin, the major plasma protein, is strongly hydrophilic and has a negatively charged cell membrane at normal blood pH. Therefore, when a negative polarity repels negatively charged cells and proteins from an area, a fluid shift will also occur.[2]

Treatment Protocol. The treatment guidelines given below are for edema due to physical disruption of blood vessels and not for edema caused by other factors.

  I. Documentation: should include, but not be limited to, the following:
    A. Measurement of the region: circumferential, volumetric, or both.
    B. Range of motion of the site and points above and below the site.
 II. Procedure
    A. Attach the active pads over the site of edema. If this is not possible, then attach the pads distally.
    B. Attach the dispersive pad proximally. The path of current flow is visualized to be sure current flows through the edematous area.

    C. The treatment can be performed in cool water.
III. Treatment parameters
    A. Polarity of the active electrodes is negative.
    B. Frequency and amplitude: A frequency between 20 and 50 pps is used to produce a tetanic muscle contraction, for muscle pumping by NMES. An on/off cycle of 1:4 or 1:5 delays onset of muscle fatigue. Amplitude is increased to patient tolerance. High frequency and amplitude subthreshold to muscle contraction are used if no muscle contraction is desired or if the patient can voluntarily perform muscle contraction.
  V. Assessment: Assessment should occur after each treatment to document the effects of treatment.

Clinical Application

Muscle Sprains and Strains. HVPC can decrease pain and edema and aid recovery. The use of ice or positive compression, in combination with NMES, is suggested for immediate treatment of sprains.

Hand Injuries. The earlier section on wound healing contains a complete description of treatment.

Postoperative. Ross and Segal describe the use of pulsed NMES for edema and pain reduction in patients following podiatric surgery.[25]

Modulation of Pain

Rationale. Several reviews exist on the mechanisms of pain and on the use of NMES for modulation of pain.[29-32] Therefore, an in-depth discussion is omitted here. However, two points will be considered: (1) the nociceptive state, in which pain originated in other tissues, responds less well to NMES than does the neurogenic or neuropathic state;[30] and (2) studies using experimentally induced tooth pulp pain prove that stimulation over the painful site is effective.[33]

Several reports exist on the use of HVPC in pain modulation. A study conducted on 25 patients with lower back pain showed no statistical difference between the use of various frequencies for pain relief. Only one treatment using a specific frequency was used in this crossover design study.[34] Replication of this study should concentrate on the effects of frequency with several treatments. As is true in examining the TENS (transcutaneous electrical nerve stimulation) literature, pain relief cannot be predicted from experimentally induced pain. Caution is exercised when extrapolating results from other pain studies. Since the normal physiological and biomechanical mechanisms for the origin of pain are not clarified, the practitioner should not insist upon one set protocol. Many different combinations of NMES exist that will modulate pain.

The fact that different combinations of waveform parameters produce pain modulation reinforces the idea of many fail-safe mechanisms to insure proper functioning of the organism.

A second report using HVPC was written by Sohn and colleagues. They described good to complete relief in 65 of 80 patients with levator ani syndrome. Reports of recurrent pain documented pain relief.[35] Morris and Newton replicated this study on 28 patients with a primary or secondary diagnosis of levator ani syndrome.[36] HVPC consisted of a 1-hr treatment with 120 pps and amplitude to patient tolerance. Patients received 3 to 10 treatments. Twenty-five percent of the patients were pain free after 4 treatments and 50 percent after an average of 7.5 treatments.

Treatment Method

I. Documentation: should include, but not be limited to, the following:
  A. Pain evaluation: An individually designed pain assessment includes a visual analogue scale, pain-rating index, and body diagram. The McGill Pain Questionnaire is an excellent assessment tool that contains these elements.[37]
  B. Pain log: A pain log documents the patient's pain by describing the pain, the activity(ies) producing pain, and methods the patient used to relieve pain.
II. Procedures
  A. General guidelines describe placement of the active electrode(s). In sequential order, the electrode sites are (1) over the painful site, (2) over the nerve trunk, and (3) paraspinally. When treating with the point-stimulator electrode, the selected site is over the painful (or trigger) area.
  B. The dispersive electrode is placed proximal to the active electrode(s). Visualization of the current path is important, because the current needs to flow through the painful area or along the nerve trunk, depending upon the location of the active electrode(s).
III. Treatment parameters
  A. Frequency: Frequencies of 4 to 80 pps are used. A trial period determines which frequency produces the greatest reduction in pain for the patient.
  B. Amplitude: Amplitude is at the level of patient tolerance but subthreshold to muscle contraction.
  C. Treatment duration: Based upon the pain log, a schedule for NMES is developed. The patient receives a predetermined number of treatments lasting for a specific period, rather than allowing the patient to use NMES for prolonged periods. Prolonged treatment periods produce accommodation in the nervous system, thereby decreasing the effectiveness of NMES.
IV. Assessment: For treatment to be effective, the time interval between treatment sessions increases.

Clinical Application. Most conditions associated with pain that respond to TENS are treatable with HVPC. Listed below are some examples of painful disorders successfully treated with NMES.

- Identification and treatment of trigger points
- Cervical or lumbar pain
- TMJ dysfunction[38]
- Cancer pain
- Postsurgical pain
- Pain associated with arthritis, with ranging joints (eg, frozen shoulders)
- Acute and chronic sprains
- Pain associated with debridement
- Phantom limb pain

TMJ. TMJ dysfunction can be treated either extra- or intraorally.[39] Assessment includes the head and neck region as well as measurements of vertical mouth opening and visual analogue scale. The patient relaxes in a supine position. Intraoral treatment consists of 50 to 80 pps frequency with amplitude to patient tolerance. A specially designed intraoral probe delivers current to the pteryoids and masseter. Treatments last several minutes per muscle. External NMES is applied with pads or a disk electrode. Treatment occurs over the TMJ and muscles of mastication. Stimulus amplitude is to patient tolerance, but subthreshold to muscle contraction. Treatment time for external application of NMES may last up to 20 minutes.

Neuromuscular Stimulation

Rationale. HVPC has been used for both muscle re-education and maintenance of muscle integrity in patients with disuse atrophy. HVPC may in some instances be used for functional electrical stimulation (FES) as described in Chapter 6.

Frequency and on/off cycle are important characteristics for NMES of intact muscle. As frequency of the electrical stimulus increases (providing amplitude and duration are appropriate), individual muscle twitches summate and incomplete tetanus occurs. Further increase in frequency results in complete tetanus. A frequency of 20 pps produces complete tetanus in some muscles. Benton and colleagues noted that a 20 to 30 pps stimulation rate was optimal for muscle contraction. Higher frequencies (50 to 100 Hz) caused faster muscle fatigue than frequencies of 20 pps.[40] The on/off cycle is another parameter that delays the onset of muscle fatigue. A 1:5 on/off ratio is the most effective, as suggested by Benton and colleagues and by Kots.[41] Benton and associates noted that a 1:1 ratio fatigued muscle more quickly than did other ratios. In summary, frequency and on/off cycle are the two most important NMES parameters to consider when developing a treatment plan.

Many techniques exist for the maintenance of muscle integrity in an immobilized muscle. To date, limited histological and biochemical analysis demonstrates an increase in muscle strength in healthy or injured muscle. Following knee surgery, a profound inhibition occurs in the quadriceps femoris muscle. This inhibition is due to disruption of the joint capsule and to profound activation of the joint receptors.[42] Voluntary exercise and HVPC may override this profound inhibition.

Since analysis of muscle tissue has not shown significant changes in either morphology or biochemical composition, alteration must be occurring at the nervous system level. With continued NMES and voluntary muscle contraction, a "motor template" forms. That is, facilitation of the activated motor units occurs when voluntary movement is performed.[2] The therapist observes an apparent increase in "strength." The evidence for such a template is indirect and is measured by an increase in force production.

Treatment Method. The technique is similar to that used in functional electrical stimulation.

I. Documentation: Appropriate assessment of the individual with neurologic or neuromuscular dysfunction is conducted.
II. Procedure
    A. Place the active electrode(s) over the motor point(s) of the muscle.
    B. Place the dispersive electrode proximally.
III. Treatment parameters
    A. Frequency: A frequency to produce muscle contraction, but below one that would produce fatigue, is used. A range of 20 to 30 pps is acceptable.
    B. Negative polarity: Erb's law states that negative polarity requires less amplitude to activate axons than does positive polarity.
    C. On/off cycle: A 1:5 on/off cycle and amplitude to produce muscle contraction is used. Due to a training effect, the "off" part of the ratio is decreased with continued treatment.[40]
    D. Train: A surged train of pulses produces a gradual buildup of amplitude. As stated earlier, a gradual buildup is beneficial in the treatment of the stroke patient, as it does not elicit a stretch reflex due to stimulation of the antagonistic muscle. A reciprocate mode is used for alternating agonist–antagonist muscle contractions.

Clinical Application. The above treatment technique has several benefits. In addition to producing muscle contraction, the waveform parameters also produce pain relief. Electrically induced muscle contractions are also used when edema is present. Documentation of treatment outcome are based on those problems being treated with NMES.

Muscle Re-education and Treatment of Innervated Muscle. Chapters 6 and 7 contain detained treatment descriptions.

Vascular System

Rationale. The last major area to discuss in this chapter is electrotherapeutic treatment to the vascular system. Activation of the muscle pump or stimulation of the sympathetic nervous system alters blood flow to a region. Lindstrom and co-workers noted that a frequency of 12 to 15 pps was more effective than an electrically induced twitch contraction for prevention of postsurgical deep-vein thrombosis.[43]

Inhibition of the sympathetic nervous system results in vasodilation and increased circulation to the wound area. Schoeler showed an increase in blood flow in a patient with Raynaud's disease. Treatment consisted of interferential current of 4 to 8 mA with a sweep frequency of 90 to 100 pps. The treatment was applied to the cervical plexus.[44]

Mohr and colleagues tested the affect of HVPC to rat hind limb muscles on blood flow.[45] A Doppler device measured blood flow velocity (BFV) changes. The purposes of their study were to examine different pulse rates, polarities, and amplitudes on blood flow. A frequency of 20 pps producing a rhythmic incomplete muscle tetanus caused the greatest change in BFV. Although both positive and negative polarity caused a significant increase in BFV, negative polarity produced the larger increase. They also found an increase in BFV with increasing amplitudes of voltage. All blood flow changes were confined to the muscles stimulated. The authors did not offer physiological mechanisms for the observed changes. This study represents a major contribution to the effects of HVPC on blood flow changes.

Contraindications

Contraindications and precautions are similar to those for other forms of NMES: patients with circulatory impairment; stimulation over the carotid sinus; stimulation across the heart, particularly in those patients who have demand pacemakers; pregnant females; and individuals prone to seizures.

SUMMARY

High-voltage pulsed current stimulation, like other forms of NMES, is used solely or with other treatments. The effectiveness of HVPC lies in the practitioner's ability to problem-solve and to select appropriate waveform characteristics based upon scientific and clinical rationales. Clinical research will increase the understanding of HVPC as an electrotherapeutic technique.

REFERENCES

1. Newton RA, Karselis TC. Skin pH following high voltage pulsed galvanic stimulation. *Phys Ther.* 63:1593, 1983

2. Newton RA. *Electrotherapeutic Treatment: Selecting Appropriate Wave Form Characteristics.* Clinton, NJ, Preston, 1984

3. Spassoff DA. *My Fabulous Life: The Story of an Athlete, Trainer, Therapist.* Boynton Beach, FL, Star, 1979:323

4. Haislip F. Personal communication, January 1984

5. Young HG. Electric impulse therapy aids wound healing. *Mod Vet Med.* Dec 1966

6. Thurman B, Christian E. Response of a serious circulatory lesion to electrical stimulation. *Phys Ther* 51:1007, 1971

7. Lehmann P. Personal communication, January 1984

8. Microdyne II, product information. Chattanooga, TN, Chattanooga Corp, 1981

9. Procacci P, Corte D, Zoppi M, et al. Pain threshold measurements in man. In: Bonica JJ, ed. *Recent Advances in Pain Therapy.* Springfield, IL, Thomas, 1974: 105–147

10. Li CL, Bak A. Excitability characteristics of the A- and C-fibers in a peripheral nerve. *Exp Neurol.* 50:67, 1976

11. Rowley BA. Electrical current effects on *E coli* growth rates. *Proc Soc Exp Biol Med.* 139:929, 1972

12. Rowley BA, McKenna JM, Chase GR, et al. The influence of electrical current on an infecting microorganism in wounds. *Ann NY Acad Sci.* 238:543, 1974

13. Barranco SD, Spadero JA, Berger TJ, et al. In vitro effect of weak direct current on *Staphylococcus aureus. Clin Orthop Rel Res.* 100–250, 1974

14. Wheeler P, Wolcott L, Morris J, et al. Neural considerations in the healing of ulcerated tissue by clinical electrotherapeutic application of weak direct current: Findings and theory. In: Reynolds DV, Sjoberg AE, eds. *Neuroelectric Research.* Springfield, IL, Thomas, 1971: 83–96

15. Pilla AA. Electrochemical information transfer and its possible role in the control of cell function. In Brighton CT, Black J, Pollack SR: *Electrical Properties of Bone and Cartilage.* New York, Grune & Stratton, 1979:455–489

16. Burr HS, Harvey SC. Bio-electric correlates of wound healing. *Yale J Biol Med.* 11:103, 1938–1939

17. Burr HA, Taffel M, Harvey WC. An electrometric study of the healing wound in man. *Yale J Biol Med.* 12:483, 1940

18. Carey IC, Lepley D. Effect of continuous direct electric current on healing wounds. *Surg Forum.* 13:33, 1955

19. Harrington DB, Meyer R, Klein RM. Effects of small amounts of electric current at the cellular level. *Ann NY Acad Sci.* 238—300, 1974

20. Bourguignon GJ, Bourguignon LYW. Electric stimulation of protein and DNA synthesis in human fibroblasts. *FASEB J.* 1:398, 1987

21. Bourguignon LYW, Wenche J, Majercik MH, Bourguignon GJ. Lymphocyte activation and capping of hormone receptors. *J Cell Biochem.* 37:131, 1988

22. Akers TK, Gabrielson AL. The effect of high voltage galvanic stimulation on the rate of healing of decubitus ulcers. In: Wachtel H, ed. *Biomedical Sciences Instrumentation.* Research Triangle Park, NC, Instrument Society of America, 1984; 20:99–100

23. Alon G, Azaria M, Stein H. Diabetic ulcer healing using high voltage TENS. *Phys Ther.* 66:775, 1986

24. Feedar JA, Kloth LC. Acceleration of wound healing with pulsing direct current. *Phys Ther.* 65:741, 1985

25. Ross CR, Segal D. High voltage galvanic stimulation—An aid to post-operative healing. *Curr Podiatry.* 19, May 1981

26. Sorenson NK. Pulsed galvanic (DC) muscle stimulation for post-op edema in the hand. Stimulus, section on clinical electrophysiology, *APTA*. 9:8, 1984

27. Sawyer P, ed. *Biophysical Mechanisms in Vascular Homeostasis and Intravascular Thrombosis.* New York, Appleton-Century Crofts, 1965

28. Williams R, Carey L. Studies in the production of standard venous thrombosis. *Ann Surg.* 149:381, 1959

29. Newton RA. Pain: Theories, evaluation and management by thermal agents. In: Michlovitz S, ed. *Thermal Agents in Rehabilitation.* Philadelphia, FA Davis, 1987: 19–48

30. Mayer DJ, Price DD. A physiological and psychological analysis of pain: A potential model of moditation. In: Pfalf D. *Physiological Mechanism of Motivation.* New York, Springer-Verlag, 1982:433–471

31. Zimmerman M. Peripheral and central nervous mechanisms of nociception, pain and pain therapy: Facts and hypotheses. In: Bonica J, ed. *Advances in Pain Research and Therapy.* New York, Raven Press, 1979; 3:3–32

32. Meyerson BA. Electrostimulation procedures: Effects, rationales and possible mechanisms. In: Bonica J, ed. *Advances in Pain Research and Therapy.* New York, Raven Press, 1983; 5:495–534

33. Anderson SA, Holmgren E. Pain threshold effects of peripheral conditioning stimulation. In: Bonica JJ, Able-Fessard D, eds. *Advances in Pain Research and Therapy.* New York, Raven Press, 1976; 1: 761–768.

34. Adams JA. *The Effects of Frequency of High Voltage Pulsed Galvanic Stimulation on the Results of Treatment for Pain in Chronic Low Back Pain Patients.* MS thesis, Medical College of Virginia, Virginia Commonwealth University, Richmond, 1983

35. Sohn M, Weinstein MA, Robbins RD. The levator syndrome and its treatment with high voltage electrogalvanic stimulation. *Am J Surg.* 44:580, 1982

36. Morris L, Newton RA. Use of high voltage pulsed galvanic stimulation for patients with levator ani syndrome. *Phys Ther.* 67:1522, 1987

37. Melzack R. The McGill pain questionnaire: Major properties and scoring methods. *Pain.* 1:277, 1975

38. Murphy GJ. Electrical physical therapy in treating TMJ patients. *J. Craniomandib Pract.* 1:67, 1983

39. Taylor K, Newton RA. Interferential current stimulation in recurrent jaw pain. In: Peat M, ed. *Current Physical Therapy.* Toronto, Decker, 1988: 203–206

40. Benton LA, Baker LL, Browman B, et al. *Functional Electrical Stimulation: A Practical Clinical Guide.* Downey, CA, Rancho Los Amigos Rehabilitation Engineering Center, 1980

41. Kots YM. Notes from Kots' (USSR) lectures and laboratory periods. Canadian–Soviet Exchange Symposium on Electrostimulation of Skeletal Muscles, December 1977

42. Newton RA. Joint receptor contributions to reflexive and kinesthetic responses. *Phys Ther.* 62:22, 1982

43. Lindstrom B, Korsan-Bengston K, Jonsson O, et al. Electrically induced short-lasting tetanus of the calf muscles for prevention of deep vein thrombosis. *Br J Surg.* 69:203, 1982

44. Schoeler H. Physical block of the sympathetic chain. *J Technik in der Medizin.* 1:16, 1972

45. Mohr T, Akers TK, Wessman HC. Effect of high voltage stimulation on blood flow in the rat hind limb. *Phys Ther.* 67:526, 1987

CHAPTER 9

Interference Current

Luther C. Kloth

Advances in electronics engineering and microprocessing during the past three decades have provided technology for development of more sophisticated, accurate, and clinically applicable electrotherapeutic instruments used in the practice of physical therapy. Among contemporary electrotherapeutic devices are those employed for ameliorating pain, augmenting strength, eliciting skeletal muscle contraction for functional purposes, facilitating osteogenesis in non-union fractures, accelerating repair of slow-healing wounds, and improving circulation to extremities affected by vasospastic disease. One electrotherapeutic current that has been and continues to be employed adjunctively in some of these applications is interference current (IFC).

In 1950 Nemec[1] applied the physical phenomenon of wave interference to conceive of and develop the first electrotherapeutic device capable of generating IFC. After years of technological refinement IFC has emerged as a documented, viable alternative for promoting positive treatment outcomes in a number of clinical conditions.

The purposes of this chapter are to (1) explain the physical principles of IFC; (2) provide rationale for the electrophysiological and clinical effects of IFC; (3) discuss clinical applications and present case studies for which this form of electrotherapy has been reported to be beneficial; (4) describe methods and protocol used in applying IFC; and (5) identify contraindications and precautions to be considered before using IFC in patient care.

PHYSICAL PRINCIPLES

Interference of Waves

When two or more sinusoidal waves originate exactly in phase from separate circuits (A and B, Fig. 9–1), they are said to be *coherent* with respect to frequency and amplitude. When the waves are superimposed, the crests of wave A add to the crests of wave B to produce a resultant amplitude summated wave (2h).

Amplitude summation produced by superimposing two sine waves that are exactly in phase is called *constructive interference*. Maximum constructive interference occurs whenever two sine waves are exactly in phase (Fig. 9–1A) or when one of the two waves is one, two, three or more wavelength(s) out of phase with the other (Fig. 9–1C). On the other hand, when one wave is any multiple of a half wavelength (eg, ½, 1½, 2½), out of phase with another wave, (Fig. 9–1B) then the upward alternation of one wave cancels the downward alternation of the other (dashed line), resulting in complete destructive interference and a sum wave amplitude of zero.[2]

A clearer conceptualization of electrical interference may be gained by making a comparison to interference of sound waves. Consider that the waves just described are sound waves originating from loudspeakers A and B (Fig. 9–2). If loudspeaker A vibrates with a frequency of 1000 pps and loudspeaker B vibrates at 999 pps, then at time t=0 the waves from both speakers are in phase, and the resulting amplified sound will represent the sum of the compression waves from the two speakers (*constructive interference*). Moments later (at t=1½ sec,) loudspeaker B, vibrating at a slightly lower frequency than

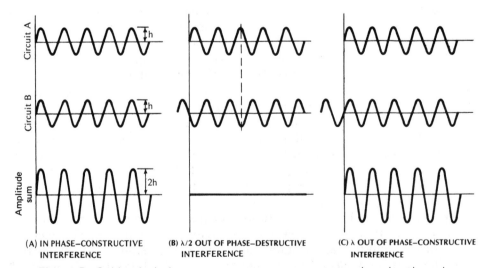

(A) IN PHASE–CONSTRUCTIVE INTERFERENCE   (B) λ/2 OUT OF PHASE–DESTRUCTIVE INTERFERENCE   (C) λ OUT OF PHASE–CONSTRUCTIVE INTERFERENCE

Figure 9–1. Identical sine waves can summate or cancel each other, depending upon their relative phase relationship. *(Adapted from Bueche F, 1965, p 278.[2])*

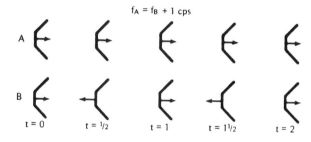

$f_A = f_B + 1$ cps

A

B

t = 0   t = 1/2   t = 1   t = 1 1/2   t = 2

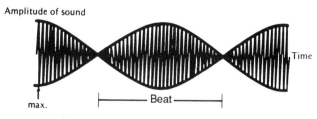

Amplitude of sound

Time

max. |——— Beat ———|

Figure 9–2. Amplitude-modulated beats result when two similar wave sources oscillate with slightly different frequencies. *(Adapted from Bueche F, 1965, p 522.[2])*

A, will begin to fall behind. At $t = 1/2$ sec, speaker A will have vibrated 500 times and will be sending out a compression wave, which increases the density of air in front of the speaker. Simultaneously speaker B, which will have vibrated 499.5 times will be exactly one-half cycle behind speaker A and will be sending out a rarefaction wave, which decreases the air density in front of the speaker. Both waves will reach the ear at the same time, but no sound will be heard because the waves will exactly cancel each other (*destructive interference*). At $t = 1.0$, speaker B will have vibrated exactly 999 times while speaker A will have vibrated 1000 times. Again both speakers are sending out compression waves that are in phase and summate to produce a sound of maximum amplitude.

Amplitude-Modulated Beats

This process will continue to repeat itself as shown in Figure 9–2. Thus, at time intervals exactly on the second the speaker sound waves will be in phase and an amplified sound is produced. However, at intervals on the half second no sound is heard because the superimposed wave phases are 180 degrees out-of-phase and cancel each other. In this illustration using two different frequencies of sound as the source of waves, the ear will hear a series of pulses or *beats* each second on the second. This phenomenon of beating also occurs when other types of sine wave oscillations from two identical sources of energy, such as alternating current, which have different frequencies are out of phase and blend (heterodyne) to produce the interference beating effect. When the beat modulations produced by heterodyned alternating currents are applied to excitable tissues, they are perceived as rhythmical sensory or motor pulsations, or both, depending on the maximum amplitude of the beat modulation.

Two-Circuit IFC. Figure 9–3 shows how heterodyned, therapeutically useful interference current beats are produced by a two-circuit IFC device when two alternating currents having slightly different frequencies are superimposed on the same time axis. In this example we may assume that alternating currents of 4100 and 4000 pps are superimposed from circuits 1 and 2, respectively, when these two currents are made to intersect. Owing to the frequency difference (100 Hz) between the two circuits there are points (A and C) along the time axes where the positive (upward) phases from each circuit add together to produce a higher-amplitude resultant wave. At point B the resultant wave amplitude is zero because a positive phase from circuit 1 cancels a negative phase from circuit 2 (destructive interference).

Thus, it may be seen that the effect of blending two alternating currents together is a rhythmical rise and fall in the current amplitude. This amplitude modulation results in a beat frequency equal to the number of times each second that the current amplitude increases to its maximum value and then decreases to its minimum value. In this example the amplitude-modulated beat frequency is the difference between the frequencies of the two alternating currents $(4100 - 4000 = 100 \text{ bps})$.

Traditionally, AC frequencies in the range of 1000 to 10,000 pps have been referred to as "medium frequencies."[3] This would lead one to assume that

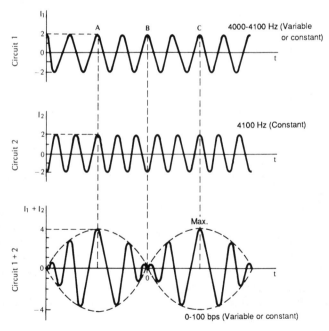

Figure 9–3. Blending of alternating currents produces a constant or variable number of amplitude-modulated beats per second (bps). *(Adapted from Nippel F: Interferential TENS: An Advanced Method in the Management of Pain. Deutsche Nemectron GmbH, Durlacher Allee 47, D-7500 Karlsruhe 1, W Germany.)*

frequencies below 1000 pps should be referred to as "low frequencies" while those above 10,000 pps would be considered "high frequencies." Unfortunately, with respect to AC frequencies used in electrotherapeutic applications, the terms *low, medium,* and *high* have assumed different meanings over the years. *Low frequency* is usually associated with the minimum frequency required for evoking tetanic muscle contractions, but has included ranges from 1 to 1000 Hz. For alternating and pulsed current, *medium frequency* is technically defined as 1000 to 10,000 Hz or pulses per second (pps); however, the extreme variability in physiological responses across these frequencies render this classification impractical. This frequency range also has been erroneously called "high" frequency. *High frequency* is technically defined as greater than 10,000 Hz and is used clinically for its thermal effects.[4] Thus the most meaningful documentation of frequency output is to state the exact numerical frequency or frequency range rather than use the descriptive terms low, medium, and high.

Constant- Versus Variable-Beat Frequencies

The amplitude-modulated current that is produced endogenously by IFC may be conducted through the target tissues in either a constant- or variable-beat frequency mode. In the constant mode there is a constant difference between the frequencies of the two circuits and this results in a constant-beat frequency. For example, if the difference in frequency between the two circuits is 40 pps, then the beat frequency will be constant at 40 bps. Most two-circuit IFC devices allow selection of any constant-beat frequency between 1 and 120 bps.

In the variable-beat mode, the frequency between the two circuits varies within preselected ranges. The time taken to vary the beat frequency through any programmed range is usually fixed by the device at about 15 sec. IFC devices often provide a choice of variable-beat frequency programs. Examples of preselectable, variable-beat frequency programs are:

- 0.1 to 1 bps
- 1 to 10 bps
- 1 to 120 bps
- 90 to 120 bps

The theoretical model shown in Figure 9–4 illustrates how the conventional quadripolar electrode arrangement from a two-circuit IFC device delivers endogenous stimulation with a variable-beat frequency of 90 to 120 to 90 bps. The beat frequency varies continuously over a range of 30 bps from 4090 to 4120 and back to 4090 pps until the treatment is terminated.

Two-Circuit Static Interference Field

Closer observation of Figure 9–4 reveals that in a homogeneous medium (such as water) the maximum IFC amplitude modulation occurs in the direction of vectors that are oriented 45 degrees to perpendicular lines extending between the electrodes. At the points within this region (shaded area) where the current

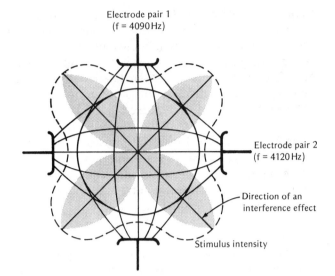

Figure 9—4. Endogenous stimulation with a variable-beat frequency of 90-120-90 bps. *(Adapted from DeDomenico G: Basic Guidelines for Interferential Therapy. Sydney, Theramed, 1981; 9.)*

lines intersect, the two currents sum by vector addition. This stationary stimulation field represents a static interference pattern (Fig. 9—5) in which the maximum amplitude modulation effect occurs at 45 degrees to perpendicular lines extending between the two pairs of electrodes. The maximum amplitude modulation effect provides the greatest variation in beat amplitude and charge quantity. From the 45-degree diagonals to the perpendicular lines between

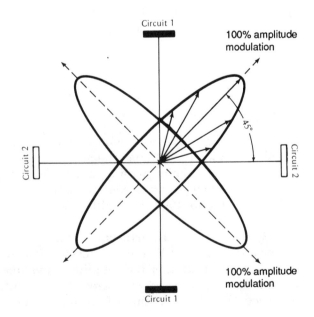

Figure 9—5. A static interference pattern. The maximum summated amplitude occurs at 45 degrees to perpendicular lines extending between electrode pairs. *(Adapted from Hansjuergens J, 1974, p 24.*[5]*)*

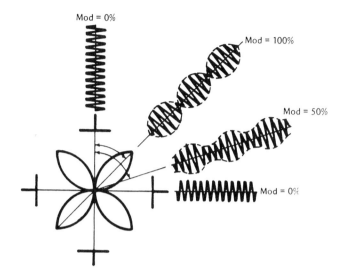

Figure 9–6. IFC amplitude modulation gradient. Maximum amplitude modulation produces a maximum stimulus amplitude at 45 degrees to perpendicular lines running between electrodes. (Mod = modulation.) *(Adapted from Hogenkamp, Mittelmeijer, Smits, Stralen: Inferential Therapy. Enraf-Nonius, 1 Rontgenweg, 2600 AL Delft, Holland, 1983: 13.)*

electrodes, a decreasing gradient for amplitude modulation and charge density occurs. Decreasing gradients for amplitude modulation and stimulus amplitude are illustrated in Figure 9–6 as a percent of maximum amplitude by arrows extending from 50 and 100 percent to zero percent.

When IFC is applied to excitable tissues in the static mode the volume of tissue stimulated by the perfusing current remains relatively constant and depends on the arrangements of the four electrodes. However, because tissues are not homogenous with regard to electrical conductivity, the amplitude-modulated beat pattern does not occur near the center of intersection of the two AC circuits as it does when alternating currents intersect in a homogeneous medium like water.

Two-Circuit Scanning Interference Field

In the early 1970s technology was developed that made it possible to scan the amplitude-modulated beat current through the conducting medium.[5] Scanning of amplitude-modulated beats through an arc of approximately 45 degrees may allow the current to conduct through a greater volume of tissue than occurs in the static mode. Compare Figures 9–7 and 9–5. When the scanning mode is selected, electronic components within the device slowly vary the current amplitude in circuit 1, between 50 and 100 percent of the maximum preset milliamperage while maintaining current amplitude in circuit 2 at 75 percent of the maximum current amplitude of the first circuit (Fig. 9–8). This variation in amplitude occurs at the intersecting current lines (Fig. 9–4). Thus, the direction of maximum-amplitude modulation that occurs at the intersecting current lines results in rhythmical clockwise and counterclockwise changes in the direction of 100 percent amplitude modulation, so that the current amplitude alternately changes position of maximum tissue stimulation. The scan-

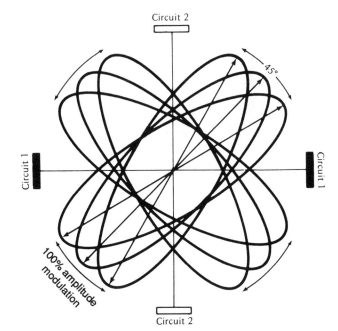

Figure 9–7. Scanning interference current. *(Adapted from the pamphlet* Nemectrodyn Model 2 Endovac Model 2. *Deutsche Nemectron GmbH, Durlacher Allee 47, D-7500 Karlsruhe 1, W. Germany.)*

ning mode may be useful when it is difficult to identify the exact focal area of the patient's symptoms.

Premodulated IFC

As previously described, the conventional method of producing IFC beats within the tissues requires the use of four electrodes (two from each circuit) positioned on the patient in a planar (single surface) or co-planar (opposing surfaces) arrangement that allows current from one circuit to intersect with current from a second (see Fig. 9–4). With this conventional delivery method the amplitude- and frequency-modulated beats are produced endogenously in the patient's tissues. An alternative method of delivering IFC premodulates the current from the two circuits exogenously within the device and delivers the

Figure 9–8. In the scanning mode, current amplitude varies in one circuit and is held constant in the other. *(Adapted from Hogenkamp, Mittelmeijer, Smits, Stralen:* Inferential Therapy. *Enraf-Nonius, 1 Rontgenweg, 2600 AL Delft, Holland, 1983; 13.)*

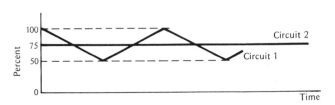

premixed amplitude- and frequency-modulated beats via two electrodes to the patient's skin. Although the premodulated bipolar method of delivering IFC is easier than the conventional, quadripolar technique, there are no controlled clinical studies in the literature that support the erroneous assumption that one delivery method is better than the other.

Three-Circuit IFC

When three amplitude-constant, sinusoidal currents of 5 kHz are superimposed in a homogeneous medium, a three-dimensional amplitude modulated interference field is created.[6] Three-circuit IFC is applied with three pairs of electrodes contained within two Y-shaped applicators that are arranged on the body to enable the three currents to intersect within the tissues (Fig. 9–9). In

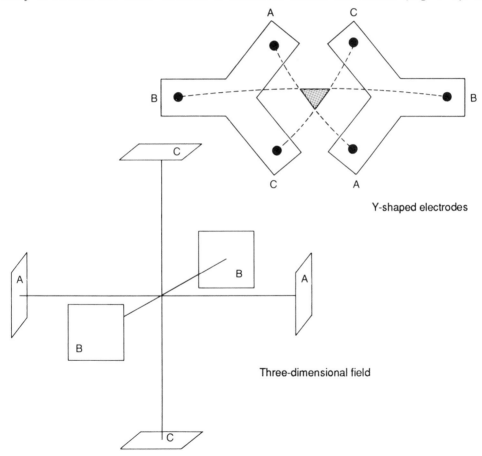

Figure 9–9. Three pairs of electrodes (A, B, C) are contained within two Y shaped applicators for delivering stereodynamic IFC to create a three-dimensional area of stimulation. *(Adapted from DeDomenico G, ed: New Dimensions in Interferential Therapy. A Theoretical and Clinical Guide. Lindfield, NSW, Australia, Reid Medical Books, 1987: 21.)*

addition to the original beat frequency produced in the tissues a second amplitude modulation of the beats is produced over a 30- to 60-sec period of time. This second amplitude modulation may be added to each of several selectable beat frequency program.

The rationale for the development of three-circuit IFC is empirically based on the principle that tissues occupy a three-dimensional space and that ions in excitable membranes and tissue fluids move in three dimensions. Although the three-circuit amplitude-modulated IFC field is intended to provide greater spatial stimulation of tissues than the two-circuit field, there are no studies in the literature to support this commercial claim.

ELECTROPHYSIOLOGICAL EFFECTS

Cutaneous and Subcutaneous Stimulation

In the previous discussion related to two-circuit IFC devices, endogenous production of the amplitude-modulated beat current was shown to require two electrodes from each circuit, for a total of four. When the four electrodes are applied to the body, the amplitude-modulated interference effect occurs when the electrodes are arranged cross-diagonally on either one or opposing body surfaces so the current delivered to the tissues from one circuit intersects and blends with the current delivered to the tissues in the opposite direction from the second. Notice in Figure 9–4 that the theoretical shape of the area of maximum subcutaneous stimulation represented by the shading occurs (in a homogeneous medium) where the current lines from the two circuits cross. It is in this region that the summated peak amplitudes of successive beats are greater than the constant amplitude of the AC carrier frequencies of 4000 and 4100 pps (Hz) applied to the skin. Therefore, somewhere within the endogenous (subcutaneous) zone, nerve fibers not only receive higher amplitude stimulation than the skin receives but in addition, because each beat is amplitude modulated, stimulated subcutaneous nerve fibers cannot accommodate.

It is important to note that the current amplitude delivered from the two circuits (eg, with conventional, quadripolar IFC) may be inadequate to elicit a nerve response. Because each circuit delivers a subthreshold, non-modulated stimulus, sensory nerve fiber excitation immediately below the electrodes is minimal. Nerve excitation from the amplitude-modulated current occurs endogenously in an unpredictable region of the tissues where the currents from the two circuits cross because of the nonhomogeneous composition of tissues. This region, dictated by the tetrapolar electrode arrangement, represents the area in and around the geometric center (Fig. 9–10) between the four electrodes where the total current is the sum of the currents from each pair of electrodes (see Fig. 9–3).

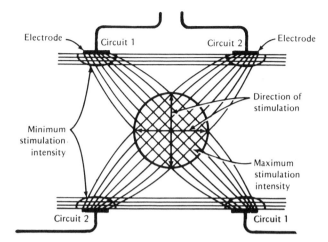

Electrode — Circuit 1   Circuit 2 — Electrode

Direction of stimulation

Minimum stimulation intensity

Maximum stimulation intensity

Circuit 2   Circuit 1

Figure 9–10. Areas of maximum and minimum stimulation. *(Adapted from Nippel F: Interferential TENS: An Advanced Method in the Management of Pain. Deutsche Nemectron GmbH, Durlacher Allee 47, D-7500 Karlsruhe 1, W. Germany.)*

Muscle Fatigue from Synchronous Recruitment of Motor Units

Under physiological conditions when a volitional muscle contraction occurs, motor neurons are asynchronously excited at different firing rates. Each motor neuron in turn maximally excites all of the muscle fibers within its motor unit, causing the excited motor units to contract and relax at different rates. For a weak willful contraction the typical firing frequency of motor units is between 5 and 15 pps.[7] During a maximum voluntary contraction, motor unit frequencies vary between 25 and 50 pps.[7] The result of the asynchronous motor unit firing rate during a voluntary contraction is a smoothly graded muscle contraction that requires less energy and is therefore less fatiguing than would be the case if motor units were recruited synchronously. In a weak volitional contraction, small motor neurons and the small, more fatigue-resistant motor units they innervate are recruited first. As the willed contraction becomes progressively more vigorous, larger motor neurons and their large, more easily fatiguable motor units are recruited.[8]

In contrast tetanizing muscle contraction elicited by transcutaneously applied pulsed, burst, or beat electrical stimulation results from synchronous excitation of many larger-diameter, lower-threshold, more excitable motor nerve fibers that innervate the larger, faster, and more easily fatiguable motor units. The smaller-diameter, more deeply located motor nerve fibers that innervate smaller, slower, more fatigue-resistant motor units are excited only if the stimulus amplitude is increased sufficiently to reach their firing threshold.[9] Thus, the tetanic contraction produced by electrical stimulation of muscle at tetanizing frequencies between 30 and 1000 pps is more fatiguing than that produced by volition.

This more fatiguing condition is partly due to the reversal in the normal pattern of motor unit recruitment as well as to the synchronous firing of motor units. In addition, recall that voluntary contractions elicit neural discharge rates between 5 and 50 pps.[7] depending on the intensity of the contraction. These physiological discharge rates allow impulse conduction along the motor nerve and periodic release of neurotransmitter substance at the neuromuscular junction. With NMES frequencies between 30 and 50 pps, the same nerve fibers are repeatedly depolarized to produce a tetanic contraction. At stimulation frequencies greater than 50 pps, the nerve fibers are repeatedly depolarized at a higher rate than occurs during a vigorous voluntary contraction. Therefore, the more rapid fatigue onset accompanying electrical stimulation may also be contributed to by a decrease in neurotransmitter released or failure of the neuromuscular synapse when NMES frequencies exceed physiological neural discharge rates.[10,11] Generally, the higher the stimulation frequency the more rapidly the muscle fatigues.[9]

Traditionally, electrotherapy devices used to stimulate innervated muscle have employed alternating or pulsed currents within the frequency range of 0.1 to 1000 pps (Hz).[12] When successive impulses within any portion of this frequency range are delivered to nerve, the largest-diameter myelinated nerve fibers respond by depolarizing at the same rate as the stimulus frequency. As the stimulus frequency increases up to 1000 pps the depolarization frequency will increase correspondingly.[12]

Every nerve fiber has a maximum depolarization frequency dictated by its refractory period.[13] When a second electrical stimulus is applied to a nerve fiber too soon after a first effective stimulus, it does not excite an action potential. The nerve is said to be in a state of *absolute refractoriness* and is inexcitable regardless of the stimulus amplitude. In A-alpha nerve fibers the duration of the absolute refractory period is approximately 1 msec.[14] This inactive period is followed by a state of *relative refractoriness*, during which time it is possible to elicit a response from the nerve if either the stimulus amplitude or the time between successive stimuli is increased from 0.5 to 1.0 msec.

This, stimulus synchronized depolarization of nerve fibers and the motor units they innervate occurs with pulsed or alternating currents having frequencies up to 1000 pps. With pulses of constant amplitude and frequencies greater than 1000 pps, successive depolarizing shocks occur within the relative refractory period of the nerve and repolarization is prevented. Additionally, the motor endplate may become fatigued and transmission of the stimulus may not occur. The loss of excitation caused by maintaining a continuous refractory state with a constant amplitude stimulus having a frequency greater than 1000 pps is called *Wedensky inhibition*.[14]

Asynchronous Recruitment of Motor Units with IFC

During NMES with AC frequencies above 1000 pps not every cycle results in a corresponding depolarization of nerve fibers as occurs with frequencies below 1000 pps. Because of Wedensky inhibition, summation of several cycles of AC is needed to depolarize even the lowest-threshold nerve fibers. In other words, the duration of the refractory period dictates how often nerve fibers can be depolarized. Thus, nerve fibers respond to AC frequencies above 1000 pps at their own depolarization frequencies. Therefore with AC frequencies greater than 1000 pps, the depolarization frequency of nerve fibers does not coincide with the frequency of the current nor with the depolarization frequency of other nerve fibers in the nerve bundle. The result, known as the *Gildemeister effect*,[3] is stimulus-asynchronous depolarization. This summation effect occurs when, according to Lullies,[13] the hypolarization influence of successive short-duration negative phases from AC frequencies above 1000 pps causes the resting membrane potential to gradually decrease over a certain effective time until threshold is reached. The higher the stimulus amplitude the shorter the effective time will be.

Typical IFC devices operate within a carrier frequency range of 3500 to 5000 pps. As previously mentioned, conventional IFC consists of frequency- and amplitude-modulated bursts or beats having an endogenous frequency between 0.5 and 200 bps. Figure 9–11 illustrates how the amplitude-modulated AC pulses (cycles) contained within individual beats of IFC summate to evoke action potentials after successive cycles are applied over an effective time. Nerve fibers depolarize at the frequency of beat interruption.

IFC and Skin Impedance. All electrical currents delivered to the tissues through cutaneous electrodes encounter opposition to the passage of currents through the skin. Several factors contribute to the impedance offered by the skin, including electrode surface area, skin temperature, dryness, thickness, and amount of skin oil and hair present. Although skin impedance may be reduced by increasing electrode surface area; by warming, wetting, and washing the skin; and by clipping excessive hair; it still remains relatively high compared to impedance of subcutaneous tissues.

When electrical current passes through tissues a force is created on electrically charged ions present at interfaces between different types of tissues and in cell membranes. Conduction of current through the tissues depends on ionic movement. When electrical currents are introduced into the body, ions accumulate at tissue interfaces and cell membranes create a charge that is opposite to the charge of the applied voltage at the electrodes. The potential

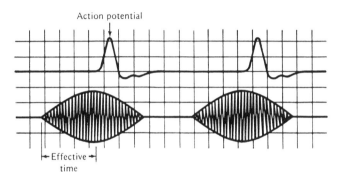

Figure ***9–11.*** Action potentials fire in response to amplitude-modulated beats of IFC.

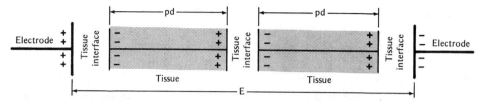

Figure 9–12. Electrolytic polarization. E is the applied voltage, and pd is the potential difference. *(Adapted from Hogenkamp, Mittelmeijer, Smits, Stralen:* Inferential Therapy. *Enraf-Nonius, 1 Rontgenweg, 2600 AL Delft, Holland, 1983: p 15.)*

difference that occurs between each electrode and the tissue is created by electrolytic polarization. This phenomenon (Fig. 9–12) occurs in living tissue, which is comparable to a conductor with capacitance. The countervoltage is called *reactance* or *capacitive impedance.* The polarizing capacitance of tissues is denoted by a constant C, which depends on electrode surface area. An electrode with a surface area of 100 cm^2 in contact with the skin has a capacitance of 1 microfarad.[15] As the frequency of AC is gradually increased to 4000 pps a pronounced decrease in capacitive skin impedance occurs (Fig. 9–13).

The following example serves to illustrate how capacitive impedance decreases when the frequency of AC is increased from 50 to 4000 pps applied transcutaneously through 10- by 10-cm electrodes. Using the formula for capacitive impedance:

$$Z = \frac{1}{C(F) \cdot 2 \pi f(Hz)}$$

where

- Z = capacitive impedance,
- C = polarization capacitance of tissue in farads (F), and
- f = frequency of the current.

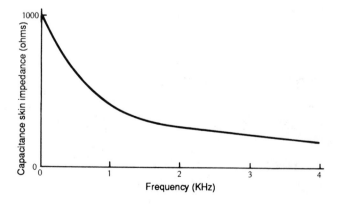

Figure 9–13. Capactive skin impedance falls as frequency increases.

For AC with a frequency of 50 pps we obtain:

$$Z = \frac{1}{10^{-6} \cdot 2\ \pi \cdot 50} = 3225\ \Omega$$

For AC with a frequency of 4,000 pps capacitive impedance is 80 times lower.

$$Z = \frac{1}{10^{-6} \cdot 2\ \pi \cdot 4000} = 40.3\ \Omega$$

The significant drop in capacitive impedance illustrated here is not unique to AC or IFC. Tissue impedance is reduced by any electrical stimulation device that allows selection of pulses having very short durations (less than 100 μsec).[16] While it is true that skin impedance decreases with increasing AC frequency, the decline occurs from the decreased pulse charge at higher AC frequencies and not from an increase in AC frequency alone. Some proponents of using IFC for treatment of deep nerve or muscle tissues explain that IFC penetrates more deeply than currents from other electrical stimulation devices and base this erroneous claim on the assumption that skin impedance only decreases in response to higher frequencies of AC. Meyer-Waarden and associates have demonstrated that IFC does permeate soft tissues and can penetrate to deep structures.[17] This explains why IFC may be effective for treating patients with either deep or superficial pain; promoting osteogenesis in delayed and nonunion fractures and pseudarthrosis; stimulating deep skeletal muscle to augment blood flow by activating the muscle pump mechanism in venous insufficiency; and depressing the activity of certain cervical and lumbosacral sympathetic ganglia in patients with increased arterial constrictor tone.

CLINICAL APPLICATIONS   *not specific studies*

During the past two and one-half decades, IFC has been reported to produce beneficial treatment outcomes in a number of clinical conditions. The most noteworthy results have been reported for individuals diagnosed with facial neuritis, with musculoskeletal and vascular conditions, as well as for urogenital dysfunction and pain.

Facial Neuritis

In 1966 Nikolova-Troeva[18] reported using IFC alone or in combination with naptha thermal pack and massage to treat 35 patients with facial nerve neuritis. The time between onset of the neuritis and initiation of treatment ranged from 15 days to 11 months. Prior to beginning treatment the electrical excitability of the involved facial nerve of each patient was evaluated with galvanic and faradic stimuli. One patient demonstrated reduced excitability to galvanic and faradic current, 29 patients showed a partial reaction of degeneration, and 5 had a complete reaction of degeneration of the involved nerve. Functional recovery was assessed by observing clinical recovery such as the ability to frown, wrinkle the brow, or close the involved eye. IFC with a rhythmical frequency of 0 to 100 bps was applied to the involved musculature of all 35 patients. Twenty patients received only IFC as treatment while 15 received IFC in combination with thermal peaks and massage. Each patient received 10 to 12 treatments for 10 min either daily or every other day.

Six patients who demonstrated inability to frown or close the involved eye and facial expression asymmetry prior to treatment completely recovered, while 20 patients showed "significant functional improvement." The remaining 9 patients showed "slight functional improvement." Electrical excitability improved in 12 patients and a return to normal excitability was observed in 2. Although Nikolova-Troeva suggests that IFC stimulation may have contributed to the favorable clinical recovery of her patients, nevertheless the results of her study are inconclusive. The inconclusiveness appears to be a result of the research design, which did not group treatment outcomes according to patients who received IFC alone versus those who received the combination treatment.

Musculoskeletal Conditions

IFC has also been credited with providing positive clinical outcomes in various orthopedic conditions. In 18 patients with chronic radial epicondylitis, Eigler[19] applied quadripolar IFC for 10 min daily with a variable frequency of 90 to 100 bps and the stimulus amplitude advanced to sensory threshold. All but one patient showed complete clinical relief of pain and other symptoms in spite of being asked to return to the activities that had caused the epicondylitis.

Nikolova-Troeva[20] treated 45 patients with joint sprains who had severe pain, edema, and restricted joint mobility. IFC at a variable frequency of 0 to 100 bps was applied 10 to 15 minutes daily with quadripolar electrodes over the affected joint. Two to 15 treatments were required to produce asymptomatic results. Clinical evaluation of patient progress focused on reduction of pain and edema and improvement in joint range of motion.

In the same study an additional 52 patients with joint sprains were treated with microwave diathermy while 70 others received diadynamic current. No mention was made of the number of applications of the latter two types of treatment. However, comparative results indicated that 75 percent of patients treated with IFC were asymptomatic compared to 56 and 36 percent for microwave and diadynamic current, respectively.

In cases of retarded callus formation following fracture as well as in Sudeck's atrophy and pseudarthroses, IFC has been reported to facilitate restoration of healing indicated by x-ray documentation. In 1969, Nikolova[21] treated 150 patients with retarded callus formation following fracture by applying IFC to the affected area at a constant frequency of 100 bps and 10 to 20 mA daily. Patients received 15 to 20 treatments lasting 15 to 20 min. Fifty of these patients also received medication. In the patients who received IFC only, x-ray showed that 73 percent had complete restoration of callus formation. Eighty percent of the patients who received IFC and medication showed completed formation of endosteal and periosteal callus.

The same IFC treatment was given to 137 patients diagnosed as having Sudeck's atrophy. In addition, 69 patients with this diagnosis received IFC and medication. Clinical healing confirmed by x-ray was achieved in 81 percent of patients who received IFC without medication. One-hundred percent of those who were treated with IFC and medication demonstrated complete recovery of bone density by x-ray documentation.

In the same report Nikolova[21] described using the same IFC treatment protocol on 22 patients with pseudarthrosis. X-ray verification of complete callus formation was noted in 32 percent of these patients while 54 percent showed extensive but incomplete callus buildup.

Other researchers have also reported that IFC augments healing in fracture complications. Ganne and associates[22] used IFC to treat 9 of 150 patients with fractured mandibles. The 9 patients all had fracture complications that predisposed them to nonunion. The treatment involved applying IFC at a frequency of 20 bps over the fracture site with a small quadripolar electrode for 20 min every 2 to 3 days. Current amplitude was adjusted to produce slight fasciculation of facial muscles beneath the electrode. The number of treatments varied from 3 to 20. All 9 patients demonstrated 100-percent healing verified by x-ray. The other 141 patients in this group also achieved satisfactory bony union. These results were compared with the healing outcomes of 10 patients who served as controls from another group of 150 patients with mandibular fractures. The 10 patients in the control group had mandibular fracture complications predisposing them to nonunion similar to the 9 patients in the treatment group. The control group did not receive IFC stimulation. Three nonunions occurred in the control group of patients. The remaining 7 patients in the control group as well as the 140 other patients in this group all proceeded to full healing. Based on 150 patients in each of the two groups the incidence of nonunion was 0 percent for the group that received IFC stimulation and 2 percent in the control group.

In studies using an animal model, Laabs and co-workers[23] investigated the influence of IFC on bone healing. A transverse osteotomy of the radius and ulna of the forelegs of 34, 6-month-old black-headed sheep was done to create a 1-mm fracture cleft. Microprobes for measuring temperature changes were inserted into the cleft of 5 animals. The fracture clefts of all animals were approximated and stabilized with a metal plate. IFC was applied for 10 min three times a week to the fracture cleft in 24 experimental animals. A control group of 10 sheep received no IFC stimulation. Part one of the study involved clinical, radiological, histological, and chemical analysis of the fracture cleft, which revealed that callus formation was accelerated by application of IFC.

In the second part of the study by Laabs and associates,[23] it was noted that temperature elevation occurred in the clefts of the five animals that had temperature probes inserted and that the temperature elevation was dependent on the mA amplitude. A similar relationship was reported for the occurrence of hydroxyprolin, an amino-acid-specific collagen that reflects increased calcification activity. Measurements of calcium and phosphorus levels in the newly regenerated bone tissue showed that full mineralization had occurred in the IFC treated animals at a much earlier date than in the untreated controls. These findings support the earlier research of Guttler and Kleditzsch[24] who reported faster callus formation in rabbits treated with IFC than in a control group that did not receive IFC.

Vascular Conditions

A few clinical studies have reported successful treatment of select vascular conditions with IFC. Using a variable frequency of 90 to 100 bps Schoeler[25] applied a scanning interference field to the neck region over the stellate ganglion of a patient with Raynaud's disease. The purpose in applying IFC in this manner was to facilitate improvement of digital circulation by physical block of the sympathetic chain. Following an eight-minute treatment with IFC at 4 to 8 mA, photoelectric plethysmographic monitoring of the digital ipsilateral pulse demonstrated a doubling of pulse volume. According to Schoeler[25], 12 to 20 sessions using this technique not only improved circulation and smooth muscle elasticity in digital blood vessels, but also decreased the number of sympathetic blocks performed by injections.

In 25 men with either first or second stage endarteritis obliterans who had no symptomatic change after treatment by medication or sympathectomy, Nikolova-Troeva[26] applied IFC to the lumbar sympathetic ganglia daily for 15 to 20 minutes. After 15 treatments all patients were discharged after objectively improving walking distance, elimination of trophic skin disturbances, improved skin temperature of the treated legs by 2°C, and improved detection of distal pulses in the lower extremities.

Similar objective findings are reported by Belcher,[27] who used IFC to treat four patients with peripheral vascular disease of the lower extremities and two patients with PVD of the upper extremities. IFC was applied daily over 10 to 16 days with vacuum electrodes positioned so the endogenous IFC field scanned through the entire limb proximal to the affected area. Each daily treatment lasted 10 min using a variable frequency of 0 to 100 bps.

Urogenital Dysfunction

The pelvic floor musculature and supporting structures in women often become lax following labor and delivery, resulting in urinary incontinence, which is defined by the International Continence Society as the loss of urine at any time unacceptable to the individual.[28] Four types of urinary incontinence are defined: stress, urge or frequency, reflex, and overflow. Stress incontinence is the involuntary loss of urine that occurs following a sudden rise in intra-abdominal pressure brought on by straining, sneezing, coughing, laughing, or other physical activities.[28] Urge incontinence is the involuntary loss of urine associated with a strong and urgent desire to void, which overcomes the voluntary ability to inhibit bladder function.[28] Patients with stress, urge incontinence, and pelvic infection have been reported to have responded very favorably following treatment with IFC. McQuire[29] used IFC to treat 21 women with stress incontinence. Combined with stress incontinence 2 patients also had urinary urge incontinence and 2 others had pelvic infection. Three additional women had urge incontinence and one of them also had pelvic infection. Symptoms had been present in these patients from several weeks to a few years and 7 patients had previous pelvic floor surgery. All 24 patients received 12 IFC treatments during a period of 1 month. Vacuum electrodes were applied to the upper medial thigh bilaterally with the second electrode of each circuit placed lateral to the navel on the contralateral side. A variable frequency of 0 to 100 bps was applied at 25 to 30 mA for 15 min to produce rhythmical contractions of the pelvic floor musculature. Prior to IFC stimulation patients were taught pelvic floor exercises; however, there was no indication that these exercises were continued during the study. One month after receiving the IFC treatments 16 of the 21 patients improved and maintained complete freedom from incontinence.

In other studies IFC was used successfully in women having partially denervated pudendal nerves, disuse atrophy, damage to sphincter muscles, and deterioration of the mucosal lining of the vagina.[30,31] IFC reportedly reduced hemorrhoidal pain, abdominal pain, and incontinence in 91 percent of patients in 12 treatments.[30] Finally, patients with excessive tension in the pelvic diaphragm (composed of the three levator ani muscles) have been reported to have improved circulation and reduced pain following treatment with IFC.[30,32,33]

Pain Conditions

One of the most common clinical uses of IFC is for treatment of pain by electroanalgesia. Although theories have been proposed to explain how IFC modulates pain,[34,35] unfortunately there is a paucity of published clinical studies that have been designed to make use of patient controls or objective methods of assessing pain suppression produced by IFC treatment. Only one publication found in a peer-reviewed journal reported results from a controlled clinical study on the placebo effect of IFC in patients with recurrent jaw pain. In that study, Taylor and associates[36] assigned 20 patients with recurrent jaw pain and reduced jaw opening to one of two groups, an IFC treatment group and an IFC placebo group. Subjects in the treatment group received three 20-min treatments to the involved temporomandibular joint and masticatory muscles with predetermined IFC stimulation characteristics. The placebo group received the exact IFC procedure as the treatment group except subjects were told that they would receive a subthreshold current sensation. Although jaw pain for both the treatment and placebo groups decreased over the three treatment sessions, the differences between the two groups were not statistically significant. Also, no statistically significant increase in jaw opening occurred between the two groups of subjects over the three treatment sessions. Thus, a short-term treatment period with IFC had no greater therapeutic effectiveness on jaw pain or jaw range of motion than a placebo procedure.

Two other studies reported positive outcomes following treatment of pain associated with osteoarthritis and vasoconstrictive disease. Burghart[37] observed relief of pain associated with osteoarthritis in 39 patients without accelerated cell sedimentation rate who had not benefited from other therapies. In her book on *Treatment With Interferential Current*, Nikolova-Troeva[38] describes various clinical applications of IFC usually in combination with other therapies but without control or placebo-treated groups. Her most convincing reports on pain relief describe the use of IFC at 100 bps for inducing sympathetic ganglion block in treating pain and symptoms associated with thromboangitis obliterans and Raynaud's disease. However, the validity of her study specifically related to IFC results is questionable because patients with both diagnoses received preliminary treatments with vasodilating drugs, novacaine block, or hydrotherapy.

Clearly additional controlled clinical studies are needed to determine whether other treatment protocols using various combinations of IFC frequency, amplitude, and duration may be more effective for treatment of pain and all of the other conditions discussed in this section. Despite the lack of controlled clinical studies, IFC is considered a viable clinical alternative to traditional transcutaneous electrical nerve stimulation (TENS) for the treatment of pain. In this regard, any electrical stimulator that delivers pulses to the body transcutaneously must be capable of delivering the pulses with sufficient and appropriate amplitude, duration, and frequencies to the involved tissues. When electrical pulses with appropriate variables pass through the target tissues, an electrical tingling paresthesia and a rhythmical muscle contraction should be perceived by the patient as occurring either simultaneously or independently.[39] These responses are produced when the stimulus has sufficient amplitude and duration and when the pulse frequency exceeds 20 pps.

The rationale for using IFC to modulate pain is based on the same electrophysiological principles that explain why traditional TENS suppresses pain. In this regard Mannheimer[40,41] and Mannheimer and Lampe[42] described four stimulation modes for producing electroanalgesia with traditional TENS that also apply to IFC devices. Although not universally effective for all pain syndromes, the most widely used and clinically effective mode used for treating acute and superficial pain syndromes as well as for chronic, deep pain syndromes is called the *conventional mode*. This mode produces non-noxious sensory level stimulation with 50 to 100 pps, a pulse duration of less than 75 μsec, and an amplitude that is low enough to produce a comfortable tingling, electrical paresthesia without muscle contraction. With stimulus variables adjusted accordingly the low pulse charge delivered to the tissues is intended to selectively excite only large-diameter afferent nerve fibers (ie, A-alpha and beta).[40-42] When only non-noxious sensory nerve fibers are excited, pain suppression is attributed to presynaptic inhibition imposed by the large-diameter sensory afferents on the transmitter cells in the dorsal horn of the spinal cord.

Pain reduction with sensory level stimulation may also be associated with activation of the analgesic neuropeptides, methionine and leucine enkephalin, which are found in various CNS structures including the substantia gelatinosa in the dorsal horn of the spinal cord.[43,44] Segmental analgesia produced by these mechanisms with stimulus variables selected for sensory level stimulation, usually occurs as soon as pulses from the TENS device are delivered to the tissue and ends within a few minutes of terminating treatment.[45-48] Based on the neurophysiological mechanisms just described, the sensory stimulation (conventional) mode is probably most appropriate for treatment of acute, superficial pain associated with inflammatory conditions, labor and delivery, musculoskeletal trauma, and postoperative incisional pain.[16,40] Electrical excitation of A-alpha and beta nerve fibers resulting in analgesia from sensory level stimulation may be achieved by alternatively using IFC between 2 and 25 bps. At these frequencies the number of cycles per beat varies from 2000 to 160 (Table 9–1), with the individual cycle duration ranging from 5 to 62.5 μsec, respectively. If the stimulus amplitude is adjusted to only produce a comfortable tingling electrical paresthesia without a muscle contraction, then primarily non-noxious A-alpha and beta afferent fibers are recruited.

The second stimulation mode described by Mannheimer[40,41] and Mannheimer and Lampe[42] for producing electroanalgesia with traditional TENS devices is called the *acupuncture-like mode*. This mode uses TENS stimulus variables and noninvasive methods that are intended to duplicate analgesia produced by electrical pulses introduced through acupuncture needles.[49,50] The pulse and phase characteristics are designed to deliver a sufficiently large charge transcutaneously to motor points or peripheral nerves that will excite high-threshold, small nonmyelinated C and A-delta fibers along with motor efferent fibers. The effectiveness of this mode is enhanced by stimulation of touch, kinesthetic, and proprioceptive receptors produced by rhythmic contractions from large and deep muscle groups without producing the sensation of tingling electrical paresthesia.[39] This is accomplished by delivering individual pulses lasting 150 to 250 usec or longer to the patient at a rate of 1 to 5

TABLE 9–1. BEAT AND CYCLE DURATIONS AS FUNCTION OF BEAT FREQUENCY (ASSUMING 4 KHz CARRIER FREQUENCY)

Beats/Sec. (bps)	Beat Duration (msec)	Cycles/Beat	Cycle Duration (μsec)
120	8.3	33.3	300.3
100	10.0	40	250
80	12.5	50	200
50	20.0	80	125
25	40.0	160	62.5
10	100.0	400	25
5	200.0	800	12.5
2	500.0	2000	5

pps and adjusting the amplitude to the highest comfortably tolerated level.[47-54] Mannheimer[39] suggested that the acupuncture-like TENS mode is most applicable for treatment of deep, aching pain of a chronic nature. Pain relief produced by this mode of TENS may be associated with elicitation of a motor response that has been shown in a few studies to promote liberation of neurohumoral analgesic substances known as endorphins and enkephalins.[55-59] Others have indicated that at least 20 to 30 min of TENS stimulation via this mode may be required to activate release of these endogenous peptides.[47,51,52] The distribution of nonsegmental analgesia produced by this mode may continue for 2 to 6 hr and sometimes longer.[47-53] This mode is probably most appropriately used for treatment of acute pain that has not responded to non-noxious sensory TENS and for chronic pain associated with degenerative joint disease, chronic inflammatory disease, and pain of neurogenic origin.[16,40]

IFC may be used as an alternative to acupuncture-mode TENS by setting the beat frequency at 5 bps, in which case the individual cycles within each beat will have a duration of only 12.5 μsec (Table 9–1). However, when delivered through small electrodes with the amplitude set at the highest comfortably tolerated level, sufficient charge will be produced endogenously within the target tissue to satisfy the electroanalgesia requirements of rhythmic muscle contractions characteristic of the acupuncture-like mode. Recall that the requirements for this mode call for stimulating touch, proprioceptive, and kinesthetic receptors by eliciting rhythmic contractions from large, deep muscles without producing a tingling electrical paresthesia. IFC applied in this manner would be very appropriate for treatment of deep, aching, chronic pain.

The third mode or TENS employs stimulus variables that combine the variables found in both the acupuncture-like and conventional TENS modes. This combination *burst mode* produces bursts or trains of pulses at low repetition (2 bursts/sec), with each burst having an internal frequency of 40 to 100 pps and burst durations ranging from 10 to 70 msec.[60-62] The concurrent delivery of low and high pulse rates produces stimulation that is perceived as a slow rhythmic electrical pulsation superimposed on a background of tingling electrical paresthesia. Selection of a low stimulus amplitude produces bursts with insufficient charge to evoke muscle contractions, and is therefore simply a modulated form of the conventional mode in which constant sensory stimulation is interrupted twice each second. Low-amplitude burst mode can substitute for conventional TENS in the treatment of acute, superficial pain syndromes. In contrast, high-amplitude burst mode delivers bursts with sufficient charge to elicit intense but comfortable, rhythmical muscle contractions at a rate of two per second on a background of strong tingling electrical paresthesia.

Thus, selection of the high-amplitude burst mode is based on both the gate theory and the endogenous opiate mechanisms.[41] When a beat frequency of 2 bps from IFC is selected and delivered to the tissues at an amplitude below that required to elicit a muscle contraction, a burst mode is produced with each burst containing 2000 cycles. This is nothing more than a modulated form of the conventional TENS in which the sensation perceived is electrical paresthesia (due to the 2000 cycles per beat) with a rhythmic sensory pulsing at 2 bps (Table 9–1). When IFC is produced in the tissues in this manner, it is appropriate for treating acute superficial or chronic, deep, aching pain. By maintaining the beat frequency at 2 bps and increasing the amplitude such that comfortable but strong muscle contractions coincide with the 2 beats per second superimposed on a moderately intense electrical paresthesia, a paradigm corresponding to high-amplitude burst mode is produced that is capable of eliciting analgesic responses produced by both conventional and acupuncture-like TENS. This combination of stimulus characteristics produces sufficient change to effectively treat pain syndromes of a chronic, deep aching nature.

The last mode of TENS described by Mannheimer is capable of exciting most sensory and motor nerve fibers to the extent that a strong continuous tingling paresthesia is perceived along with either tetanic or fascicular muscle contractions.[39] This least tolerable of the four TENS paradigms, the *brief-intense mode*, is delivered to the tissues at a frequency of 100 to 150 pps, with long-duration pulses of 150 μsec to 10 msec and the amplitude adjusted to the highest tolerable level of comfort. A stimulus with these characteristics is capable of producing profound analgesia within 1 to 15 min, which makes this mode appropriate for applications requiring rapid onset of pain suppression. In fact, a profound level of analgesia may be achieved in that time period that allows procedures such as painful joint mobilization, surgical wound debridement, deep transverse friction massage, and some vigorous stretching techniques to be performed.[55,56] One explanation for the analgesic efficaciousness of brief-intense TENS is conduction block, which may be attributed to chemical, anodal, or ischemic mechanisms.[63–65] To mimic the brief-intense mode of traditional TENS with IFC, beat characteristics that correspond to traditional TENS must be used. Selecting a beat frequency between 100 and 120 bps produces a beat duration between 10 and 8 msec. If the amplitude is adjusted to the highest-tolerated output, a strong continuous tingling paresthesia combined with mild to moderate muscle fasciculation or tetany will be produced. Because this technique may induce analgesia within 15 min, one should be aware that muscle ischemia may also occur, especially if tetanic contractions are maintained. As previously mentioned, the rapid-onset analgesia produced by this combination of IFC stimulus variables may be used to allow performance of procedures such as painful surgical wound debridement and deep transverse friction massage.

Thus, IFC may be as effective as traditional TENS in suppressing acute or chronic, superficial or deep, pain from various tissue origins.

METHODS OF APPLICATION

Quadripolar Method
The previous discussion has indicated that two-circuit IFC is generated by a device having two isolated oscillator circuits that produce AC in the vicinity

of 4 kHz. With the quadripolar method, current from each circuit is delivered to two electrodes; therefore four electrodes must be applied to the body in a crisscross arrangement to allow mixing of the two currents and formation of the endogenous amplitude-modulated beats. This method of applying IFC may utilize either four individual electrodes composed of metal or carbonized rubber covered with sponges (Fig. 9–14) or one nonconductive rubber pad with two fabric-covered electrodes from each circuit laminated into the pad in a cross-diagonal arrangement (Fig. 9–15). The four individual electrodes may be applied cross-diagonally to the body in either a planar arrangement (all electrodes on one surface) as shown in Figure 9–16A, or a co-planar arrangement (electrodes from both circuits on opposing surfaces).

Optimum production of endogenous IFC beats requires that the individual electrodes in a quadripolar arrangement be positioned on the skin to allow optimum heterodyning (mixing) of currents near or within the desired target tissue area. To achieve this the therapist must observe that electrode leads for many conventional IFC devices are color coded. One circuit may have red leads and the other circuit white leads. In addition, both ends of the leads that connect to the device and the electrode are also color coded. To optimize the

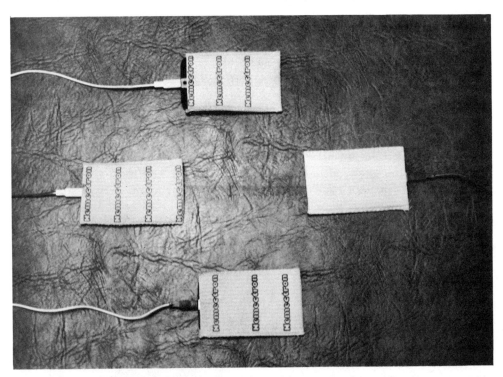

Figure 9–14. Four individual electrodes with sponges in a criss-cross arrangement. *(From Deutsche Nemectron GmbH, Durlacher Allee 47, D-7500 Karlsruhe 1, W. Germany, with permission.)*

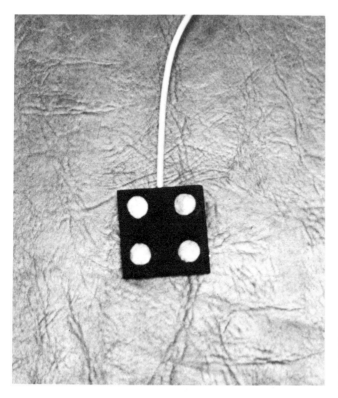

Figure 9–15. A rubber pad applicator with two electrodes for each circuit for quadripolar applications.

endogenous beating effect, the terminals of the connecting leads that are closest together should be the same color (Fig. 9–17). This color arrangement applies to the use of four individual pad or vacuum electrodes. The rubber pad with two electrodes from each circuit laminated into it cross-diagonally, is applied to the body in a planar arrangement. If the pad is split, the two halves may be applied in a co-planar arrangement so that the two circuits are oriented in a cross-diagonal alignment (Fig. 9–18).

The four individual electrodes are also available as separate vacuum electrodes, each consisting of a metal sponge-covered plate contained within a rubber suction cup attached to a vacuum pump and the IFC generator by a hollow tube. A single rubber-cup vacuum electrode in a variety of sizes, containing four small metal plates (two for each circuit) covered by a sponge, may also be available for more localized applications (Fig. 9–19). Vacuum electrodes are held to the patient with negative pressure created by a vacuum pump. The vacuum pump usually allows selection of continuous or pulsed vacuum modes. The magnitude of the vacuum should be adjusted so the least amount of suction is used to keep the electrodes on the skin. Vacuum electrodes are easy to apply because no straps are required. In addition, the negative pressure within the electrode draws cutaneous capillary fluid closer to the

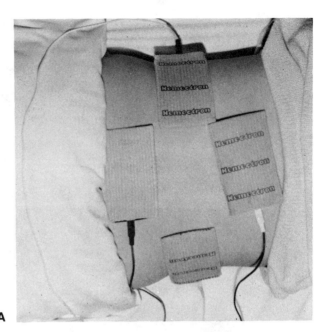

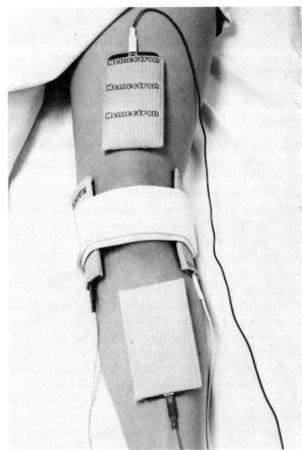

Figure 9–16. Quadripolar planar (**A**) and co-planar (**B**) electrode application techniques. *(From Deutsche Nemectron GmbH, Durlacher Allee 47, D-7500 Karlsruhe 1, W. Germany, with permission.)*

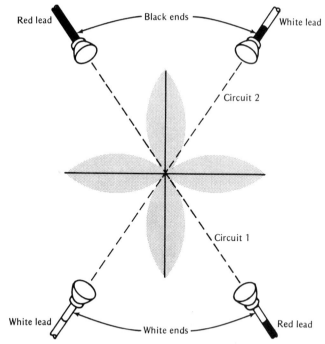

Figure 9–17. For optimum endogenous interference effect, electrodes must be positioned by colorcoding. *(Adapted from DeDomenico G. Basic Guidelines for Interferential Therapy. Sydney, Theramed, 1981: 10)*

skin surface, which serves to enhance conductivity of current across the skin. If vacuum pressure is too high a superficial hematoma with petechiae may be observed when electrodes are removed. Therefore, it is not advisable to use vacuum electrodes on patients with fragile skin or on skin that is vulnerable to ecchymosis. A soft moistened sponge is inserted into each suction cup to contact the metal plate and enhance conductivity. The smallest self-contained quadripolar applicator has four very small electrodes (two from each circuit)

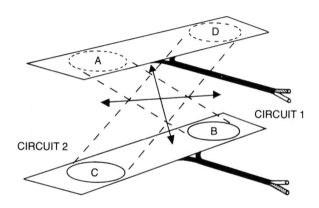

Figure 9–18. Split quadripolar electrode pads arranged for co-planar application. *(From DeDomenico G, ed. New Dimensions in Inteferential Therapy. A Theoretical and Clinical Guide. Lindfield, NSW, Australia, Reid Medical Books, 1987:76, with permission.)*

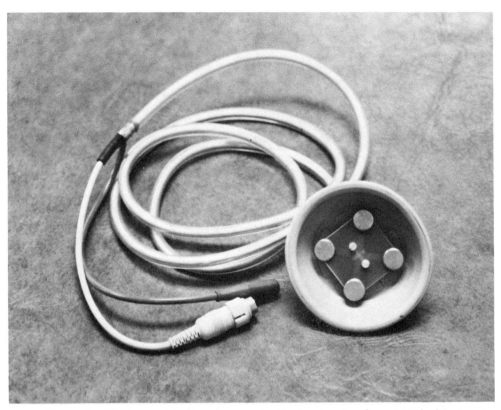

Figure 9–19. A quadripolar vacuum electrode showing four metal plates over which a moist sponge is inserted.

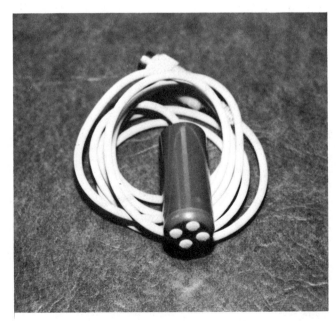

Figure 9–20. A quadripolar probe applicator used for stimulation of trigger or acupuncture points.

embedded into one end of a plastic cylinder having a diameter of 3 cm (Fig. 9–20). This applicator is sometimes referred to as a *quadripolar probe*, which is intended for transcutaneous stimulation of trigger or acupuncture points. For certain quadripolar applications it is also possible to combine two pad electrodes with two vacuum electrodes in cross-diagonal arrangements (Fig. 9–21).

Bipolar Method

The bipolar method is used to deliver premodulated IFC via two electrodes from only one of the two available circuits (in a two-circuit IFC device) while the other circuit remains open. The bipolar application method may utilize two sponge-covered metal plate electrodes, two vacuum electrodes, or a probe applicator with two electrodes built into the tip. Figure 9–22 shows two sponge-covered carbonized electrodes applied to a lower leg and ankle in a bipolar arrangement.

Recall that with the bipolar method the beats are pre (amplitude) modulated within the device and are delivered directly to the skin, unlike the quadripolar method in which the AC arriving at the skin–electrode interface is unmodulated. Thus, the bipolar method by which premodulated IFC is applied does not provide endogenously formed IFC beats because the two alternating currents are mixed inside the device. In practice, it is easier to apply two electrodes with the bipolar method than four with the quadripolar method except when a single four-electrode pad or vacuum electrode is used. In theory the premodulated beats delivered to the skin with the bipolar method may be perceived as feeling more intense than the unmodulated AC delivered to the skin with the quadripolar method.

Hexipolar Method

The use of six electrodes is required when IFC is generated by three-circuit devices. Just as is the case for two-circuit devices, two electrodes are required for each circuit. As previously mentioned in the section on physical principles, the three pairs of electrodes are contained within two Y-shaped pad or vacuum applicators, which must be applied to the skin so the three currents can mix and form amplitude-modulated beats within the tissues. (Fig. 9–9).

Scanning Versus Static-Field IFC

Whenever it is clinically difficult to identify the exact site of tissue involvement, such as the site of pain origin, the scanning IFC mode is preferred over the static mode. In theory when IFC is scanned through the tissues a larger volume of tissue is stimulated by the current than occurs with the non-scanning (static) mode. This allows the position of the areas of maximum stimulation to shift to-and-fro, which increases the probability that the involved tissues will receive stimulation. Static-field IFC is more appropriately used when the target tissue is well defined or localized.

A.

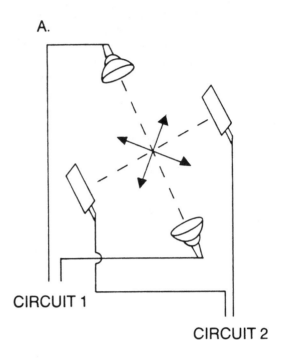

CIRCUIT 1

CIRCUIT 2

B.

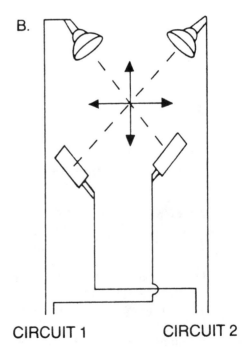

CIRCUIT 1   CIRCUIT 2

Figure 9–21. A quadripolar combination of pad electrodes in one circuit and vacuum electrodes in the other (**A**) and pad and vacuum electrodes in both circuits (**B**). *(From DeDomenico G, ed:* New Dimensions in Inteferential Therapy. A Theoretical and Clinical Guide. *Lindfield, NSW, Australia, Reid Medical Books, 1987:76, with permission.)*

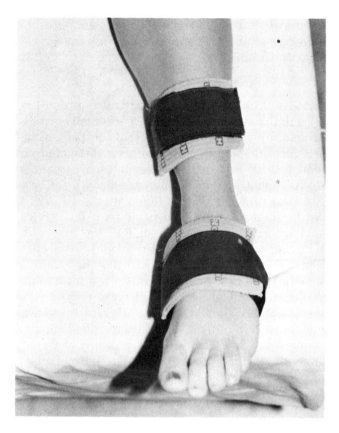

Figure 9–22. Two pad electrodes showing a bipolar application for premodulated IFC.

Constant Frequency Versus Variable-Beat Frequency Modulation

Although few reports were found in the literature related to advantages or disadvantages of constant- or variable-beat frequency, clinical practice has shown that less accommodation of nerve fibers occurs when IFC is applied in the variable-beat frequency mode. Examples of variable-beat frequency programs were presented in an earlier section of this chapter. According to DeDomenico[35] a variable beat frequency between 80 and 100 bps produces better and longer-lasting analgesia than a constant frequency of 100 bps.

CLINICAL DECISION MAKING

In the previous discussion related to clinical applications of IFC, four main areas were mentioned for which there are some clinical studies supporting IFC as an efficacious electrotherapeutic intervention. In this section clinical decision-making paradigms will be used to illustrate how IFC may be used to treat select dysfunctions associated with the four areas: orthopedic, vascular, urogenital, and pain conditions. However, because there is a paucity of published results from controlled clinical studies in which IFC has been used, the reader should realize that the suggested clinical applications and methods of treatment presented are empirically based.

Paradigm 1

A 47-year-old male with a diagnosis of delayed union fracture of the right first metatarsal shaft was referred 3 months after his podiatrist performed a wedge osteotomy to correct a bunion deformity. Despite the fact that the patient had been ambulating with crutches since the surgery and had been instructed not to bear weight on his right foot, he still experienced constant aching pain in the medial aspect of the foot. Treatment of the osteotomy site with IFC was begun immediately according to the protocol of Nikolova[21] discussed earlier. Four small pad electrodes (two from each circuit of a two-circuit IFC device) were applied in a cross-diagonal arrangement along the shaft of the first metatarsal with the osteotomy site lying within the zone spanned by the criss-crossed electrode arrangement. Using a frequency of 100 bps and a sub-motor-stimulus amplitude of 10 to 20 mA, treatment was given for 20 min, 5 days a week for 6 weeks. X-rays taken at weekly intervals confirmed a gradual buildup of callus at the osteotomy site. At 6 weeks, IFC treatment was discontinued because sufficient callus had formed to make the site stable and the patient's symptoms were markedly reduced. Additional x-rays revealed that callus continued to form until healing was complete at the end of an additional 3 weeks, at which time the patient was instructed to ambulate with a partial weight-bearing gait.

Paradigm 2

Question: Could one expect that patients with deficient arterial circulation, such as occurs in Raynaud's disease, would derive benefit from stimulating the cervical sympathetic chain with IFC?

Answer: Based on the previous reference to Schoeler's[25] work on stimulation or the stellate ganglion, a positive outcome may be expected by placing a small quadripolar pad electrode posterior to the belly of the ipsilateral sternocleidomastoid muscle and adjusting the beat frequency to vary between 90 and 100 bps at an amplitude of 4 to 8 mA for 8 min. Additionally, the current amplitude must excite the cervical plexus, causing the scapula to be elevated and the head turned toward the side of stimulation. According to Schoeler, previously depressed or absent digital pulse volume in the ipsilateral hand becomes measurable following 6 to 8 minutes of IFC stimulation, suggesting that electrical block of the stellate ganglion has occurred. After 12 to 20 treatment sessions, circulation to the involved extremity may be improved, and may continue improvement so that the number of ganglion injection blockade procedures may be reduced considerably.

Question: Could one expect that patients with venous insufficiency, venous thrombosis, or orthostatic hypotension would derive benefit from stimulating leg musculature with IFC to promote venous return?

Answer: Based on case studies by Kaindl and associates,[66] who used venograms to study blood flow, rhythmical contractions of leg muscles produced by IFC improves the emptying of leg veins. In addition. Martella and colleagues[67] used electrical stimulation to elicit 20 contractions per min in leg muscles of 350 patients during the postoperative period immediately following various surgical procedures. They reported that none of the patients developed thrombosis or embolism. Thus, IFC applied with either quadripolar or bipolar electrodes to leg (pre- and posttibial) muscles at 5 to 15 bps is appropriate treatment to facilitate the muscle pump mechanism in patients with venous circulation problems.

Paradigm 3

Neuromuscular electrical stimulation using various techniques has been shown to be effective in the treatment of urinary stress incontinence (incompetence of the urethral sphincter mechanism), which is more common in women than in men. According to reports from various sources,[29,34,68] at least 50 percent of patients treated for stress incontinence with IFC respond very favorably, with virtually complete freedom from incontinence. According to Laycock and Green,[68] the keys to producing optimum inhibition to the involuntary loss of urine in females with quadripolar IFC is to position the electrodes so that (1) they are in close proximity to the pudendal nerve; (2) current flows through the path of least resistance; (3) current spread to muscles outside of the pelvic floor is minimized; and (4) the patient is comfortable.

From experiments using vaginal sensors to determine optimum current flow and pelvic muscular contraction during IFC stimulation with different electrode positions, Laycock and Green[68] determined that the criteria listed above are best met by using the following quadripolar electrode positions. Using pad electrodes, one electrode from each circuit is placed just medial to the ischial tuberosity on each side of the anus (to stimulate the pudendal nerves) and the other two electrodes from each circuit are placed in criss-cross arrangement over the obturator foramina 1.5 to 2.0 cm lateral to the symphysis pubis. The dimension of the electrodes is 8 by 6 cm. The patient, in a semi-sitting position, sits on the two electrodes that are placed medial to the ischial tuberosities while the other two electrodes are held in place with light sandbags. The IFC stimulus variables found by Laycock and Green[68] to be most efficacious for stimulation of the pudendal nerves and pelvic floor musculature include a frequency sweep from 10 to 50 bps and a maximum current level within a range of 35 to 60 mA adjusted according to the patient's tolerance for 15 min, followed by 15 min at 50 bps and an amplitude set to patient tolerance also within the range of 35 to 60 mA. Although daily treatments of 20 min has been suggested by Plevnik and associates,[69] Laycock and Green[68] report obtaining good results with three 30-minute treatments per week for a total of 12 treatments. In addition, patients are taught to do pelvic floor exercises in a home program.

Paradigm 4

Question: Can IFC be used as a substitute for traditional TENS to produce analgesia in patients who present with acute, superficial or chronic, deep aching pain?

Answer: In reviewing the literature no controlled clinical studies published in refereed journals were found that directly support this premise. However, if the stimulus variables described in numerous traditional TENS studies[48,49,55,60,70] can be produced by IFC devices, then these devices can also deliver the desired quantity of charge to the target nerve(s), allowing the clinical response of electroanalgesia to be achieved. Alon and co-workers[71] reported producing adequate stimulation with a prototype stimulator capable of providing phase and pulse variables with variable voltage ranges. They concluded that physiological responses are similar as stimulus variables change from "low" to "high" voltage above 150 volts.

Thus, for a TENS device (all electrotherapeutic devices are TENS devices) to most efficaciously suppress pain, it is essential that the device deliver electrical pulses with sufficient amplitude, duration, and frequency to the target tissues so that electrical, tingling paresthesia and rhythmical muscle contraction responses are produced simultaneously or independently.[39] According to Mannheimer[40,41] and Mannheimer and Lampe,[42] conventional mode TENS, although not universally effective for all pain syndromes, is the most widely used and clinically effective mode used for treating acute and superficial pain syndromes as well for chronic, deep pain. The stimulus variables for tradition TENS in the conventional mode produce non-noxious sensory stimulation. Primarily A-alpha and beta afferent fibers are recruited with a pulse rate of 50 to 100 pps, a pulse duration of 30 to 75 μsec, and an amplitude that is low enough to produce a comfortable tingling, electrical paresthesia without muscle contraction.[40–42] The same nerve fibers may be recruited and the same electrical paresthesia produced with IFC if a constant-beat frequency of 25 bps is selected, in which case each beat would contain 160 cycles each having a duration of 62.5 μsec. Thus, IFC applied in this manner would be appropriate for treating acute superficial or chronic, deep aching pain.

Other Muscle-Stimulation Applications

Muscle stimulation with IFC for restoring purposeful or volitional movements is difficult because of the rhythmical quality of contractions produced. IFC devices operated in either the static or variable-frequency mode and applied to a group of agonistic muscles with quadripolar or bipolar electrodes will not elicit a physiological-like contraction that results in functional movement of a skeletal lever. Likewise for muscle strengthening; a gradual buildup to a sustained vigorous contraction with a gradual decline in contractile force cannot be achieved with conventional IFC. However, some IFC devices are equipped with a selectable mode that delivers AC at a frequency of 2000 pps modulated in bursts 50 times per second. This current applied from bipolar electrodes produces a muscle contraction response similar to that produced by devices that deliver 50 bursts per second with a carrier frequency of 2500 pps. This current is not interference current.

TREATMENT CONSIDERATIONS

Preparation for Treatment
To optimize patient compliance to treatment and obtain positive treatment outcomes, steps must be taken to avoid potential dangers when IFC is administered by making the following preparations. Each patient should receive a thorough evaluation to determine if the integument and neural pathways that convey cutaneous sensation for pain and temperature are intact. To further improve patient compliance, the skin where electrodes will be applied should be washed to remove any nonconductive skin oil and briefly warmed with a superficial heating agent to decrease skin impedance and improve conductivity. Excessive hair present on the skin where electrodes will be applied may also increase resistance. Close clipping of hair, but not shaving, may make treatment more comfortable. Electrodes should not be placed over cuts, abrasions, scratches, or denuded skin because current density tends to concentrate in these areas and discomfort may occur. When electrodes are applied they should all be of equal size, and pad electrodes should be secured to the patient with pressure evenly distributed over the entire electrode surface. Absorbent sponges should be thoroughly and evenly moistened with tap water but not saturated, to facilitate conductivity. Patient evaluation will provide information enabling the therapist to choose the appropriate type, size, and position of electrodes. As mentioned earlier, vacuum electrodes may cause temporary hematoma or ecchymosis when used on fragile skin. When vacuum electrodes are used the vacuum should be adjusted to provide only enough suction to hold the electrodes in place. Electrodes should be positioned to allow optimum conduction of IFC to the target tissues. Because IFC is alternating current, no electrolytic effects are produced on the skin or in tissues lying adjacent to orthopedic metallic implants.

In preparing the patient for treatment, explain clearly what IFC is and the intent of the treatment. Caution the patient not to touch or adjust the electrodes or the equipment during treatment and to call for assistance if at any time the treatment becomes painful or any adverse reaction begins to occur. During the first few treatments the initial milliamperage should be adjusted relatively low, and then advanced as required to offset accommodation.

Contraindications
Conditions for which IFC is contraindicated are generally similar to those cited for most other types of therapeutic electrical stimulation. Asthenic individuals and children with small body mass should not receive IFC to the rib cage because electrical current may tend to be conducted into or through vital

organs and interfere with their function. Patients with demand-type cardiac pacemakers should not receive IFC to the rib cage, because the electrical field may cause erratic functioning or malfunctioning of the pacemaker, leading to asystole or ventricular fibrillation. A similar danger exists for patients who have advanced cardiac disease. Patients with severe hypertension or hypotension may react adversely to IFC owing to increased anxiety and psychogenic responses. Blood pressure regulation may be altered in these cases either when IFC stimulates the autonomic nervous system in the extremities or when the sympathic chain is stimulated in the cervical or lumbosacral regions. One must be especially observant of undesirable vascular responses to treatment when IFC is applied to the neck to stimulate the stellate ganglion. Care must be taken in this case to avoid stimulating the carotid sinus.

Patients with arterial or venous thrombosis or thrombophlebitis are at risk of developing embolism when IFC is applied over or adjacent to the vessels containing the thrombus. Emboli may break off from the thrombus secondary to mechanical squeezing of blood vessels from contraction of surrounding muscles or direct stimulation of smooth muscle in arteries. Following trauma or when tissues are vulnerable to hemorrhage or hematoma, IFC should not be used over the involved area. IFC is contraindicated over dermatological diseases such as psoriasis and dermatitis.

Conditions in which the temperature of the body is elevated or a disease process produces an increase in local cellular metabolism are also contraindicated for IFC application. Muscle contraction evoked by IFC causes increased local and general metabolism, which in turn may cause exacerbation of conditions such as neoplasm, tuberculosis, infection, and fever.

IFC should not be applied to the abdominal, lumbosacral, or pelvic areas of pregnant women because of the risk that the current may induce uterine contractions or adversely affect the developing fetus.

Patients who are senile or confused should not receive IFC therapy because of their inability to comprehend why the treatment is being given. In addition, these patients are often unable to remain relaxed or quiescent during a treatment period and may pull electrodes or lead wires off.

Finally, whenever a patient is receiving another type of electrotherapeutic treatment such as traditional TENS, or has indwelling electrodes, lead wires, or transmitters for electrophrenic pacing or cerebellar or urinary bladder stimulation, IFC should not be applied in such a way that its current crosses the path of the device, its lead wires, or its electrodes. If IFC is applied to a patient within 15 feet of a shortwave diathermy device that is in operation, the electrode leads of the IFC unit may act as an antenna and collect the radiant frequency energy from the shortwave device. This may not only adversely effect the operation of the IFC device but may also produce undesirable surging of the stimulus the patient is receiving.

SUMMARY

Interference current is produced by mixing two or three independent circuits of alternating current with pulses of 3900 to 5000 Hz. When the current from these circuits mixes within the tissues, an amplitude-modulated beat is produced where the currents intersect. The frequency of the beat current may be held constant at any value between 1 and 120 bps, or it may be continuously varied over this range or segments of this range in 15-sec repetitions. Conditions IFC has improved clinically include delayed and nonunion fracture, vasospastic disease, urinary stress incontinence, venous insufficiency, and acute superficial and chronic deep pain.

REFERENCES

1. Nemec H. Electromedizinischer Apparat patent number 163979. Patent document number 165657. Published by the Austrian Patent Office, April 11, 1950
2. Bueche F. *Principles of Physics*. New York, McGraw-Hill, 1965
3. Gildemesiter, M: Untersuchungen uber die Wirkung der mittelfrequenzstrome auf den Menschen. *Pfluger's Arch Ges Physiol*. 247:266, 1944
4. American Physical Therapy Association. *Standard Terminology of Electrotherapy: Report of the Electrotherapy Standards Committee of the Section of Clinical Electrophysiology* (in press)
5. Hansjuergens A. Dynamische Interferenzstromtherapie. *Physik Med Rehabil*. 15:24, 1974
6. Szehi E, David E. The stereodynamic interferential current—new electrotherapeutic technique. *Electromedica*. 48: 13, 1980
7. Goodgold J, Eberstein A. *Electrodiagnosis of Neuromuscular Diseases*. Baltimore, Williams & Wilkins, 1978
8. Mountcastle VB, (ed). *Medical Physiology*, 13th ed. St. Louis, CV Mosby, 1974: 1
9. Benton L, Baker L, Bowman B, et al. *Functional Electrical Stimulation—A Practical Clinical Guide, 2nd ed*. Downey, CA, Rancho Los Amigos Hospital, 1980
10. Krnjevic K, Miledi R. Failure of neuromuscular propagation in rats. *J Physiol*. 140:440, 1958
11. Brown G, Burns B. Fatigue and neuromuscular block in mammalian skeletal muscle. *Proc Roy Soc*. 136:182, 1949
12. Wyss O. Die Reizwirkung sinusformiger Wechselstrome untersucht bis zur oberen Grenze der Niederfrequenz (1000 Hz). *Helv Physiol Acta*. 21:419, 1963
13. Lullies H, Trincker D. Taschenbuch der Physiologie. Stuttgart, Fischer, 1970:2
14. Selkurt E, ed. *Physiology, 2nd ed*. Boston, Little, Brown, 1966
15. Dumoulin J, de Bisschop G. *Electrotherapie*. Paris, 1966. In: Edel H. *Fibel der Elektrodiagnostik und Electrotherapie*, 3rd ed. Auflage, Dresden, Steinkopf, 1975, 126
16. Alon G. *High Voltage Stimulation: An Integrated Approach to Clinical Electrotherapy*. Chattanooga, TN, Chattanooga Corp, 1987: 17

17. Meyer-Waarden K, Hansjuergens A, Friedman B. New research results—Demonstration of interferential current in deep biological structures. *Biomed Technik.* 25:295, 1980
18. Nikolova-Troeva L. The effect of interference current in facial nerve neuritis. *Arztliche Praxis.* 13:520, 1966
19. Eigler E. Success achieved by treatment with interferential current on patients with epicondylitis humeri. Read at the 84th congress of the German Society of Physical Medicine and Rehabilitation, Hannover, 1979
20. Nikolova-Troeva L. Interference current therapy in distortion, contusions and luxations of the joints. *Med Wochenschrift (Munich).* 109:579, 1967
21. Nikolova L. Physiotherapeutic rehabilitation in the presence of fracture complications. *Med Wochenschr (Munich).* 111:592, 1969
22. Ganne JM, Speculand B, Mayne LH, et al. Inferential therapy to promote union of mandibular fractures. *Aust NZ J Surg.* 49:81, 1979
23. Laabs W, May E, Richter K, et al. Knochenheilung und dynamischer interferenzstrom (DIC)—Erste vergleichende tier experimentelle studie an schafen. Teil I: Experimentalles vorgchen und histologische ergebnisse. Teil II: Physikalische und chemische ergebnisse. *Langenbecke Arch Chir.* 356:219, 1982
24. Guttler P, Kleditsche J. Die Anregung der Kallusbildung durch Interferenzstrome. *Deutsch Gesund Wesen.* 34:91, 1979
25. Schoeler H. Physikalische Grenzstrangblockade. *Tech Med.* 1, 1972
26. Nikolova-Troeva L. The modern electrotherapeutic methods in the therapy of endarteritis obliterans. *Ther Gegenwart.* 102:190, 1966
27. Belcher J. Interferential therapy. *NZ J Physiotherapy.* 6:29, 1974
28. Palmer M. *Urinary Incontinence.* Thorofare, NJ, Slack, 1985
29. McQuire W. Electrotherapy and exercise for stress incontinence and urinary frequency. *Physiotherapy.* 61:305, 1975
30. Chirarelli P, O'Keefe D. Physiotherapy for the pelvic floor. *Aust J Physiother.* 27:4, 1981
31. Wharton L. The non-operative treatment of stress incontinence in women. *J Urol.* 69:511, 1953
32. Millard R. The conservative management of urinary incontinence. *Aust Physiother Ob/Gyn Bull.* 3:30, 1982
33. Haag W. Practical experience with interference current therapy in gynecology. *Frauenarzt.* 1:1, 1979
34. DeDomenico G. Pain relief with interferential therapy. *Aust J Physiotherapy.* 28:14, 1982
35. DeDomenico G. Treatment Techniques. In: DeDomenico G, ed. *New Dimensions in Interferential Therapy. A Theoretical and Clinical Guide.* Lindfield, NSW, Australia, Reid Medical Books, 1987: 96–100
36. Taylor K, Newton RA, Personius W, et al. Effects of interferential current stimulation for treatment of subjects with recurrent jaw pain. *Phys Ther.* 67:346, 1987
37. Burghart W. Behandlung mit dem Nemectron. *Wien Med Wochenschri.* 101:999, 1951
38. Nikolova-Troeva L. Surgical Conditions. In: *Treatment with Interference Current.* New York, Churchill Livingstone, 1987: 95–98
39. Mannheimer JS. Transcutaneous electrical nerve stimulation: Its uses and effectiveness with patients in pain. In: Echternach JL, *Pain.* New York, Churchill Livingstone, 1987: 220

40. Mannheimer JS. Electrode placement for transcutaneous electrical nerve stimulation. *Phys Ther.* 58:1455, 1978
41. Mannheimer JS. *Optimal Stimulation Sites for TENS Electrodes.* Trenton, NJ, Hibbert, 1980
42. Mannheimer JS, Lampe GN. *Electrode placement sites and their relationships.* In: *Mannheimer JS, Lampe GN, eds. Clinical Transcutaneous Electrical Nerve Stimulation.* Philadelphia, FA Davis, 1984: 249–329
43. Bishop B. Pain: its physiology and rationale for management, parts I, II, and III. *Phys Ther.* 60:13, 1980
44. Barker JL, Groul DL, Guang LM, et al. Enkephalin: pharmacologic evidence for diverse functional roles in the nervous system using primary cultures of dissociated spinal neurons. *Dev Neurosci.* 4:87, 1978
45. Woolf CJ, Mitchell D, Myers RA, et al. Failure of naloxone to reverse peripheral transcutaneous electroanalgesia in patients suffering from acute trauma. *S Africa Med J.* 53:179, 1978
46. Burton C, Maurer DD. Pain suppression by transcutaneous electrical stimulation. *IEEE Trans Biomed Eng.* 21:81, 1974
47. Linzer M, Long DM. Transcutaneous neural stimulation for relief of pain. *IEEE Trans Biomed Eng.* 23:341, 1974
48. Andersson SA, Holmgren E, Roos A. Analgesic effects of peripheral conditioning stimulation II. Importance of certain stimulation parameters. *Acupunc Electrother Res.* 2:237, 1977
49. Andersson SA, Holmgren E. Analgesic effects of peripheral conditioning stimulation III. Effect of high frequency stimulation: Segmental mechanisms interacting with pain. *Acupunc Electrother Res.* 3:23, 1978
50. Holmgren E. Increase of pain threshold as a function of conditioning electrical stimulation: An experimental study with application to electroacupuncture for pain suppression. *Am J Clin Med.* 3:133, 1975
51. Andersson SA, Holmgren E. Pain threshold effects of peripheral conditioning stimulation. In: Bonica J, Albe-Fessard D, eds. *Advances in Pain Research and Therapy.* New York, Raven Press, 1976:6; 761
52. Chapman CR, Wilson ME, Gehrig JD. Comparative effects of acupuncture on dental pain: Evaluation of threshold estimation and sensory decision therory. *Pain.* 3:2131, 1977
53. Chapman CR, Chen AC, Bonica JJ. Effects of intrasegmental electrical acupuncture on dental pain: Evaluation of threshold estimation and sensory decision theory. *Pain.* 3:2131, 1977
54. Eriksson MBE, Sjolund BH. Acupuncture-like electroanalgesia in TNS resistant chronic pain. In: Zotterman Y, ed. *Sensory Functions of the Skin.* Oxford, Pergamon Press, 1976: 575
55. Eriksson MBE, Sjolund BH, Neilzen S. Long term results of peripheral conditioning stimulation as analgesic measure in chronic pain. *Pain.* 335, 1979
56. Sjolund BH, Terenius L, Ericksson MBE. Increased cerebrospinal fluid levels of endorphin after electro-acupuncture. *Acta Physiol Scand.* 100:382, 1977
57. Sjolund BH, Ericksson MBE. Electro-acupuncture and endogenous morphine. *Lancet.* 2:1035, 1976
58. Akil H, Richardson DE, Barchas JD, et al. Appearance of beta-endorphin-like immunoreactivity in human ventricular cerebrospinal fluid upon analgesic electrical stimulation. *Proc Nat Acad Sci.* 75:170, 1978

59. Fox EJ, Melzack R. Transcutaneous electrical stimulation and acupuncture: Comparison of treatment of low back pain. *Pain.* 2:141, 1976

60. Mannheimer C, Carlsson CA. The analgesic effect of transcutaneous electrical nerve stimulation (TNS) in patients with rheumatoid arthritis: A comparative study of different pulse patterns. *Pain.* 6:329, 1979

61. Mannheimer JS, Lampe GN. Pain and TENS in pain management. In: Mannheimer JS, Lampe GN, eds. *Clinical Transcutaneous Electrical Nerve Stimulation.* Philadelphia, FA Davis, 1984: 7

62. Mannheimer JS, Lampe GN. Electrode placement techniques. In: Mannheimer JS, Lampe GN, eds. *Clinical Transcutaneous Electrical Nerve Stimulation.* Philadelphia, FA Davis, 1984: 331, 562

63. Ignelzi RJ, Nyquist JK. Excitability changes in peripheral nerve fibers after repetitive electrical stimulation: Implication in pain modulation. *J Neurosurg.* 51:824, 1979

64. Mannheimer JS, Lampe GN. Factors that hinder, enhance and restore the effectiveness of TENS: Physiologic and theoretical consideration. In: Mannheimer JS, Lampe GN, eds. *Clinical Transcutaneous Electrical Nerve Stimulation.* Philadelphia, FA Davis, 1984: 529

65. Ignelzi RJ, Nyquist JK. Direct effect of electrical stimulation on peripheral nerve evoked activity. Implication for pain relief. *J Neurosurg.* 45:159, 1976

66. Kaindl F, Schuhfried F, Thurnher B, et al. Elektrische Reizung der Wadenmuskulatur und venöser Blutstrom. *Wien Klin Wochenschr.* 65:340, 1953

67. Martella J, Cincotti J, Springer W. Prevention of thromboembolic diseases by electrical stimulation of leg muscles. *Arch Phys Med.* 35:34, 1954

68. Laycock J, Green RJ. Interferential therapy in the treatment of incontinence. *Physiotherapy.* 74: 161, 1988

69. Plevnik S, Janez J, Vrtacnik P, et al. Short-term electrical stimulation: Home treatment for urinary incontinence. *World Urol.* 4:24, 1986

70. Shealy CN. Six years experience with electrical stimulation for control of pain. *Adv Neurol.* 4:475, 1974

71. Alon G, Allin J, Inbar GE. Optimization of pulse duration and pulse charge during transcutaneous electrical stimulation. *Aust J Physiotherapy.* 29:195, 1983

Transcutaneous Electrical Nerve Stimulation for Pain Management

John O. Barr

Pain has been recognized as the symptom that most commonly causes people to seek health care. In the United States alone, the economic impact of health care and lost productivity associated with chronic pain has recently been estimated to be greater than $80 billion annually.[1] Clinicians who are challenged by a wide range of clinical pain problems will find that transcutaneous electrical nerve stimulation (TENS) can be an important component of many treatment programs for pain management. Although this chapter is introductory in nature, the reader will be encouraged to critically assess factors influencing the efficacy of TENS. The chapter begins with a historical perspective on TENS. Details of commercial equipment are then reviewed and suggestions are made for improving equipment-related performance. Critical elements of clinical decision making with TENS are reviewed and key steps in implementing a successful treatment program are presented. The theoretical bases for pain management with TENS are next highlighted. Finally, the clinical effectiveness of TENS is assessed.

HISTORICAL PERSPECTIVE

The first recorded use of electricity for pain relief appeared in *Compositiones Medicae*, written in 48 A.D. by Scribonis Largus, a Roman physician. A live torpedo fish (also called the electric ray) was used for the treatment of gout and headache, its electrical discharge being used to shock the affected body part into numbness.[2] In the 1760s, John Wesley wrote specifically about the use of static electricity for pain relief. With Faraday's discovery of alternating current in the 1830s, further interest was directed toward the ability of electricity to relieve a variety of painful conditions by the late 1800s.[3,4] The early 1900s saw a proliferation of questionable therapeutic applications. This proliferation, coupled with an upsurge of promotion by both paramedical and occult practitioners, brought about federal and medical society reaction such that many manufacturers of crude stimulators were forced out of business.[5] However, electrical analgesia continued to be described in the literature into the 1950s.[3] In 1967, Wall and Sweet tested a central hypothesis of the recently proposed gate control theory of pain.[6] They reported temporarily abolishing chronic pain by electrically stimulating peripheral nerves via electrodes on the surface of the skin; the technique soon became known as *transcutaneous electrical nerve stimulation (TENS)*.[7]

For the 20-year period from 1967 to 1987, Nolan compiled a bibliography of over 300 papers concerning TENS from clinical and basic science literature.[8] In addition, a journal special issue[9] and books[10-12] have been devoted to the topic. A number of health professionals, including physical therapists, nurses, physicians, and dentists, have employed TENS for a wide range of acute and chronic pain conditions. For example, TENS for acute pain management has been utilized in the emergency room,[13] during minor surgical procedures,[14] for postoperative pain,[15] during labor and delivery,[16] with acute spinal cord injuries,[17] and for athletic injuries.[18] Quite commonly TENS has been employed for treatment of chronic back pain[19] and headache,[20] but it has also been used for chronic pain associated with a wide range of diagnoses including angina pectoris,[21] cancer,[22] causalgia,[23] Guillain-Barré syndrome,[24] reflex sympathetic dystrophy,[25] rheumatoid arthritis,[26] multiple sclerosis,[27] and phantom limb.[28] Recently, Robinson and Snyder-Mackler found that 92 percent of the physical therapists responding to their survey on electrotherapeutic modalities utilized TENS, 67 percent at least once a week.[29]

COMMERCIAL EQUIPMENT

As has been pointed out by Alon in Chapter 3, all forms of electrical nerve stimulation done through electrodes on the skin's surface represent transcutaneous electrical nerve stimulation. Quite commonly the terms TENS (transcutaneous electrical nerve stimulation), TNS (transcutaneous nerve stimulation), or TES (transcutaneous electrical stimulation) are used interchangeably to denote such a technique used for pain management.[30] (In contrast, percutaneous electrical stimulation is done through needle electrodes or surgically implanted wires.) Since 1974, when the Food and Drug Administration (FDA) classified transcutaneous electrical nerve stimulators as Class II devices, numerous domestic and foreign-made stimulators have become available. Currently there are more than 60 TENS manufacturers registered with the FDA.[31] Recently, some transcutaneous stimulators used for pain management have been classified as Class III devices (eg, "cranial electrotherapy stimulators"), and their manufacturers have enjoyed this distinction in the marketplace. Although the present discussion of commercial equipment will primarily focus on portable battery-powered Class II stimulators, similar concepts can be applied to the wide range of neuromuscular electrical stimulators used for pain control.

Contemporary TENS systems are usually marketed as a "kit" consisting of the TENS unit, a battery power source, lead wires, electrodes, instruction manual, carrying case, and possibly electrode coupling gel and adhesive patches (Fig. 10–1). The TENS unit, a small portable electrical pulse generator, may be secured by a clip to a patient's belt or clothing, or it can be carried in a pocket.

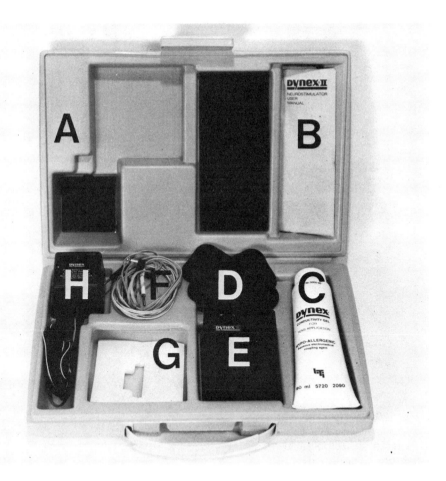

Figure 10–1. Typical TENS unit kit. Components: **A** = storage/carrying case; **B** = instruction manual; **C** = electrode gel; **D** = electrodes; **E** = TENS unit; **F** = lead wires; **G** = adhesive patches; **H** = battery charger.

TENS Units

Most units produce an electrical output having one characteristic waveform, usually of the symmetrical or balanced asymmetrical biphasic type with zero net current to minimize skin irritation. The optimal waveform for pain management has yet to be determined.[32,33] Typically, units can be operated in one or more stimulation modes (eg, conventional, strong low-rate, brief-intense, pulse-burst, modulated, or hyperstimulation). Various arrangements of control dials, switches, or buttons on the unit may allow for regulation of power (on/off), mode, and electrical stimulation characteristics (eg, amplitude, pulse duration and frequency) for one or two output channels (Fig. 10–2). As discussed

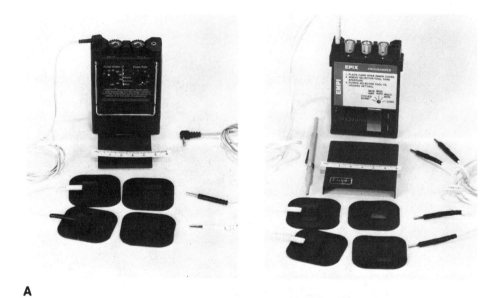

A

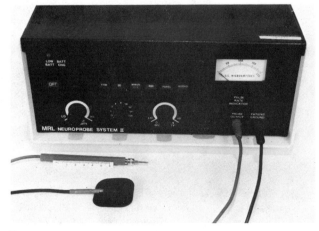

Figure 10–2. Sample of some commercially available TENS units. **A** = portable dual-channel units and attachments; **B** = stationary single channel unit (note the small-diameter electrode used for hyperstimulation).

B

in Chapter 2, numbers listed on the controls often are nonlinearly related to the actual stimulator output characteristics, which makes it difficult to predict the amount of stimulation a patient will receive. The controls themselves are usually recessed, and they may be internally located to prevent accidental movement or to limit patient access. The unit may have one or more lights to indicate that the unit is turned on, the battery charge is low, or there is a lead wire or electrode malfunction. Although two output channels would seem to provide more versatility and greater likelihood of clinical success than just one,[11] this assumption has been challenged.[34] Some units with independent channels permit asynchronous channel activation, or allow two different TENS modes to be used simultaneously.

The power source is most often a rechargeable battery pack or a long-life disposable battery. Although initially more expensive, rechargeable batteries are more economical for repeated use if properly maintained. It is especially important that a rechargeable battery be largely discharged before attempting to recharge it. If not, a "memory" develops that limits acceptance of a full charge.[34] It has been recommended that these batteries be fully discharged at least once per week, and then recharged using a slow "trickle charger," which may take 12 hours.[11] Disposable batteries are favored where reliablity is critical or for long periods of continuous stimulation, as in postoperative applications. Battery life is inversely related to the number of stimulating channels employed, stimulator output characteristics (eg, amplitude, pulse duration and frequency), and duration of stimulation. New disposable or fully recharged batteries should be stored in a cool location to better maintain shelf-life.

Lead Wires and Electrodes

Lead wires are attached to unit output channel jacks by a variety of connectors, but most commonly with subminiature phono plugs. The fit of jacks and plugs should be firm enough to prevent accidental disconnection during patient activities, yet connectors should allow for separation with minimum effort when desired by clinicians and patients. Single and paired lead wires come in various lengths. Paired wires may be attached by common separable insulation, movable plastic sleeves, or both, which limits tangling of the leads. The unit lead wire most commonly ends in a metal tip connector, which is inserted directly into a receptacle on the back of an electrode. Care must be taken not to drive the tip through the electrode surface, thus placing the tip in direct contact with the skin. This problem can be avoided by using electrodes with snap connectors or their own short leads with insulated receptacles. Tip-to-snap converters are available for various brands of lead wires. Some TENS units permit electrodes to be "piggybacked" so that more than two electrodes may be connected to an output channel. Conductive metal connectors should not come in contact with a patient's skin during treatment as high-current density will produce local irritation or burns.

TENS unit output channel jacks are often marked with symbols such as + (positive) and − (negative), and related lead wire connectors are frequently color coded. Lack of industry definitions and standardization have resulted in confusion. For example, one manufacturer refers to its red-coded connectors as being negative! Given that most contemporary TENS units have symmetrical or balanced asymmetrical biphasic waveforms that produce zero net current, and thus no polar effects, coding referenced to polarity makes no sense. Yet, based upon other waveform characteristics (eg, rapid rise or decay times for one phase), such units may have a lead or electrode that is more "active" than its paired partner. Units having monophasic or unbalanced asymmetrical biphasic waveforms can produce polar effects associated with active and "indifferent" electrodes, and thus might benefit from such coding.

Clinical effects of polarity or relative electrode activity on pain treated with TENS are not well documented.[11] In order to standardize lead and electrode orientation for each output channel, the following technique is suggested for determining if one lead is more active than its paired partner.[35] Two equal-sized electrodes are prepared and secured to the clinician's skin, one over a known motor point and the other over a bony prominence. Lead wires from one output channel are then carefully attached to the electrodes. Using a low frequency (eg, 2 pps) and narrow pulse duration (eg, 50 μsec), the amplitude control is slowly advanced to the point of initial sensation and then to initial muscle contraction. Amplitude dial settings at these two points are noted, as are differences in qualities of sensation and contraction at the electrodes. The unit is then turned off, and the lead wires are reversed at the electrodes while the electrodes themselves remain in place. Stimulation amplitude is increased to the previous settings and observations are again documented. This process can be repeated a number of times in order to discern if a difference in lead or electrode activity exists, as opposed to effects resulting from the different electrode sites. If one lead is found to be more active, its output jack and connectors can be distinctively marked with paint or durable tape. To standardize technique, the more active lead or electrode is placed distal to its paired partner during treatment.

As noted in Chapter 2, a wide variety of electrodes can be utilized for TENS (Fig. 10–3). In selecting the appropriate electrode for a given pain-management problem a number of factors should be considered, initial versus long-term cost, durability, ease of preparation and application, and potential for skin irritation. Electrodes come in a variety of sizes, and many can be cut to different sizes and shapes. Electrodes that are reusable or disposable, and non-sterile or pre-sterilized, are available for specific applications. Typically, reusable non-sterile electrodes are employed for long-term repeated use as with chronic pain, while disposable presterilized electrodes are used for acute post-operative pain.

Carbonized silicone rubber electrodes, which are relatively low in cost, come with most TENS unit kits. They require a conductive medium, which may be either water-based (eg, electrolytic gel, and moist conductive or karaya gum pads) or dry (eg, a conductive adhesive "tac gel"). Conductive media should completely cover the electrode surface in order to avoid focal areas of

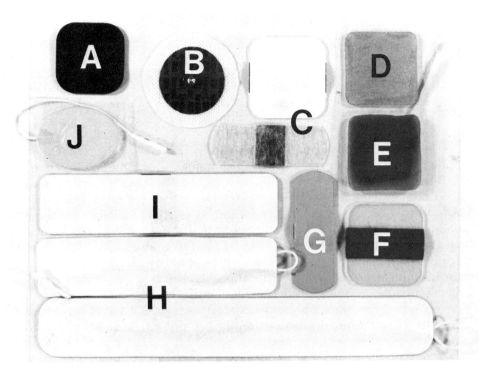

Figure 10–3. Sample of TENS electrodes. **A** = carbonized silicone rubber; **B** = pregelled self-adhering, with snap connector; **C** = disposable self-adhering; **D** = karaya gum pad; **E** = karaya gum electrode; **F** = reusable synthetic; **G** = resuable high heat/humidity; **H** = sterile postoperative; **I** = nonsterile postoperative; **J** = polymer gel.

high-current density or of high resistance that can produce skin irritation or burns. Drying out of water-based conductive media can cause areas of high-current density. If too much of the medium (water or gel) is used, it can ooze from under an electrode which may render tape or other adhesives useless to secure the electrode; or the medium may "bridge" between two electrodes in a manner that effectively shorts them out. Maintenance of the conductive medium is enhanced by attaching a lead wire to the electrode prior to placing the medium on the electrode. With a little practice, a dab of gel (quantity depending on electrode size) can be thinly, completely, and quickly spread on an electrode. Adequacy of coverage can be confirmed by reflecting room light onto the gelled electrode surface.

Carbonized rubber electrodes are commonly secured to the skin with surgical tape, or with a variety of commercial paper or foam adhesive patches. While such patches are often more convenient than tape, they are considerably more expensive. Electrode placement belts, which hold a pair of electrodes so that they can be secured in difficult to reach locations (such as the lower back), are also commercially available. At the conclusion of each treatment, siliconized carbon rubber electrodes should be washed with mild soap and warm water, thoroughly rinsed, and patted dry with a soft towel. Alcohol should not be used as a cleansing agent, as this breaks down the electrode. Over a period of months, some electrodes loose their flexibility and demonstrate increased electrical resistance, which renders them ineffective. Thus, some authorities have suggested that this type of electrode be replaced at 6-month intervals.[11]

A few TENS kits come with electrodes made of sponge rubber over a metallic base that is encased in a nonconductive backing. While such electrodes lack the glamour of other electrodes, they are inexpensive, durable, and easy to prepare and maintain. Tap water is used as the conductive medium. These electrodes can be quickly repositioned as they are often hand-held by the clinician or patient, or are secured with fishnet surgical stockinet (note: solid stockinet or elastic bandages can become wet, also creating a conductive bridge between electrodes). Impressed with the utility of this type of electrode in determining optimal electrode locations for treating pain, some clinicians have described how these electrodes can easily be fabricated at low cost.[11,36] The electrode sponges should be periodically removed if possible and washed with mild soap, thoroughly rinsed, gently compressed to remove most of the water, and air dried on a flat surface.

More expensive self-adhering electrodes are usually purchased separately from the TENS kit. While very convenient to apply, they are not without limitations. Made from reinforced karaya gum or synthetic polymers, some of these electrodes (or the skin itself) must be moistened with a few drops of water to maintain or restore conductivity and self-adhesion. Too much water, however, will turn their surfaces to non-adhering mush. Some of the most recent polymer-gel electrodes should not be moistened additionally. Between treatments, reusable models must be positioned on a nonporous backing and placed in an airtight container to prevent the conductive surface from drying out. Various self-adhering electrodes are also available for single-use applications. Unfortunately, skin irritation and burns at higher stimulation amplitudes have been noted with some karaya[37] and polymer-gel electrodes.[38] Despite having self-adhesive properties, some electrodes require additional fixation in order to withstand motion from patient activities. Because their adhesive surfaces may harbor infective organisms, these electrodes should only be used on an individual patient.

Adverse Skin Reactions

Prevention of adverse skin reactions is especially important with TENS since electrodes may remain in place for hours to days. The incidence of adverse skin reactions has been widely cited to be quite low, with 4 to 5 percent of the population having reactions to electrolytic gels, for example.[39] Eriksson and colleagues reported a 12 percent occurrence of skin irritation in their long-term study.[40] A nationwide survey of 196 physical therapy departments reported that 79% of respondents saw some side effects associated with TENS, of which the most common (68 percent) was skin irritation.[41] Noting that such reactions are the primary reason that otherwise successful TENS programs are discontinued, one electrode manufacturer has identified contributing allergic, chemical, electrical, and mechanical factors.[42] Regular inspection of patient's skin and use of alternate electrode sites may minimize the occurrence of irritation from most of these factors. Although electrodes and related materials (conductive media and adhesives) are usually made from nonirritating or hypoallergenic compounds, instances of localized skin reactions have been noted.[38,39] Rubber electrodes containing mercaptobenzothiazole or having metal components made of nickel, gels containing silicon oxide or propylene glycol, and alkaloids in karaya gum have been implicated. In such cases, different types or brands of electrodes and related materials should be utilized. Skin at electrode sites should be cleaned with mild soap and water before and after treatment. All residues, including those from operative site preps, soaps, gels, and adhesives, should be removed in order to minimize chemical reactions.

Prior to treatment, electrode sites should be inspected for cuts and abrasions, which can become focal paths of low impedance that produce high-density electrical currents. Undesirably high current density is a primary electrical factor causing skin irritation, which can be minimized by using larger electrodes that are not placed too close together (ie, at least one electrode diameter apart).[11] Griffin has reported that direct current densities of less than 1 mA / cm^2 will limit likelihood of skin irritation.[43] Under conditions of extremely intense stimulation (85 mA, 500 μsec, and 185 pps), it has been noted that electrodes larger than 4 cm^2 will prevent burns and those larger than 16 cm^2 will avoid stimulating nociceptors.[44] Overly dry skin at intended electrode sites can be hydrated by rubbing in a small amount of nonabrasive electrode gel, which overcomes undesirably high skin impedance.

Mechanical reactions are thought to be largely related to poor technique in affixing electrodes to the skin. Electrodes should be positioned to accommodate body movement. Lead wire pins or connectors should be aligned perpendicular to the plane of body segment motion, which allows the electrode to be more flexible in this orientation. A similar alignment should be used for tape, which will stretch and slacken less, thereby minimizing shear forces in the skin. For a similar reason tape, adhesive patches, and electrodes should not be stretched as they are placed on the skin. Long lead wires can be coiled and taped together at some distance from electrodes in order to provide a relief for tension pulling on the electrodes. Adhesive electrode materials should be removed by slowly lifting them as the underlying skin is held down to prevent skin stripping.

Critical Evaluation of TENS Units

Unfortunately, only a few publications have critically evaluated specific brands of either domestic or foreign-made TENS units since the mid-1970's.[19,34,45,46]

Apparently only battery-powered units were assessed; no disposable postoperative models were included. Mason tested TENS unit electrical output characteristics and effectiveness in alleviating pain.[19] Using a simulated body impedance circuit, three out of the five units demonstrated changes in current output as resistive loads were varied from 500 to 5000 Ω. Noticeable changes in the sensation produced by TENS were also related to current variations based on different electrode preparations. On one unit, simultaneous adjustment of amplitude and frequency controls from mid to maximum settings resulted in a 37 percent decrease in output pulse duration. Such lack of independence between unit control settings and other output characteristics is usually not apparent when lower settings are used.[47] Present standards require that a given control not change by more than 5 percent of its adjusted value when the remaining controls are adjusted over their range in any combination.[48] All five units were able to produce some degree of pain relief in certain instances. Ultimately, two of the units (Stim-Tech EPC and Avery TNS) were recommended for use in Veterans Administration Prosthetic Center Clinics.

The clinical and engineering staff of Health Devices conducted extensive consumer-oriented tests on 18 TENS units.[34] These tests included measurement of various electrical output characteristics, assessment of functional controls, minimization of startle response, safety related to output characteristics, labeling and warning legends, battery life and insertion, construction quality, effects of drops and fluid spills, damage from open- and short-circuit conditions, ease of use, indication of on/off status, quality of operator's manual, and cost of the TENS unit kits. Interestingly, warranties and service on equipment were not addressed. Most units were judged as being approximately equal and received "acceptable" ratings. Some of the evaluated units had controls that were difficult to see clearly or to adjust which could present a significant problem to some elderly or disabled patients. Two units (Bio-Instrumentation TENS-1 and Koken Kogyo Health Point) were not recommended. Although two of the units (Electreat 250 and Koken Kogyo Health Point) exceeded the 75 μC charge per pulse maximum limit proposed in the Association for the Advancement of Medical Instrumentation (AAMI) Standard for Transcutaneous Electrical Nerve Stimulators (1980), they were not seen to pose a risk greater than that associated with most of the other units. (Instead, the Health Devices staff challenged the validity of the testing circuit load used with the 1980 AAMI standard.) Given the generally high cost of TENS units, manufacturers were encouraged to review their pricing policies. Although efficacy of the TENS units was not evaluated, it was suggested that clinicians consider having more than one brand of unit available in order to improve the possibility of determining the most effective unit for a given patient.

Stamp briefly summarized the evaluation of 18 TENS units marketed in Britain during 1980 and 1981.[46] Recommended design features were reviewed. Breakage of electrode cables and battery connector wires from mechanical stress were the two most common equipment failures. Although concern for the cost of TENS units was expressed, it was noted that product quality was usually related to unit price.

Campbell assessed the electrical output characteristics of 10 TENS units that were commercially available in the United Kingdom.[45] Some of the measurements were conducted with resistive loads varying between 1000 and 5000 Ω, values that had been derived from actual electrode preparations. None of the units was determined to have either true constant current or constant voltage outputs over this load range. Nonlinear relationships were seen between control settings and output characteristics of amplitude, frequency, and pulse duration for most units. The test load used for establishing the AAMI Standard for Transcutaneous Electrical Nerve Stimulators (revised, 1981) was criticized, but this time in reference to the 25 μC charge per pulse threshold for a required label warning against transthoracic use. The more expensive units did not necessarily have the most reliable output characteristics. Several suggestions were given for improvements in TENS unit design.

Equipment-related factors can play a significant role in the success or failure of any clinical treatment with TENS. Practical details discussed above and cited sources of information, including the American National Standard for Transcutaneous Electrical Nerve Stimulators (1985),[48] should prompt those utilizing TENS to be more critical consumers of this equipment. Indeed, little effort would be required to develop an equipment rating form that can be referred to when discussing equipment with colleagues, distributors, manufacturers, and regulatory groups.

CLINICAL DECISION MAKING

The clinician needs to make a number of important decisions prior to, during, and after implementing a TENS program in order to insure safe and successful pain management. Treatment must be based upon a thorough evaluation of the patient's pain and related dysfunction. Indications and contraindications for treatment must be disclosed, taking into account information from the patient's health history and physical examination. The optimal TENS mode, with unique neuromuscular electrical stimulation (NMES) characteristics and electrode placements, must be determined for each patient. Related decisions will be guided by an understanding of the theoretical basis for pain relief by TENS. In order to carry out successful treatment with TENS, the treatment protocol may need to be modified in order to provide effective pain relief or to handle problems that may develop. Ideally, the patient will be actively involved in the treatment after appropriate instruction.

Evaluation of Patient and Response to Treatment

Both initial and ongoing evaluations of the patient are important to any treatment program. A wide range of clinical problems present pain as a major symptom. It is critical that an accurate assessment be made concerning the underlying basis for pain, and aggravating factors should be fully explored. Other sources should be consulted for detailed information about physical and psychological testing procedures.[11,49,50] Although the initial evaluation is primarily diagnostic in character, and may require more than one session, it provides valuable baseline information. Importantly, the evaluation allows review of indications and contraindications to treatment, and guides the clinician in selection of TENS modes and electrode sites. The clinician should also be able to arrive at a prognosis for success in managing pain with a comprehensive program that combines TENS with other relevant treatments (eg, joint mobilization, strengthening exercises, and instruction in body mechanics or ergonomic principles). The patient history should include information about medication use or abuse, and about treatments previously used successfully or unsuccessfully for pain management. Ongoing evaluations conducted during each session allow the clinician to determine if the patient is progressing adequately or if the treatment program requires modification. In many cases, a multidisciplinary approach to evaluation and treatment of pain may be most beneficial.[51,52] Ultimately, it is important for the clinician to recognize if the patient's response is based upon effective treatment, or if a positive outcome represents a natural resolution of the clinical problem, a placebo effect, or both.[53]

The complexity of the pain experience is well known and has prompted numerous attempts to define pain. In an abstract manner, *pain* has been defined in terms of a multidimensional space comprising several sensory and affective dimensions.[54] Simply, pain has been described as a hurt that we feel.[50] Pain of less than 4 to 6 months in duration is often termed *acute*, while pain of longer duration is called *chronic*.[55] Acute pain, which occurs with conditions such as trauma and active inflammation, is frequently associated with sympathetic nervous system ("fright/flight") responses. Chronic pain, however, may be associated with a decrease in autonomic factors and an increase in psychological factors, particularly depression.[50]

Historically, attempts to measure clinical pain have been confounded by its private and subjective character.[56] The manner in which a person expresses pain has been found to be related to factors of personality, past pain experiences, age, gender, behavioral needs, ethnic membership, and cultural heritage.[50,54] A variety of methods have been developed to permit assessment of clinical pain. In the past 20 years, investigators have been increasingly concerned with the validity, reliability, and objectivity of pain assessment techniques.

An assortment of "behavioral indicators," which are demonstrable patient pain behaviors, can be documented by the clinician during the patient interview and physical examination.[50] For example, it is possible to qualify facial expression. The patient's verbal complaint of pain can provide information concerning the quality, distribution, and duration of pain, and can disclose aggravating or relieving factors. The quality and distribution of pain may be charted by the patient on a body diagram.[57] Other verbal indicators may include crying and changes in mood. Requests for pain medications, including frequency, type, and amount, may be documented. For purposes of comparison, a wide range of pain medications may be converted to a standard "morphine equivalent dose."[58] Automated techniques for quantifying functional aspects of movement, such as "uptime"[59] and activity patterns,[60] have been described. Various indexes and scales have been employed to evaluate functional activities in relation to pain, but lack of sensitivity or limited correlation to changes in pain have been apparent for some measures.[61-63]

A number of physical signs may be assessed in relation to pain. In association with acute pain, Sternbach has observed increases in pulse rate, systolic blood pressure, and respiratory rate, as well as dilated pupils, perspiration, nausea, and pallor.[50] Physical characteristics of posture,[64] gait,[66] joint range of motion,[66-68] muscle strength[69,70] and endurance,[70] duration of joint loading time,[26] pressure threshold and tolerance,[71,72] tissue compliance,[71] skin temperature,[73,74] and pulmonary functions[15,75] have also been evaluated in conjunction with pain.

Pain rating scales have been developed in an attempt to quantify pain that patients are experiencing or have experienced in the past. The *pain estimate* requires the patient to rate his or her pain intensity on a scale of 0 to 100. Zero indicates no pain, while 100 represents "pain so severe you would commit suicide if you had to endure it more than a minute or two."[76] In less suggestive terms, 100 might be taken to represent the worst pain that a patient could ever imagine. With the *verbal rating* scale, the patient selects one of five or more words that best describes pain (eg, none, mild, moderate, severe, unbearable).[77] The *visual analogue* scale utilizes a 100-mm line, with verbal anchors "no pain" next to the line at the left and "pain as bad as it could be" at the right. Pain is rated by the patient placing a mark in one location on the line.[77-80] A visual analogue scale can also be used to assess pain relief by employing anchors of "complete pain relief" and "no pain relief".[81] The *graphic rating* scale combines features of the verbal rating and visual analogue scales, such that word descriptors (eg, mild, moderate, severe) are placed along the analogue line with anchors as previously described.[80] To date, a number of comparative studies have been done with these scales.[77,79,82,83] Although these scales can be quickly administered, patients who have trouble with abstract thinking may have difficulty with some scales (eg, visual analogue).[79] These scales have also been criticized for focusing primarily on the intensity of pain, for lacking sensitivity in some situations, and for being used with inappropriate mathematical analyses.[84]

Various sensory matching tests have been introduced in the attempt to improve the accuracy of pain assessment. Sternbach[76] has advocated use of the *submaximal effort tourniquet technique* originally developed by Smith and colleagues.[85] Essentially, the procedure involves using a blood pressure cuff on the nondominant arm to induce ischemic pain after submaximal isometric exercise. The patient first notes the point at which the induced pain matches the intensity of the clinical pain. Some time later, the patient indicates when the ischemic pain is the maximum that can be tolerated. The time elapsed to the clinical match is divided by the time to reach maximum tolerance, this ratio is multiplied by 100, and the result is termed the "tourniquet pain ratio."

Some procedural aspects of this approach have been modified by Moore and associates to improve standardization.[86] *Cross-modalilty* matching procedures have also been employed, whereby input to another sensory modality is matched to some characteristic of clinical pain. The intensity of an auditory tone,[87,88] grip strength,[84] and color matching[89] have been utilized, and comparative studies have been performed.[87]

A number of more comprehensive approaches to assessing pain, sometimes in conjunction with function, have recently been summarized by Echternach.[90] The McGill Pain Questionnaire[57] is probably the most often utilized of these techniques. The questionnaire seeks information relative to the location of pain via a coded body diagram, characterizes the qualities of pain via the Pain Rating Index (PRI), determines how the pain changes with time, and assesses pain intensity through the Present Pain Intensity (PPI) scale. Derived measures have been shown to be sensitive to a number of therapeutic interventions including TENS.[91–94] Although the original form of the questionnaire required 5 to 10 min to administer, a newer short-form reportedly takes only 2 to 5 min.[95] My experience, and that of others,[94] is that patients have difficulty understanding pain descriptors used in the original format. Other pain assessment techniques have been compared to this questionnaire.[96]

Indications, Contraindications, and Precautions

As there are a number of sources of information in both professional literature and commercial publications concerning TENS indications, contraindications, and warnings or precautions, the American National Standard for Transcutaneous Electrical Nerve Stimulators (1985)[48] is relied upon as the main reference. The primary indication for TENS has been described as the "symptomatic relief and management of chronic pain or as an adjunctive treatment or both in the management of post-surgical and post-traumatic acute pain."[48] Such wording cautiously implies that TENS should not be viewed as curing the pathology or injury that has given rise to the pain. However, there is mounting evidence that externally applied electrical currents can affect tissue repair, which may be associated with pain relief.[97–100] Although many types of pain can be effectively treated, some conditions have historically failed to respond well. Long[101] has noted that patients with peripheral nerve injuries respond more than 70 percent of the time, and that those with postherpetic neuralgia or acute musculoskeletal syndromes also regularly benefit. In contrast, patients having metabolic peripheral neuropathy with hyperesthesia or serious sensory loss, or those with "central pain states" associated with spinal cord injury and thalamic syndrome, generally do not benefit from TENS. Patients who have psychosomatic pain or drug addiction, or who are involved in situations where secondary gain is important, are also rarely helped by TENS.[101] Johansson and colleagues determined that patients with psychogenic or somatogenic pain had significantly poorer results than those with neurogenic pain, and that pain in the extremities was significantly better controlled with TENS than that located on the face, neck, or trunk.[102] However, as exceptional responses can be found despite these general trends, it would seem prudent to permit most pain patients a trial evaluation period with TENS.

The use of TENS with some patients having demand-type (synchronous) cardiac pacemakers has been recognized as the sole contraindication for this modality.[48] Eriksson and colleagues assessed the effects of TENS having a pulse duration of 200 μsec, and frequencies of 10 to 100 pps pulsed at 1 to 10 pps.[103] Four ventricular-inhibited synchronous pacemakers were blocked with stimulation at 1 to 3 pps, and in one instance at frequencies up to 6 pps. The current amplitude required for this effect was 5 mA with electrodes on the thoracic wall, and 10 mA with electrodes on the lumbar-sciatic region. No blocking was produced with the electrodes distal on the lower extremity, or with modulating frequencies above 6 and not greater than 10 pps. One ventricular-triggered synchronous pacemaker was activated to reach its upper limit (130 beats per minute) using TENS at frequencies above 2 pps. An atrial synchronous pacemaker was triggered by unspecified TENS characteristics to operate at its maximum rate of 150 beats per minute. Electrode position was not noted in these latter two cases. The proper functioning of two asynchronous (fixed-rate) pacemakers were not interfered with when using any of the frequencies at maximum current amplitude.

Long observed that although TENS should not be used "in the proximity" of demand pacemakers, it could be used on other areas of the body.[101] Shade noted no interference with a temporary demand pacemaker using a dual-channel TENS unit (pulse duration 20 μsec, frequency 35 pps, amplitude not specified) with electrodes simultaneously positioned on the upper thorax in paraspinal and midaxillary locations on one patient monitored in an intensive care unit over a period of days.[104] Most recently, Rasmussen and associates evaluated TENS effects on 51 patients having 20 models of permanent cardiac pacemakers.[105] Two electrodes from one TENS unit channel alternately stimulated four sites (cervical, lumbar, left leg, and forearm ipsilateral to the pacemaker) for 2-min periods. TENS characteristics included a pulse duration of 40μsec, frequency of 110 pps, and an amplitude initially producing discomfort that was readjusted to a comfortable level. In no case was there evidence of pacemaker interference, inhibition, or reprogramming. However, it was admitted that the electrodes had not been placed in what was likely the most hazardous configuration, parallel to the pacemaker electrode vector (eg, for a unipolar pacemaker, one electrode over the right ventrical and the other near the pacemaker).

TENS has been safely done on body areas close to fixed-rate (asynchronous) pacemakers and remote from demand-type (synchronous) pacemakers. However, the range of hazardous stimulation characteristics and electrode positions has yet to be competely determined. In order to ensure safety, and to alleviate both patient and clinician anxiety, it would be appropriate to monitor all pacemaker patients during at least the initial application of TENS. Monitoring devices themselves may require special filters to prevent interference from TENS.[11]

Specific warnings and precautions for TENS use have been identified. It has been recommended to manufacturers that these warnings should be specified in clinician and patient information that is part of the TENS kit.[48] The above-noted use with demand-type cardiac pacemakers should be acknowledged as being hazardous. Some have suggested that electrodes not be placed on the anterior chest wall of patients with histories of any cardiac problems.[11] Stimulation over the carotid sinus, which may reflexly induce slowing of the heart, a fall in blood pressure, or fainting, should also be recognized to be hazardous. Despite a number of studies that have documented safe TENS use during labor and delivery,[16,106,107] it has been felt that the safety of TENS during pregnancy and delivery has not been established. It should be noted that TENS may suppress the sensation of pain in a manner that deprives the patient of this protective mechanism against acute injury, although this could be questioned.[108] The use of TENS in the presence of skin irritation should be warned against, and improper use (eg, prolonged use or contact with metal lead wire tips) should be recognized to be associated with skin burns.

As a precaution, TENS should be used with caution for undiagnosed pain syndromes. (TENS may provide a reduction in pain and related muscle spasm, which permits more specific evaluation and diagnosis.) TENS is more effective for pain of peripheral than of central origin. Furthermore, the treatment outcome can be influenced by the patient's psychological state and by the use of drugs. Specific drugs such as diazepam, codeine, corticosteroids, and other narcotics, and drug addiction, have been reported to limit success with TENS.[11] As discussed previously, TENS should be acknowledged to be of no known curative value. Finally, a TENS unit must be kept out of the reach of children. TENS is recommended for use only under supervision of or referral from a physician, which is not consistent with contemporary practice of other licensed health care professionals.

Aside from these precautions presented in the 1985 American National Standard,[48] suggestions from other groups merit some consideration.[11,43,101,109] Intense stimulation, especially that associated with muscle contraction, may lead to the disruption of fractures, sutures, and other fragile tissues. Stimulation over the eyes and internally on mucosal membranes has been seen likely to produce irritation or other damage. Stimulation in proximity to the larynx might lead to restriction of the airway. Effects on patients with cerebral vascular accidents, transient ischemic attacks, epilepsy and seizure disorders, or stimulation on the head or upper cervical regions, are not well established, and thus close monitoring is required. Special precautions will be necessary if attempting to treat the confused or incompetent patient (eg, it may be necessary to cover unit controls to prevent readjustment or to ensheath the device in protective padding). Manufacturers have traditionally cautioned against the use of TENS units while operating a motor vehicle or other hazardous equipment where unanticipated stimulation might produce a startle response or uncontrolled muscle contraction. As there is always a probability that a patient will encounter an adverse reaction to treatment, even after some delay, it is important that the clinician provide a follow-up and document the response to treatment.[110]

Overview of TENS Modes

Six primary types or modes of TENS have been discussed with regularity in the literature.[11] Although descriptive labels have been used in an attempt to classify each mode (conventional, strong low-rate, brief-intense, pulse-burst, modulated, and hyperstimulation), this has led to some confusion. Essentially, each mode is distinguished by unique stimulator output characteristics (Fig. 10–4), and sometimes also by electrode placements and other protocol details. In order to improve communication in clinical notes and publications, it is recommended that such detailed information always be specified when describing a TENS mode. To date, some studies have assessed the optimal stimulation characteristics for pain relief within a given TENS mode,[32,94,108,111] while others have attempted to determine the most effective TENS mode for given pain management problems.[26,112,113] The following overview will introduce common TENS modes based largely upon stimulation characteristics.

The majority of publications dealing with clinical TENS have been concerned with the *conventional* mode, which is generally characterized by a high-rate frequency and low amplitude (Fig. 10–4A).[7,11,15,23,44,108,13] Conventional TENS utilizes frequencies in the range of 10 to 100 pps and an amplitude intensity that produces comfortable cutaneous stimulation without muscle contraction.[41] As a sensation of distinct paresthesia is usually desired, a frequency approaching 30 pps is required before individual electrical impulses will perceptually fuse. Research has indicated that frequencies approximating 60 pps are optimal for producing pain relief with this mode.[32,108,111] Frequencies in the range of 80 to 200 pps have been reported to worsen pain for some patients.[108] Where separate linear unit control adjustments are possible, perception of amplitude is based upon a narrow pulse duration (typically 50 to 100 μsec) and low to mid-range amplitude (eg, a minimum of 24 mA has been seen as necessary for excellent pain relief).[111] A narrow pulse duration favors preferential stimulation of large-diameter myelinated afferent neurons, the purported target of conventional TENS.[114] As patients treated with this mode often accommodate to the stimulation, amplitude must be periodically increased in order to maintain adequate perception of electrical paresthesia. There have been reports of this mode being done with amplitude purposefully adjusted to just below that required for sensory perception, a "subthreshold" setting.[108,113] Neuronal stimulation has been documented at this low amplitude.[115]

The *strong low-rate* mode (also called "acupuncture-like") is characterized by a high amplitude and low frequency (Fig. 10–4B).[11,113,116] The stimulating frequency is below 10 pps, most commonly in the range of 1 to 4 pps. Pulse duration typically ranges from 100 to 300 μsec, which can be at mid to maximal control settings. Amplitude is adjusted to produce visibly strong and rhythmical muscle contractions. The beating of these contractions is uncomfortable, but within the patient's tolerance to discomfort. This mode and other

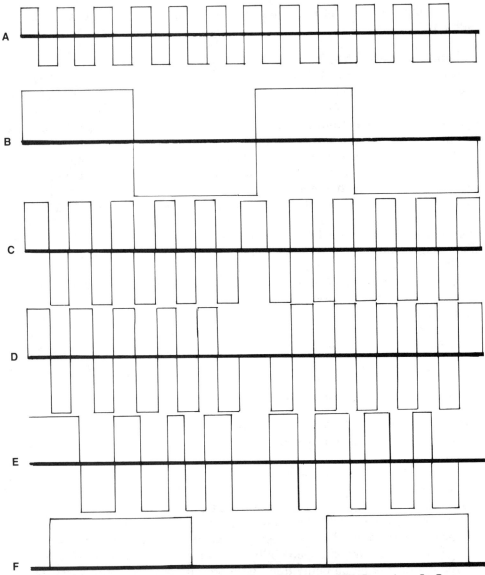

Figure 10–4. Schematic representation of common TENS modes. **A.** Conventional low-amplitude high-rate frequency. **B.** Strong low-rate. **C.** Brief-intense. **D.** Pulse-burst. **E.** Modulated (pulse duration). **F.** Hyperstimulation.

high-amplitude modes are thought to be more resistant to perceptual accommodation.

Some confusion has been associated with the specifications for the *brief-intense* mode of TENS. Commonly denoting stimulation with a high amplitude and high-rate frequency (Fig. 10–4C),[26,113,116] considerably lower amplitudes are sometimes used.[11]   Unfortunately, the term "brief-intense"[91,92] has also been used to define TENS with output characteristics most similar to another contemporary mode ("pulse burst"). Typical stimulating frequency is from 60 to more than 150 pps, a range that has been seen to produce significant muscle fatigue with continuous stimulation.[117] Pulse durations of 50 to 250 μsec are commonly employed. Amplitude is adjusted to produce muscle contraction, with high settings yielding uncomfortable tetanic muscle contractions and low settings giving nonrhythmic muscle fasciculations. Either amplitude should also yield a sensation of paresthesia.

The *pulse-burst* mode (also called "burst," "pulse-train,"[11] and even "acupuncture-like"[41] TENS) is depicted in Figure 10–4D.[26,118] It has been utilized in the attempt to improve patient acceptance of high-amplitude stimulation, as some patients have had difficulty tolerating muscle beating associated with the strong low-rate mode.[41,116] This mode is characterized by high frequency (eg, 60 to 100 pps) modulated by a low-frequency carrier (eg, 0.5 to 4 pps). Pulse durations may range from 50 to 200 μsec. Again, both high- and low-amplitude settings have been utilized.[11] High-amplitude stimulation produces intermittent tetanic muscle contractions and paresthesia, but low amplitude provides just a sensation of pulsating paresthesia.

Although the *modulated* mode has been advocated by some manufacturers and authors to prevent accommodation to stimulation or to improve patient tolerance,[11] few studies have specifically examined this TENS format.[119,120] TENS units with this feature automatically change (modulate) one or more output characteristics (pulse duration, amplitude, or frequency) by a given percentage from an initially set level. Affected characteristics may be modulated in a manner that decreases their values by up to 60 percent one to two times each second. Figure 10–4E illustrates modulation of pulse duration alone. Output parameters characteristic of the modes discussed above can thus be altered in a manner that may enhance patient acceptance and pain management.

The TENS mode of *hyperstimulation,* also called "noninvasive electroacupuncture,"[11] has received limited but promising assessment.[25,68,121,123] Undeniably the most noxious form of TENS, it is the only mode which regularly utilizes either direct or monophasic pulsed currents (Fig. 10–4F). This mode relies upon high current density to produce very noxious cutaneous stimulation that is sharp and burning in character, without resultant muscle contraction. This noxious stimulation is achieved by using a very small probe-type stimulating electrode, with a tip that may be only 1 to 3 mm in diameter, and a very long pulse duration (eg, 500 msec) in some TENS units. Because of these factors, required current amplitude may not need to be higher than 50 μA with some equipment. Although the pulsed frequency can exceed 100 pps, the range of 1 to 4 pps enjoys the greatest empirical use. Progressively higher frequencies become more noxious because the total current per unit time is increased.

Electrode Placement Options

Effects ascribed to the various TENS modes are not based solely upon NMES characteristics. A variety of electrode placement options permit specific neuro-muscular structures to be targeted and help to assure the efficacy of stimulation. Previously, a technique was described for discerning if one electrode is more "active," and the suggestion was made to standardize placement distal to its paired partner. Discussion will now focus on electrode placement relative to the location or distribution of pain. These placement options may be used as initial or alternative electrode sites. For the sake of simplicity, discussion will begin with placements using just two electrodes from a single TENS unit channel.

Electrodes can be positioned relative to a localized site of painful trauma or inflammation, so that stimulation occurs primarily via cutaneous afferents. There are at least four options that exist for electrode placement when using just two electrodes (Fig. 10–5). First, both electrodes may be placed just proximal to the site of pain. This placement is useful if pain arises from a distal extremity location. Second, the electrodes can be positioned just outside the proximal and distal margins of the painful region, in a manner that "brackets" the area. Third, one electrode may be placed on the painful area while the other is situated adjacent to the spine over the related spinal nerve root. The second and third options may not provide sufficient current density to stimulate adequate sensory perception if the electrodes are situated too far apart. Finally, both electrodes may be placed distal to the site of pain. Such distal stimulation, however, has been reported to have more limited effectiveness than the first and second options.[124]

It is critical that the site to be stimulated be sentient, in order to assure that NMES is being conveyed to the nervous system. For example, a body region may become denervated from accidental trauma, or a surgeon may purposefully cut an intercostal nerve in the attempt to minimize incisional pain. However, high-amplitude stimulation may still be capable of producing pain relief in the absence of cutaneous sensation.[112] Generally it appears important that conventional TENS, and possibly low-amplitude formats of other modes, be done so that stimulation occurs at a site segmentally related to tissues that are giving rise to pain,[11] but conflicting observations have been reported.[108] As illustrated in Figure 10–6, dermatomes used as sites for stimulation may not spatially overlap painful myotomes or sclerotomes that share the same segmental innervation.[49,125]

Specific peripheral nerves that innervate a painful region can be targeted for stimulation, especially where located superficially. Picaza and colleagues produced more than a 50 percent reduction in pain for 55 of 100 patients in whom peripheral nerves were stimulated.[108] The electrodes from one channel may be placed at varying distances apart along the course of a nerve. Also, the two electrodes can be used to simultaneously stimulate two peripheral nerves (eg, ulnar and median nerves at the wrist). Quite commonly, pain is associated with injury to the peripheral nerve itself. In such cases, Long has recom-

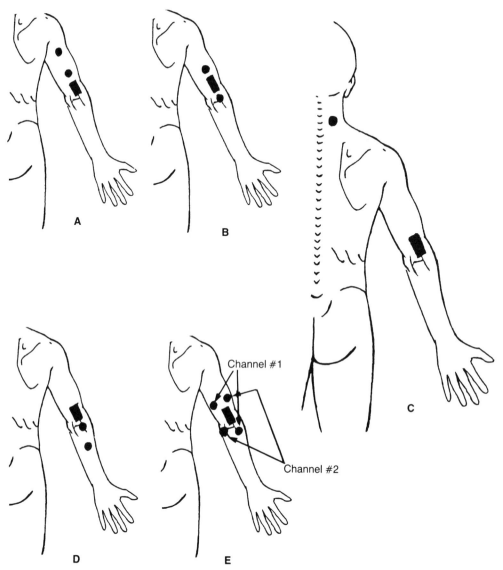

Figure 10–5. Electrode site options for localized pain. **A.** Both electrodes proximal to area of pain. **B.** Electrodes bracketing painful area. **C.** One electrode over site of pain, the other paraspinally over nerve root. **D.** Both electrodes distal to area of pain. **E.** Crisscross placement.

mended that stimulation be done proximal to the site of nerve injury and that hyperesthetic areas be avoided.[101] Stimulation of peripheral nerves "remote" (not segmentally related) to painful areas has been reported to relieve pain in some instances. In 42 of 280 tests done by stimulating remote nerves, Picaza and associates documented pain suppression, but it was variable and generally

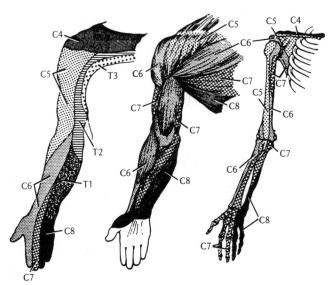

Figure 10–6. Segmental innervation of right upper extremity, anterior view. **A.** Dermatomes. **B.** Myotomes. **C.** Sclerotomes. *(From Inman VT, Saunders JB: Referred pain from skeletal structures. J Nerv Ment Dis. 99:660, 1944, with permission.)*

weak. Remote stimulation tended to be positive if stimulation of nerves directly innervating the area was successful.[108]

A motor point can be physiologically identified as a specific location on the skin that requires the lowest amplitude of NMES to produce excitation of an underlying innervated muscle. Anatomically this area of skin has been found to transversely overlie a muscle's neurovascular hilus, which contains sensory, motor, and autonomic axons, and the zone of innervation, where branches of motor axons terminate on individual muscle fibers.[126,127] Such points would seem well suited to afford input to the central nervous system, permit efficient stimulation of muscle contractions, and influence circulatory control, all of which are desired outcomes for specific TENS modes. Although motor points have been suggested as sites for TENS electrodes,[11] no studies were found that specifically assessed TENS done at these locations.

Trigger points exist as hyperirritable foci in skin, fascia, muscle, tendon, ligament, and periosteum.[128] They are painful upon compression and produce a characteristic pattern of referred pain and related signs. The zone of referred pain often does not follow a segmental pattern. TENS electrodes may be positioned relative to a trigger point or relative to its zone of referred pain.[92] Also, one electrode may be placed over the trigger point while the other is located at the reference zone. Travel and Simons have cautioned against using high-amplitude TENS that produces muscle contraction that can aggravate a myofascial trigger point.[128]

Acupuncture points, tender sites on the body surface utilized for pain management in traditional Chinese acupuncture,[129] can also be used in TENS. Currently, there are two approaches popularly used for treating these points.[130] One approach involves treating a predefined sequence of acupuncture points for a given pain problem. The other approach involves treating successive points of low pain threshold along the acupuncture "meridian" that passes through the painful area, points on the auricle of the ear in locations related to the pain, or both. Electrodes are placed directly on a single point or on multiple points simultaneously. Fox and Melzack produced greater than a 33-percent reduction in chronic lower back pain in 8 out of 12 patients using high-amplitude pulse-burst TENS at three predetermined acupuncture points for a total of 30 min.[118] The duration of pain relief averaged 23 hr. Treatment with TENS at appropriate acupuncture points, as opposed to inappropriate points, has resulted in significant pain relief.[92] Recently, Lein and associates reviewed a number of other studies that used somatic or auricular acupuncture points, or both, for pain control with TENS.[121] However, the basis for and effectiveness of treatment at auricular points is controversial.[131–134]

Mannheimer and Lampe have comprehensively summarized the relationships between motor, trigger, and acupuncture points.[11] All of these points can be spontaneously painful or tender to palpation. Palpation can also produce referred pain. These points often present resistance to manual pressure, which may sometimes be associated with fibrositic components. The locations of these points[135,136] and the distributions of their referred pain are very similar.[136] Often these points are situated over superficial nerves or dense groupings of sensory end organs. Electrically, these points demonstrate locally increased conductivity, and therefore decreased impedance. Taken as a whole, these relationships seem to indicate that motor, trigger, and acupuncture points represent the same entity,[11] although dissent has been voiced.[128]

The preceeding discussion has been referenced to single-channel TENS treatment given ipsilateral to a painful body region or related target such as a dermatome, peripheral nerve, motor point, trigger point, or acupuncture point. In some situations it may be desirable to add a second channel of stimulation or to "piggyback" additional electrodes. Under certain circumstances it may be appropriate to stimulate contralateral to a painful region, as in the case of limited sensation, skin irritation, herpes zoster, postherpetic neuralgia, or causalgia.[11,137] Bilateral placement of electrodes should provide even greater input to the central nervous system. Although both clinical and experimental pain can be decreased with bilateral electrode placements, results may not be superior to unilateral treatment alone.[138] Electrodes from two separate TENS channels may be crisscrossed so that stimulating current intersects in the painful area (see Fig. 10–5E). When such a setup is done without using a true interferential stimulator, this approach has been called the "modified interferential" technique. Additional electrode placement arrangements are discussed in other publications.[11,137]

Except where limited by TENS unit hardware features (eg, limited adjustment of output characteristics, single channel, inability to piggyback electrodes, or electrodes that are too large or too small), any of the above electrode site options might be used with any TENS mode. However, as a given TENS mode is characterized by the presence (or absence) of particular perceptual, neural, and muscular responses, certain electrode placements have come to be favored for each mode. Some of this information has already been mentioned earlier in this section. Conventional TENS and low-amplitude formats of pulse-burst and modulated modes can be done using all of electrode sites. Generally, pain relief is better if the sensation of electrical paresthesia is felt throughout the painful area, but exceptions have been noted.[108] Higher-amplitude modes (strong low-rate, brief-intense, pulse-burst, and modulated), which involve muscle contraction, must stimulate the muscle via a peripheral nerve or motor point. Perhaps pain relief is more effective if these sites also represent acupuncture points. Although high-amplitude stimulation that produces muscle contraction at painful trigger points has been warned against,[128] further investigation of this precaution is warranted. Hyperstimulation TENS produces a very noxious sensation through stimulation of cutaneous entities such as nerves and acupuncture, trigger, and motor points. The sensation is not nearly as noxious if stimulation is not provided at these low-impedance points. Current density below the skin is not adequate to significantly stimulate muscle at peripheral nerves or motor points with this mode at amplitudes that will be tolerated.

As might be anticipated, various electronic devices have been marketed to assist in the precise location of motor, trigger, and acupuncture points based upon their conductive or amplitude characteristics. These devices are sometimes incorporated within a TENS unit. However, the validity of relying only upon such measurements to locate points is questionable, as Mann has noted many low-impedance sites that do not correspond to acupuncture points.[129] Furthermore, the reliability of such devices has not been adequately documented in the literature. In fact, the small sharp metal tips on some of the electrodes used to probe the skin can produce minor abrasions that actually lower the measured impedance. It would seem important to use tips that are smooth, and spring-loaded to standardize the pressure of application. The precision with which points can be located becomes a more critical factor when small-diameter electrodes will in turn be used for TENS, as in the hyperstimulation mode.

Berlant has suggested an alternative approach to locating superficial peripheral nerves or related acupuncture points,[139] which warrants further assessment for reliability and safety. Using a single TENS channel, one electrode is placed on the palm of a patient's hand while the other electrode is held by the clinician in the hand used for testing. TENS unit pulse duration is set low and frequency is adjusted within the range of 30 to 50 pps. The clinician then probes the patient's skin with the tip of the index finger in the vacinity of a likely peripheral nerve or acupuncture point, while slowly advancing the TENS amplitude. Peripheral nerves and acupuncture points are located at sites where the patient perceives the strongest sensation of radiating paresthesia. It has been my experience that the clinician also feels stronger paresthesia in the tip of the index finger when these sites are found. Furthermore, it is recommended that electrode position in this technique be modified to limit unnecessary current flow through the thorax of the patient being assessed (ie, place the electrode on the extremity being tested).

Theoretical Bases for Pain Relief with TENS

An understanding of the theoretical basis for pain relief with TENS will guide the clinician in various aspects of decision making (eg, selection of TENS modes and electrode sites). The clinician will also be better prepared to respond to questions from patients and colleagues, and to anticipate patient response to treatment and likely treatment outcomes. Additionally, research may be encouraged to further clarify the bases for the effects of TENS. This section briefly reviews a number of mechanisms by which TENS has been suggested to act. For a more detailed discussion of theory concerning the basis for pain itself, the reader is referred to a number of excellent resources,[11,53,54,128,140–144] including the series *Advances in Pain Research and Therapy*, edited by Bonica and associates, and *Pain*, the journal of the International Association for the Study of Pain.

One action of TENS might be to change the sensitivity of peripheral receptors or free nerve endings responsible for the transduction of nociceptive stimuli. However, evidence for these mechanisms remains limited.[101] Enhanced blood flow in the skin[145] and deeper tissues[146] in response to stimulation producing intermittent muscle contraction[147] (as with strong low-rate, pulse-burst, or modulated TENS) may supply required oxygen and rid the area of stimulating or sensitizing chemical mediators. Similarly, fatigue of muscle spasm produced by sustained muscle contraction[43] (as with brief-intense TENS) may subsequently lead to improved blood flow. Both low[97,147,25] and high-amplitude stimulation that does not produce muscle contraction may also be associated with improved blood flow.

TENS may block transmission of impulses in afferent nerves (eg, A-delta and C) conveying nociceptive information. Blocking of potassium has been implicated as a possible mechanism.[101] Taub and Campbell assessed averaged compound action potentials from the median nerve during noxious pinprick.[148] High-amplitude TENS (100 pps with pulse duration of 500 μsec) was delivered in two forms. Continuous stimulation (most like brief-intense or high-frequency hyperstimulation), which finally became painless after about 20 min, produced analgesia to pinprick and a preferential decrease in the A-delta component of the compound potential. In contrast, bursted stimulation (0.5 sec bursts every 30 sec) was painful throughout, induced no analgesia, and did not produce a change in the compound potential. Using painful NMES in the range of 0.5 to 10 pps through intradermal needle electrodes, Torebjörk and Hallin observed decreases in induced pain, and increased latencies and blocking of averaged C-fiber responses.[149] Similar changes were reported in averaged

A-delta fiber responses, but not usually at frequencies below 20 to 30 pps. Ignelzi and Nyquist, however, used stimulation at 15 pps to produce the most dramatic decreases in the A-delta component of compound action potentials from isolated cat peripheral nerves, although changes were also seen in A-alpha and A-beta components.[150] In 30 percent of the experiments there was an enhancement of both the amplitude and conduction velocity of these components after initial poststimulation depression. Devor and Wall determined that ongoing neural activity in experimentally produced neuromas could be stopped by high-amplitude antidromic stimulation (square wave frequency 100 pps, pulse duration 100 μsec).[151] However, an explanation for the effect of stimulation that can be tolerated by subjects or patients, based solely on peripheral mechanisms, has been challenged.[152]

TENS may also exert an effect on the autonomic nervous system through peripheral or central mechanisms. Jenkner and Schuhfried employed high-amplitude monophasic pulses to produce an electrical block of the stellate ganglion, which was best associated with increased circulation in the arm or head when using a frequency of approximately 100 pps modulated by an 8-Hz carrier.[153] These stimulation characteristics were also effective for relieving chronic pain. The effect of TENS on angina pectoris was examined by Mannheimer and associates.[21] The chest wall was stimulated using a frequency of 70 pps, pulse duration of 200 μsec, and an amplitude just below that producing pain. In a short-term 4-day series, 10 patients experienced significantly increased maximum work capacity and decreased ST segment depression. In a long-term series, 11 TENS-treated subjects had significantly better outcomes than 10 control subjects both during and after a 10-week experimental period with respect to frequency of anginal attacks, nitroglycerin consumption, recovery time, and ST segment depression. These studies used high-amplitude stimulation similar to pulse-burst and brief-intense TENS modes, respectively.

Since the late 1960s, Melzack and Wall's "gate control" theory of pain[6] has been utilized as the standard explanation for pain relief via TENS, especially that of the low-amplitude conventional mode. This theory has been credited with rekindling interest in electrical control of pain[154] and inspiring research with important scientific and clinical ramifications.[155] An essential tenet of this theory is that large-diameter A-beta afferents excite interneurons in the dorsal horn of the spinal cord, producing inhibition of nociceptive input from smaller-diameter A-delta and C fibers. Descending inhibitory influences from higher centers are also accounted for. This theory has been subjected to critical analyses and experimentation[155–157] and has undergone the revisions expected of any theory.[152] However, exact mechanisms of the theory remain to be elucidated.[101,152]

More recently, attention has focused on the relationship between TENS and the production of endogenous opiates (eg, endorphins and enkephalins). Most currently, Mayer and Price have critically examined the evidence for endogenous opiate analgesia in man.[144] In only two of ten studies using high-rate frequency TENS were there indications of endorphin involvement. In contrast, five of eight studies using low-rate frequency TENS demonstrated endorphin involvement either directly or indirectly. Furthermore, they noted that these studies collectively indicate that it is low-frequency high-amplitude TENS that is associated with endogenous opiate mechanisms. Langley and Sheppeard reviewed mechanisms of TENS and placebo therapy.[158] They concluded that intense "acupuncture-like" (i.e.: pulse-burst) and intense low-frequency (eg, 1 to 4 pps) TENS both act through descending pathways involving endorphins. Intense high-rate frequency TENS, however, was not seen to be endorphin mediated. In addition, placebo effects were found to be based on both endorphin and non-endorphin mechanisms.

Possible reflex-based effects of TENS have also been examined. Chan and Tsang assessed the lower-extremity flexion reflex induced in healthy subjects.[159] Conventional TENS (square waveform, frequency 100 pps, pulse duration 1 msec, amplitude two to three times perception threshold) to the L4–S1 region paraspinally for 30 min was associated with significant inhibition of the reflex both during and after stimulation The time to maximum effect took 20 to 30 min for select muscles, and the effect persisted for as much as 50 min after stimulation. Similar changes were not seen in subjects treated with sham TENS. Of particular interest is the fact that Facchinetti and associates also demonstrated inhibition of the flexion reflex that was correlated with an increase in endogenous opiates (Beta-lipotropin and Beta-endorphin) after conventional TENS.[160] Effects of TENS on yet other reflexes have also been described.[89,161]

Carrying Out Successful TENS Treatment

After completing appropriate evaluation procedures, ruling out potential contraindications, and determining that TENS is indeed indicated, the clinician should discuss treatment goals with the patient and proceed with treatment. Although TENS is typically but one component in a comprehensive pain management program,[11,162] it alone will be the topic of discussion here.

When introducing the concept of TENS to a patient, steps should be taken to minimize anxiety about NMES. Emphasis on use of a small battery-powered unit with well-controlled output may be helpful. Avoid referring to stimulation as "electrical shocks," no matter how low the amplitude is described to be. It is often helpful to let the patient experience the sensation of stimulation on a noninvolved body part prior to the actual treatment. However, demonstration at the intended site of an operation is usually used as a part of preoperative patient education.

Patients are naturally interested in the probability of a successful treatment outcome, although some are skeptical of "high-tech" interventions. A straightforward and nontechnical explanation of both the basis of and plan for treatment is effective with most patients. The clinician should also be aware that confidence and competance, conveyed by both verbal and nonverbal means, can positively shape patient expectation in a manner that enhances treatment outcome.[53] With many patients it is possible that significant pain relief can occur as a result of nonspecific factors, including the psychological framework, related to treatment.[163] Recently, Fields has noted (p. 309) that "placebo analgesia occurs when some aspect of the treatment situation causes the patient to expect pain relief and the patient's expectation of relief, rather than any specific action of the treatment, triggers a neurally mediated reduction in pain."[53] Although any patient will respond under the right conditions, the placebo effect is actually enhanced by patient stress and anxiety, and by more severe pain.[53,163,164] Some authorities have suggested that the placebo effect from a given treatment regimen becomes limited after 1[5] or 2 weeks.[55] Thus, the placebo effect may be employed to help establish a successful result from initial TENS treatments.

While appreciating the concerns of others,[11] it is my belief that pain medications should be continued during initial TENS treatments as long as they are not impairing a patient's cognitive function. This is done so that a reduction in pain medications might be documented as a measurable treatment outcome. Similarly, the patient should maintain pretreatment activity levels unless a decrease in mechanical stress is warranted (eg, through the use of cane in osteoarthritis of the hip, or cessation of jogging for shin splints). However, during the initial part of a TENS treatment the patient should be positioned for comfort, stability, safety, and good access to intended electrode sites. Most often this involves using a recumbent position for the patient. As pain relief is progressively induced during a treatment session, the affected body part should be carefully tested in order to assess if pain relief is due to TENS or to rest from function.

Unfortunately, the clinician must deduce the appropriate TENS mode with which to commence treatment. Presently there is not an adequate number of comparative studies to determine the optimal TENS mode for a given pathology or diagnosis associated with pain. A few studies have examined patient acceptance or tolerance of TENS modes.[112,119,165] As might be anticipated, patients generally find low-amplitude conventional TENS, and lower-amplitude formats of other modes (brief-intense, pulse-burst, and modulated), to be most acceptable. Not considering lower-amplitude formats of established modes, it has been my experience that patients are most acceptive of TENS modes in the following rank order: conventional > modulated > pulse-burst > strong low-rate > brief-intense > hyperstimulation. Some studies have suggested that TENS using a low amplitude and high frequency produces a rapid onset of pain relief, while stimulation with high-rate amplitude and low-rate frequency gives longer carryover of pain relief.[41,166] Exceptions to these observations, however, have been noted.[23,26,121] Some patients with peripheral nerve injury or radiculopathy require higher stimulation amplitudes to produce satisfactory pain relief.[94] Greater stimulation amplitude, based upon a longer pulse duration or higher amplitude, or both, may also be required to stimulate deep peripheral nerves, especially if there is intervening fat or scar tissue. As initial patient acceptance and likelihood of successful outcome are critical to proceeding with treatment, conventional TENS (at a frequency of 60 pps, short pulse duration, and amplitude producing distinct paresthesia in the area of pain) is usually the TENS mode of first choice.[32,111]

Once the initial TENS mode and electrode sites have been selected, the electrodes are prepared and placed on the patient, based upon previously discussed rationale. Regardless of the TENS mode to be used, it is advisable to preset the unit's pulse duration and frequency, and then to turn the unit on and advance the amplitude to the desired setting. Although durations of stimulation for clinical pain have ranged from 2 min[7,23] to continuous for up to 5 days,[67] the typical duration of TENS is probably 20 to 60 min. Stimulation with the high-amplitude modes of strong low-rate, brief-intense, and pulse-burst tend to be on the short end of this range due to limited patient tolerance. Hyperstimulation is often done twice for 15 to 30 sec to multiple acupuncture points.[130]

It is advisable that the patient be continually monitored during treatment for such things as changes in vital signs, adequacy of stimulation, and patient acceptance of treatment. Minor readjustments of stimulation characteristics within the initial TENS mode may be necessary. At approximately 10 to 30 min into the period of stimulation, the patient's pain should be reevaluated and the effect of body movement (via active range of motion, gait, and deep breathing and coughing) should be assessed as appropriate. If the patient is experiencing some pain relief, the period of stimulation may be continued. If the patient becomes distraught or intolerant of the treatment, it may be necessary to terminate the treatment session for the day in a dignified manner, and to plan a new approach for another session with the patient's willing participation. If the patient is bothered by the sensation of NMES or is not getting any pain relief, it is advisable to proceed with one of the following options. First, further readjust the parameters within that TENS mode. Was the pulse charge, a resultant of amplitude and pulse duration, too high or too low? Was the frequency optimal? For example, I have had patients complain of "a terrible sensation of bugs on my skin" at 60 pps that disappeared when 10 pps was used instead. Second, relocate the electrodes to an alternative site, with some forethought as to which sites would also be optimal for another TENS mode. Third, select another TENS mode. Stimulation should then be continued for another 10- to 30-min period. At the end of the 20- to 60-min stimulation period, reevaluate pain, range of motion, and other functional activities. Depending on outcome, other components of the comprehensive pain management program may be instituted at this time.

Assuming that significant pain relief has been attained, next determine if there is any treatment carryover. This carryover is accomplished by turning off the TENS unit and monitoring the length of time it takes pain to return to a significant level. Either the patient can be questioned at the next session, or a more formal log of pain ratings at regular time intervals can be kept (eg, every 2 waking hours). Although very unlikely, it is not impossible that pain will be totally relieved, never to return. Usually there is a slow return to a level of significant pain over a period of hours, at which point TENS can be resumed. In some instances, pain will immediately return to a significant level as soon as the unit is turned off. This may warrant almost continuous TENS use. It is important that the patient be taught how to operate the TENS unit, and even to troubleshoot problems with electrodes and batteries. Through such activity, the patient will gain a greater sense of controlling the pain. Similar instruction should also be given to other members of the health-care team who are vital to the success of postoperative or home health pain management programs.

Generally, acute pain responds more rapidly to treatment than chronic pain, although significant relief of chronic pain has been observed with as little as 2 min of conventional low-amplitude TENS.[7,23] In treating acute pain, the primary aim is to decrease pain and related muscle spasm as rapidly as possible. Continuous application of TENS may be warranted, for example, with postoperative pain.[15,67,75] Although the clinician is concerned with eliminating chronic pain, one should recognize that the patient may become dependent on the TENS unit as an external symbol of pain that evokes a reaction from others. Where chronic pain behaviors are a problem, it may be necessary to administer TENS "by the clock" at fixed time intervals rather than at patient request.[167]

Most commonly it will be necessary for the patient to continue TENS treatment as part of a home pain management program. The clinician should be sure that the individual is attaining significant pain relief through two or more treatment/education sessions, either as an inpatient or as an outpatient, before switching to a home program and periodic outpatient reassessment. Patients seen only for one session of "TENS evaluation and treatment" do not seem to respond as well to TENS. Wolf and colleagues found that only 10 out of 114 patients with chronic pain had their best results during the first treatment.[94] In fact, up to 1 month of TENS use may be necessary to determine if treatment will be effective.[101] Some insurance plans require a trial TENS unit rental period of 1 month before a unit can be purchased. Both verbal and written home program instructions should include a number of features to assure patient understanding and compliance. It also may be important to educate other family members. Information should clarify and go beyond that provided in the TENS kit's manual. The schedule for TENS use, be it intermittant or continuous, should be specified. Details of skin and electrode preparation should be outlined. Special electrodes or methods of attachment may be required. Primary and alternate electrode sites can be noted on a body diagram. All unit controls should be reviewed, and adaptations utilized as needed. For example, some small control knobs are slotted, which permits the patient to turn them with the edge of a coin. The TENS mode and stimulation characteristics that have proven optimal for the patient should be noted. Battery replacement and recharging, and other unit maintenance procedures, should be reviewed. The TENS unit itself should not be cleaned with solvents that might damage its case (eg, acetone). All warnings and precautions should be summarized and reviewed, and instructions should be provided for care of skin irritation. Finally, an acceptable procedure should be adopted for recording and reporting the patient's response to ongoing and long-term treatment. This may include return-mail pain and function ratings, or questionnaires, the use of which the patient should clearly understand. It has been suggested that specific reevaluations be conducted at intervals of 1, 3, and 6 months, and periodically thereafter.[11] It is desirable to decrease or eliminate the patient's pain medications if adequate relief with TENS permits. Ultimately, the patient should be weaned from TENS as intervals of significant pain relief become longer.

Healthcare professionals should be strongly discouraged from simply sending patients to a medical supply house or pharmacy for instruction in TENS. Aside from risking ineffective treatment and patient injury, legal and ethical questions arise if the practitioner is an owner of such a facility.[168] Additionally, some healthcare professionals have allegedly been involved in selling TENS units directly to patients, or in benefitting from sales. While such practices have drawn fire from those in the durable medical equipment industry,[169,170] they also have legal and ethical consequences.

EFFECTIVENESS OF TENS FOR CLINICAL PAIN MANAGEMENT

Numerous reports in the literature give credence to the efficacy of TENS in the treatment of both acute and chronic pain. In a series of approximately 300 patients with acute pain, Cohen reported that more than 80 percent of the time patients treated with TENS had no need for narcotics.[5] Vander Ark and McGrath determined that 77 percent (47 out of 61) of patients with acute postoperative pain had a significant reduction in pain.[171] However, results with chronic pain have not appeared to be as successful. Long and Hagfors surveyed five pain treatment centers with a caseload of 3000 patients and found that 25 to 30 percent of patients formerly incapacitated by pain had significant pain relief with TENS alone.[154] It has been reported that approximately 25 percent of nearly 1000 chronic pain patients treated with TENS by Cohen had their pain relieved to the point where no other therapy was necessary, while this result was seen in 39 percent of a series of 500 patients treated by Long.[5] In 1976, Long noted that of over 900 cases reported in the literature, satisfactory pain relief was noted with TENS alone 35 percent of the time.[172] By 1984, Long's 10-year experience with TENS allowed him to conclude that one third of patients with chronic pain attained pain relief and decreased muscle spasm, with most patients using TENS indefinitely.[101]

The assessment of long-term pain relief with TENS has been difficult. Not only are studies hard to conduct, but researchers have used varying criteria to judge successful pain relief. Stonnington and colleagues noted that of 81 patients who purchased TENS units, 72 percent had partial pain relief and 6 percent had complete pain relief at 3 months.[173] Long determined that of 104 chronic pain patients using TENS for an average of 9 months, 68 percent were able to maintain satisfactory pain relief, 63 percent decreased or eliminated pain medications, and 46 percent significantly increased activity levels.[174] Loeser and associates found that 68% of 198 unselected chronic pain patients had significant initial pain relief;[175] yet approximately 1 year later only 13% had continued effective pain relief. Eriksson and colleagues reported that of 123 chronic pain patients, 41 percent continued to use TENS after 1 year. Of this group, 72 percent had significant pain relief, 44 percent significantly decreased their analgesics, and 50 percent had increased social activities. After 2 years, 31 percent of the patients continued to employ TENS, with 79 percent of this group achieving significant pain relief. Keravel and Sindou noted that in following patients with deafferentation pain for a period of 1 to 3 years, 80 percent of those with peripheral nerve lesions most commonly attained partial pain relief.[176] However, only 25 percent of patients with postherpetic pain found stimulation of benefit after 1 year.

Recently, Fields indicted TENS and other nondrug methods of pain control as not being established as effective for controlling chronic nonmalignant pain.[53] Furthermore, he has claimed that a specific analgesic effect for TENS has not been proven. Both of his arguments relate to a need to demonstrate that TENS is superior to placebo treatment under a double-blind methodology. Beecher determined that an average of 35 percent of patients obtain satisfactory pain relief from placebo (eg, sugar pill) treatment,[164] although a later review noted up to a 69 percent response.[177] A double-blind methodology requires that neither the patient nor the clinician know which treatment (active or placebo) is being given.[178] Obviously it is impossible to disguise some treatments so that the clinician remains unaware of which is the active or placebo treatment. In such instances, it may be sufficient to assure that whomever performs the patient assessment after treatment is unaware of which treatment has been given.[178] Others have suggested that the double-blind technique is actually invalid if the perception of stimulation is necessary for pain relief.[179]

A chronological sampling of 15 studies that have examined the effectiveness of TENS by including some type of control procedure in their experimental design is described in Table 10–1. Unfortunately, only 6 out of 15 studies are described in enough detail to permit adequate understanding of key methods and procedures. Although only 2 appear to be true double-blind studies,[91,180] additional studies may possibly be so.[92,181] Three other studies have employed a variant of the double-blind procedure.[158,182,183] Of these 15 studies, only the one by Langley and associates[158] failed to support the superiority of active TENS treatments over placebo or other control interventions in clinical trials. The placebo treatment in this study incorporated a strong suggestion and a focus of attention not utilized in the other studies, which merits further examination. Additionally, Langley and colleagues have suggested that crossover trials may be inappropriate as the patient can easily distinguish active from inactive TENS.[158,182]

TABLE 10-1. CHRONOLOGICAL SURVEY OF STUDIES CONCERNED WITH EFFECTIVENESS OF TENS

Researchers	Subjects	Design	TENS Mode[a]	Electrode Sites[b]	Treatment Duration/ Frequency	Comments	Outcome
Melzack (1975)[92]	N = 53, chronic pain[c]	Only part is double-blind[d]	"BI" (really PB: 60 Hz modulated at 3 or 10 Hz; intensity to toler- ance)	TP, PN, AP for all subjects	20 min, most used 1–3 x/wk (varied days to months)	Used negative response sites as control (N = 15). "Vanagas" stimulator, no output (N = 7) but strong suggestion. Assessed with McGill (PRI and PPI).	(1) Across pain syndromes: 0–74% decrease in PRI, 0– 75% decrease in PPI. (2) Sig decrease PRI at positive vs negative points. (3) Sig pain relief true TENS > "Vanagas", which had no lasting effect.
Coopermann et al (1975)[183]	N = 50, upper abdominal surgery, age 20– 74	Single-blind, random assignment to active (N = 26) and sham	Stim Tech EPC; unspecified output	On either side of incision	Apparently continuous for 5 days	Pain relief without negative side effects suggested to all	(1) Based on comfort and medica- tion use: 77% with active (Continued)

TABLE 10–1. (Continued)

Researchers	Subjects	Design	TENS Mode[a]	Electrode Sites[b]	Treatment Duration/Frequency	Comments	Outcome
		TENS (no current, N = 24)				patients.	TENS vs 33% with sham TENS had good to excellent results. Difference significant. (2) No differences in incidence of ileus atelectasis, pneumonia, or ICU stay.
Thorsteinsson et al (1978)[180]	N = 93, chronic pain,[c] mean age = 49	Double-blind, crossover, with random assignment to active and placebo TENS (no current)	Unspecified output	Center of pain, related nerve, and unrelated nerve	Three active and three placebo treatments in succession; follow-up home use of active unit (N = 44)	All informed that study double-blind. Expectation of positive outcome not given.	(1) During Tx sig better effect was obtained by active vs placebo with stim of pain center and unrelated nerve. (2) Subsequent to Tx sig better

Study	Subjects	Design	Stimulation parameters	Tx conditions	Duration	Comments	Results
							effect by active at pain center. (3) Complete pain relief with home treatment at 3 mo in 7% and at 6 mo in 2%.
Jeans (1979)[91]	N = 16, chronic pain,[c] mean age = 47.4	Double-blind, crossover, 4 Tx conditions (see electrode sites)	"BI" (really PB: sine waveform at 60 Hz, in trains 2–3/sec)	4 Tx conditions: (1) PA; (2) distant TP or AP; (3) sham Tx ("Vanagas" unit); (4) distant NRPs	Two sessions/day for 4 consecutive days	Technician convinced "Vanagas" (placebo) was effective. Pain assessed by McGill pre/post Tx.	Descriptive results: Tx #1 produced substantially greater decrease in pain than #2–4.
Long et al (1979)[184]	N = 150 in first series of unselected patients with chronic pain[c]	Crossover	Unspecified output, treatment for all patients at (1) suprathreshold intensity; (2) subliminal	Unspecified	Duration unspecified; 3 successive days (one type each day); Tx continued to 1 yr	Results rated as "satisfactory" if patients satisfied with pain relief (possibly not complete) and no alter-	(1) "Successful" pain relief at 1 mo: suprathreshold = 35%, subliminal = 8%, no battery = 11%. (2) At 1 yr: (Continued)

295

TABLE 10–1. (Continued)

Researchers	Subjects	Design	TENS Mode[a]	Electrode Sites[b]	Treatment Duration/ Frequency	Comments	Outcome
			intensity; (3) without battery			nate treatment.	suprathreshold = 34%, subliminal, no battery = 0%.
Ali et al (1981)[185]	N = 40, elective cholecys-tectomy	Assignment to 1 of 3 groups: (1) active TENS (N = 15); (2) sham TENS (no stimulation, N = 10); (3) no TENS (N = 15)	CONV, GR	On either side of incision	Treatment begun in OR; TENS continuous, 48 hr postop; then on demand to 5th day	All had postop PT (deep breathing, coughing, exercise, and ambula-tion) Pain not directly assessed.	(1) Compared to other 2 groups, active TENS had: (a) sig less medication thru day 3 (b) sig higher vital capacities thru day 5 (c) sig higher functional residual capacity thru day 5 (d) sig higher pO_2 thru day 5 (e) no postop complications.

Study	Sample	Design	Treatment		Schedule	Methods	Results
							(2) No differences between sham and control.
Hansson and Ekbolm (1983)[186]	N = 62 acute orofacial pain[c] age 19–54	Random assignment to 1 of 3 groups: (1) high-freq TENS (N = 22); (2) low-freq TENS (N = 20); (3) placebo TENS (N = 20)	Cefar SIII unit; monopolar square wave; (1) high freq = Conv: 100 Hz, 200 μsec, intensity at constant tingling; (2) low freq = PB: 71 Hz train, 84 msec long, at 2 Hz, intensity = nonpainful muscle contraction; (3) placebo TENS = no stim	PA	Schedule unspecified	Avoided suggestion of pain relief. Placebo group advised that stim might not be felt. Verbal pain ratings pre/post Tx.	(1) Nonsig difference in pain relief and induction times of high-vs low-freq TENS. (2) Muscle contractions of low-freq uncomfortable. (3) 38% active TENS vs 10% placebo had pain relief >50%. (4) 74% active TENS vs 40% placebo had "some" pain relief.

(Continued)

TABLE 10–1. (Continued)

Researchers	Subjects	Design	TENS Mode[a]	Electrode Sites[b]	Treatment Duration/ Frequency	Comments	Outcome
							(5) 52% active TENS vs 20% placebo rated TENS superior to prior analgesic medications.
Abelson et al (1983)[182]	N = 32 rheumatoid arthritis with chronic wrist involvement, age 35–72	Double-blind,[e] crossover, random assignment to active or placebo TENS (no stim)	Cyrax Mark II; "high intensity" at 70 Hz	Dorsal and ventral wrist	15 min × 1/ wk for 3 wk	Anti-inflammatory analgesics stopped 12 hr prior to treatments. Neutral statement of antici-pated effects. Unit indicator light on. Eval pre/ post Tx, including visual	(1) Only active TENS showed: (a) sig improvement in resting and grip pain (b) sig improvement in power and work log ratios. (2) Placebo effect assessed to be 17%.

Lewis et al (1984)[181]	N = 28, osteoarthritis with knee pain, age 40–83	Double-blind[d] crossover, active vs placebo TENS (no stim)	RDG Tiger Pulse; 70 Hz	4 APs simultaneously on knee.	After instruction, did home program 30–60 min × 3/day for 3 wk	Unit indicator light on. Standard meds available. Assessed weekly, including visual analog scale.	(1) Median duration of pain relief sig different, active (151 min) vs placebo (110 min). (2) Sig improvement in pain relief after 3 wk active, not placebo. (3) Sig improvement in "pain index" (knee ROM and weight-bearing scores) and decreased meds—both groups. (4) 46% "response rate" to active vs 43% to placebo TENS.

(Continued)

TABLE 10–1. (Continued)

Researchers	Subjects	Design	TENS Mode[a]	Electrode Sites[b]	Treatment Duration/ Frequency	Comments	Outcome
Langley et al (1984)[158]	N = 33, rheumatoid arthritis and chronic hand involvement	Double-blind[e] non-crossover, random assignment to 1 of 3 matched groups: (1) high-freq TENS; (2) acupuncture-like TENS; (3) placebo TENS	Grass S48; monophasic waveform; (1) high freq: 100 Hz, 200 μsec; (2) acupuncture-like 100 Hz train for 70 msec × 2/sec (#1 & #2 at highest tolerated intensity shown on oscilloscope); (3) placebo = no current, but saw TENS waveform on oscilloscope	Volar and dorsal wrist	20 min	Initial neutral instructions to all. Strong suggestion provided to placebo group. Meds stopped 24 hr prior to study. Assessment at 15 min intervals post Tx, including visual analog scale.	(1) All groups had sig decreased resting and grip pain, nonsig group diffs. (2) Nonsig diffs between groups in "overall" pain relief, total joint tenderness or number of tender joints. (3) Mean power and work scores with no sig change for any group. (4) Positive placebo response rated at

Study	Sample	Design	Device/Parameters	Electrode placement	Duration	Procedure	Results
							55% for pain relief.
Solomon and Gulielmo (1985)[20]	N = 58, migraine and/or muscle contraction headaches	Random assignment to 1 of 3 treatments: (1) TENS at perception; (2) subliminal TENS; (3) placebo TENS (no stimulation)	Pain Supressor; GR	Active electrode, PA Indifferent electrode opposite active or on hand.	15 min on 1 day	All informed that Tx might be placebo. No meds. in prior 24 hr. Pain estimate pre/post Tx.	(1) "Improvement" in 55% with TENS at perception, 28% with subliminal TENS, 18% with placebo TENS. (2) Perceived TENS sig better than placebo.
Smith et al (1986)[93]	N = 18, caesarian section surgery, mean age = 29	Single-blind, random assignment to 1 of 2 groups: (1) active TENS (N = 9); (2) placebo TENS, no current (N = 9)	Medtronics Comfort-burst (#7718); 85 Hz, 80 μsec ≤ tingling sensation	On either side of incision	Continuous from recovery room through 3 days	Unit indicator light on. Equivalent instructions suggestive of pain relief. Meds permitted. Pain assessed up to 3 × day w/ McGill.	(1) Active TENS sig less cutaneous movement-associated and constant pain. Nonsig diff on day 3. (2) Active TENS, less constant deep incisional

(Continued)

TABLE 10–1. (Continued)

Researchers	Subjects	Design	TENS Mode[a]	Electrode Sites[b]	Treatment Duration/ Frequency	Comments	Outcome
							pain, and uterine pain, but nonsig diff. (3) Nonsig diff in gas pain. (4) Active TENS with nonsig fewer doses of analgesic meds. (5) TENS less effective in pts with epidural anesthesia.
Ordog (1987)[13]	N = 100, acute trauma outpatients (sprains, lacerations, fractures, hematomas with contusions)	Random assignment to 1 of 4 groups: (1) function-ing unit; (2) non-functioning unit (3) function-	TENS-PAC; unspecified output	Over or close to injury site	As needed, including continuous	Subjects informed that some would get nonfunctioning units. Both active and placebo units gave slight hum	(1) Sig decreased pain at day 2 for functional vs nonfunc-tional TENS, nonsig diff at day 30.

	ing unit + Tyelenol 3; (4) nonfunctioning unit + Tyelenol 3		and vibration. Graphic rating scale used to assess pain. Tylenol 3 = acetaminophin + codeine.				(2) Nonsig diff in pain for functioning TENS vs Tyelenol group at day 2 or 30. (3) 10% using meds, but 0% TENS at day 30. (4) Side effects noted with Tyelenol 3, but not TENS.
Finsen et al (1988)[187]	N = 51, amputations (Symes, below and through knee), age 39–92	Random assignment to 1 of 3 groups: (1) active TENS (N = 17); (2) sham TENS (no stim) (N = 19); (3) sham TENS +	Tenzcare; PB (100 Hz, 90 μsec in bursts of 7 pulses, × 2/sec, amplitude to discomfort)	2 at femoral nerve and 2 at sciatic nerve	30 min × 2/ day × 2 wk postop	Unit indicator light on. Analgesic meds on demand. Limited assessment of analgesic effect.	(1) At 2 wk: analgesic effect in all active TENS and 50% of sham. (2) Nonsig diff in analgesic intake in first 4 wk. (3) Sig more

(Continued)

TABLE 10–1. (Continued)

Researchers	Subjects	Design	TENS Mode[a]	Electrode Sites[b]	Treatment Duration/ Frequency	Comments	Outcome
		chlorpromazine (N = 15)					healed below knee amputations at 6 and 9 wk with active TENS. (4) Sig fewer incidents of phantom pain in active TENS (10%) than in sham (36%) or sham + chlorpromazine (58%) at 16 wk, but not 1 yr later.
Hargreaves & Lander (1989)[183]	N = 75, abdominal surgical wounds, age 18– 89	Partial-blind,[f] random assignment to 1 of 3 groups: (1) active	Grass SD9; 100 Hz 400 μsec intensity just below discomfort	Adjacent to incision	15 min prior to and during wound cleaning and repack-	TENS naive subjects. Each group had pain meds. Pain rated on	Active TENS with sig lower pain level than placebo or no TENS

TENS;
(2) placebo
TENS (no
current);
(3) no TENS

ing, 2 days
after
surgery

visual
analogue
scale.

groups.

[a] CONV = conventional; BI = brief-intense; PB = pulse-burst; GR = only general range of output characteristics given.
[b] AP = acupuncture point; NRP = non-related points; PA = painful area; PN = peripheral nerve; TP = trigger point.
[c] A variety of diagnoses.
[d] Not specific enough information in paper to determine if a true double-blind study.
[e] Patient blinded to treatment; separate therapist and evaluator.
[f] Patient blinded to treatment; therapist rated pain before patient assignment; patient independently rated pain after treatment.

We conducted a controlled study of pain management in the elderly, the results of which were recently reported.[61] Twenty-two residents of life-care communities (mean age 74 ± 10 years) with chronic musculoskeletal pain consented to participate. All subjects were informed that TENS had the potential to produce temporary pain relief, and that three forms of TENS were being used in this study. In a crossover design, subjects received each of three randomized treatments for 30 min every 48 hr during 1 week. Treatments consisted of control (conventional TENS for only 10 sec, then unit turned off); conventional TENS (pulse duration 40 μsec, frequency 60 pps, amplitude producing paresthesia); and pulse-burst TENS (pulse duration 40 μsec, frequency 110 pps, bursts at 2/sec, amplitude to produce maximum tolerated muscle contraction) using a Dynex II stimulator. Electrodes from a single channel were placed so that stimulation occurred within the area of pain. Visual Analogue Pain and Function scales were used to assess pain and related functional limitations prior to and at intervals after treatment. One clinician performed initial assessments and treatments, while another (blinded to whom received what treatment) carried out assessments immediately after treatment and assisted the patient with self-evaluation as needed. Results were analyzed by MANOVA (significance-$P < 0.05$). The control treatment demonstrated significantly less immediate pain relief (19.5 percent for control, 32.5 percent for conventional, and 33.9 percent for pulse-burst TENS). Significant placebo effects were seen through 6 hr for pain and 8 hr for function. Both active treatments had equal efficacy through 30 hr for pain and function. When compared to control, however, active treatments had significant effects through 8 hr for pain, but no significant differences were found through 30 hr for function. It was concluded that TENS was effective for decreasing pain, but not for increasing function as defined by this study.

Long, a pioneer in TENS therapy and research, has observed (p. 327) that "it is probable that transcutaneous electrical stimulation represents the single most effective physical entity yet introduced in the management of chronic pain."[101] Greater insight is being gained as to which acute and chronic conditions are amenable to treatment with TENS, and optimal TENS treatment procedures are being more specifically defined. Although most studies have focused on pain management, appropriate functional assessment in relation to pain relief clearly remains a major challenge to those involved in patient care or research.

REFERENCES

1. Bonica JJ. Management of pain. Lecture as visiting professor, Department of Anesthesiology, College of Medicine, University of Iowa, Iowa City, December 7, 1988
2. Kellaway P. The William Osler medal essay: The part played by electrical fish in the early history of bioelectricity and electrotherapy. *Bull His Med.* 20:112, 1946
3. Kane K, Taub A. A history of local electrical analgesia. *Pain.* 1:125, 238, 1975

4. McNeal DR. 2000 years of electrical stimulation. In: Hambrecht FT, Reswick JB, eds. *Functional Electrical Stimulation: Applications in Neural Prostheses.* New York, Marcel Dekker, 1977:3–35
5. Kohen IJ, ed. A new approach to pain. *Emerg Med.* 6:241, 1974
6. Melzack R, Wall PD. Pain mechanisms: A new theory. *Science* 150:971, 1965
7. Wall PD, Sweet WH. Temporary abolition of pain in man. *Science.* 155:108, 1967
8. Nolan MF. A chronological indexing of the clinical and basic science literature concerning transcutaneous electrical nerve stimulation (TENS) 1967–1987. Section on Clinical Electrophysiology, Alexandria, VA, American Physical Therapy Association, 1988
9. Wolf SL, ed. Transcutaneous electrical nerve stimulation (special issue). *Phys Ther.* 58:1441, 1978
10. Ersek RA. Pain control with transcutaneous electrical neuro stimulation (TENS). St. Louis, Warren H Green, 1981
11. Mannheimer C, Lampe GN. *Clinical Transcutaneous Electrical Nerve Stimulation.* FA Davis, Philadelphia, 1984
12. Tapio D, Hymes AC. *New Frontiers in Transcutaneous Electrical Nerve Stimulation.* Minnetonka, MN, Lec Tec Corp, 1987
13. Ordog GJ. Transcutaneous electrical nerve stimulation versus oral analgesic: A randomized double-blind controlled study in acute traumatic pain. *Am J Emerg Med.* 5:6, 1987
14. Strassburg HM, Krainick JU, Thoden U. Influences of transcutaneous nerve stimulation (TNS) on acute pain. *J Neurol.* 217:1, 1977
15. Tyler E, Caldwell C, Ghia JN. Transcutaneous electrical nerve stimulation: An alternative approach to the management of postoperative pain. *Anesth Analg.* 61:449, May 1982
16. Bundsen P, Peterson LE, Selstam U. Pain relief during delivery, an evaluation of conventional methods. *Acta Obstet Gynecol Scand.* 61:289, 297, 1982
17. Richardson RR, Meyer PR Jr, Cerullo LJ. Transcutaneous electrical neurostimulation in musculoskeletal pain of acute spinal cord injuries. *Spine.* 5:42, 1980
18. Roeser WM, Meeks LW, Venis R, et al. The use of transcutaneous nerve stimulation for pain control in athletic medicine. A preliminary report. *Am J Sports Med.* 4:210, 1976
19. Mason CP. Testing of electrical transcutaneous stimulators for suppressing pain. *Bull Prosthet Res.* spring 1976, pp 38–54
20. Solomon S, Guglielmo KM. Treatment of headache by transcutaneous electrical stimulation. *Headache.* 25:12, 1985
21. Mannheimer C, Carlsson CA, Vedin A, et al. Transcutaneous electrical nerve stimulation (TENS) in angina pectoris. *Int J Cardiol.* 7:91, 1985
22. Avellanosa AM, West CR. Experience with transcutaneous electrical nerve stimulation for relief of intractable pain in cancer patients. *J Med.* 13:203, 1982
23. Meyer GA, Fields HL. Causalgia treated by selected large fiber stimulation of peripheral nerve. *Brain.* 95:163, 1972
24. McCarthy JA, Ziganfus RW. Transcutaneous electrical nerve stimulation: An adjunct in the pain management of Guillain-Barre syndrome. *Phys Ther.* 58:23, 1979
25. Leo KC. Use of electrical stimulation at acupuncture points for the treatment of reflex sympathetic dystrophy in a child. A case report. *Phys Ther.* 63:957, 1983
26. Mannheimer C, Carlsson CA. The analgesic effect of transcutaneous electrical nerve stimulation (TENS) in patients with rheumatoid arthritis. A comparative study of different pulse patterns. *Pain* 6:329, 1979

27. Winter AW. The use of transcutaneous electrical stimulation (TENS) in the treatment of multiple sclerosis. *J Neurosurg Nurs.* 8:125, 1976

28. Gessler M, Struppler A. Relief of phantom pain following modification of phantom sensation by TENS. In: Bonica JJ, Lindbolm U, Iggo A, eds. *Advances in Pain Research and Therapy.* New York, Raven Press, 1983; 5:591–594

29. Robinson AJ, Snyder-Mackler L. Clinical application of electrotherapeutic modalities. *Phys Ther.* 68:1235, 1988

30. *Standards of Electrotherapeutic Terminology.* Electrotherapy Standards Committee of the Section on Clinical Electrophysiology, American Physical Therapy Association, Alexandria, VA, July 1988

31. Witters D, Hinkley S, Lapp A. Electrical output performance tests on transcutaneous electrical nerve stimulation devices. Section on Clinical Electrophysiology. *Am Phys Assoc.* 4:15, 1989

32. Barr JO, Nielsen DH, Soderberg GL. Transcutaneous electrical nerve stimulation characteristics for altering pain perception. *Phys Ther.* 66:1515, 1986

33. Lampe GN. Introduction to the use of transcutaneous electrical nerve stimulation devices. *Phys Ther.* 58:1450, 1978

34. Mosenkis R, ed. Transcutaneous electrical nerve stimulator (TENS) units. *Health Devices.* 10:179, 1981

35. Barr JO. *The Effect of Transcutaneous Electrical Nerve Stimulation Parameters on Experimentally Induced Acute Pain.* Master's thesis, University of Iowa, Iowa City, 1980

36. Lamm KE. Optimal placement techniques for TENS: A soft tissue approach. Workshop on TENS, Tucson, AZ, 1986

37. Ronnen M, Suster S, Kahana M, et al. Contact dermatitis due to karaya gum and induced by the application of electrodes. *Int J Dermatol.* 25:189, 1986

38. Henley EJ. Pain suppression device is explained: Henley responds (letter). *PT Bulletin.* Dec 7, 1988, p 8

39. Fisher AA. Dermatitis associated with transcutaneous electrical nerve stimulation. *Cutis.* 21:24, 1978

40. Eriksson MBE, Sjolund BH, Nielzen S. Long term results of peripheral conditioning stimulation as an analgesic measure in chronic pain. *Pain* 6:335, 1979

41. Paxton SL. Clinical uses of TENS: A survey of physical therapists. *Phys Ther.* 60:38, 1980

42. *TENS, The Path to Pain Control: Skin care.* St. Paul, Medical Products Division/ 3M, F-TCBR (421) II

43. Griffin JE, Karselis TC. *Physical Agents for Physical Therapists,* 2nd ed. Springfield, IL, Charles C. Thomas, 1982

44. Shealy CN, Maurer D. Transcutaneous nerve stimulation for control of pain—A preliminary note. *Surg Neurol.* 2:45, 1974

45. Campbell JA. A critical appraisal of the electrical output characteristics of ten transcutaneous nerve stimulators. *Clin Phys Physiol Meas.* 3:141, 1982

46. Stamp JM. A review of transcutaneous electrical nerve stimulation (TENS). *J Med Eng Technol.* 6:99, 1982

47. Barr JO. *Evaluation of Transcutaneous Electrical Stimulation Unit Output.* Unpublished report, December 9, 1976

48. *American National Standard for Transcutaneous Electrical Nerve Stimulators.* ANSI/AAMI NS4-1985. Arlington, VA, Association for the Advancement of Medical Instrumentation, 1986

49. Cyriax J. *Textbook of Orthopaedic Medicine*, 6th ed. *Diagnosis of Soft Tissue Lesions*. Baltimore, Williams & Wilkins, 1975; 1
50. Sternbach RA. *Pain—A Psychophysiological Analysis*. New York, Academic Press, 1968
51. McCombs D. Current opinions on electrotherapy. *Rehabil Manage*. 2:35, 1989
52. Stieg RL, Williams RC, Gallagher LA. Multidisciplinary pain treatment centers. *J Occupat Med*. 23:94, 1981
53. Fields HL. *Pain*. New York, McGraw-Hill, 1987
54. Melzack R. *The Puzzle of Pain*. New York, Basic Books, 1973
55. Sternbach RA. Evaluation of pain relief. *Surg Neurol*. 4:199, 1975
56. Chapman CR. Measurement of pain: Problems and issues. In: Bonica JJ, ed. *Advances in Pain Research and Therapy*. New York, Raven Press, 1976; 1:345–353
57. Melzack R. The McGill pain questionnaire: Major properties and scoring methods. *Pain*. 1:277, 1975
58. Olin BR, Hunsaker LM, Covington TR, et al. *Drug Facts and Comparisons*. St. Louis, JB Lippincott, 1989: 242–244
59. Sanders SH. Toward a practical system for the automatic measurement of "uptime" in chronic pain patients. *Pain*. 9:103, 1980
60. Follick MJ, Ahern DK, Laser-Wolston N, et al. Chronic pain: Electromechanical recording device for measuring patient's activity patterns. *Arch Phys Med Rehabil*. 66:75, 1985
61. Barr JO, Forrest SE, Potratz PE, Reed VL. Effectiveness of transcutaneous electrical nerve stimulation (TENS) for the elderly with chronic pain. *Phys Ther*. 69:165, 1989 (abstract)
62. Burton KE, Wright V. Functional assessment. *Brit J Rheumatol*. 22(suppl):44, 1983
63. Huskisson EC, Jones J, Scott PJ. Application of visual-analogue scales to the measurement of functional capacity. *Rheumatol Rehabil*. 15:185, 187, 1976
64. Zacharkow D. Posture: Sitting, standing, chair design and exercise. Springfield, IL, Charles C. Thomas, 1988
66. Ducroquet R, Ducroquet J, Ducroquet P. *Walking and limping: A Study of Normal and Pathological Walking*. Philadelphia, JB Lippincott, 1968
67. Birkhan J, Carmon A, Meretsky P, et al. Modification of TENS by constant-energy stimulation delivered through multiple electrodes: Method and evaluation. In: Bonica JJ, Liebeskind JC, Albe-Fessard DG, et al, eds. *Advances in Pain Research and Therapy*. New York, Raven Press, 1979; 3.
68. Paris DL, Baynes F, Gucker B. Effects of the neuroprobe in the treatment of second-degree ankle inversion sprains. *Phys Ther*. 63:35, 1983
69. Hoke B, Howell D, Stack M. The relationship between isokinetic testing and dynamic patellofemoral compression. *J Orthop Sports Phys Ther*. 4:150, 1983
70. Smidt GM, Herring T, Amundsen L, et al. Assessment of abdominal and back extensor function. A quantitative approach and results for chronic low-back pain patients. *Spine*. 8:211, 1983
71. Fisher AA. Advances in documentation of point soft tissue pathology. *J Fam Med*. Dec 1983, pp 24–31
72. Fischer AA. Pressure algometry over normal muscles. Standard values, validity and reproducibility of pressure threshold. *Pain*. 30:115, 1987
73. Pochaczevsky R. Assessment of back pain by contact thermography of extremity dermatomes. *Ortho Rev*. 12:45, 1983
74. Pochaczevsky R, Wexler CE, Meyers PH, et al. Liquid crystal thermography of the

spine and extremities. *J Neurosurg.* 56:386, 1982

75. Rooney SM, Jain S, McCornack P, et al. A comparison of pulmonary function tests for post-thoracotomy pain using cryoanalgesia and transcutaneous nerve stimulation. *Ann Thorac Surg.* 41:204, 1986

76. Sternbach RA, Murphy RW, Timmermans G, et al. Measuring the severity of clinical pain. In: Bonica JJ, ed. *Advances in Neurology.* New York, Raven Press, 1974; 4:281–289

77. Ohnhaus EE, Adler R. Methodological problems in the measurement of pain. A comparison between the verbal rating scale and the visual analogue scale. *Pain.* 1:379, 1975

78. Carlsson AM. Assessment of chronic pain I. Aspects of the reliability and validity of the visual analogue scale. *Pain.* 16:87, 1983

79. Kremer E, Atkinson JH, Ignelzi RJ. Measurement of pain. Patient preference does not confound pain measurement. *Pain.* 10:241, 1981

80. Scott J, Huskisson EC. Graphic representation of pain. *Pain.* 2:75, 1976

81. Huskisson EC. Visual analog scales. In: Melzack R, ed. *Pain Management and Assessment.* New York, Raven Press, 1983; 33–37

82. Downie WW, Leatham PA, Rhind VM, et al. Studies with pain rating scales. *Ann Rheum Dis.* 37:378, 1978

83. Jensen MP, Karoly P, Braver S. The management of clinical pain intensity: A comparison of six methods. *Pain.* 27:117, 1986

84. Gracely RH. Psychophysical assessment of human pain. In: Bonica JJ, Liebeskind JC, Albe-Fessard DG, eds. *Advances in Pain Research and Therapy.* New York, Raven Press, 1979; 805–824

85. Smith GM, Lowenstein E, Hubbard JH, et al. Experimental pain produced by the submaximal effort tourniquet technique: Further evidence of validity. *J Pharm Exp Ther.* 163:468, 1968

86. Moore PH, Duncan GH, Scott DS, et al. The submaximal effort tourniquet test: Its use in evaluating experimental and chronic pain. *Pain.* 6:375, 381, 1979

87. Adams J. The reliability of some techniques utilized in quantifying the intensity of clinical pain. *Pharmacol Ther.* 4:629, 1979

88. Peck RE. A precise technique for measurement of pain. *Headache.* 6:189, 1967

89. Francini F, Maresca M, Procacci P, et al. The effects of non-painful transcutaneous electrical nerve stimulation on cutaneous pain threshold and muscular reflexes in normal subjects with chronic pain. *Pain.* 11:49, 63, 1981

90. Echternach JL. Evaluation of pain in the clinical environment. In: Echternach JL, ed. *Pain. Clinics in Physical Therapy,* vol 12. New York, NY, Churchill Livingstone, 1978:39–72

91. Jeans ME. Relief of chronic pain by brief, intense transcutaneous electrical stimulation: A double blind study. In: Bonica JJ, Liebeskind JC, Albe-Fessard DG, eds. *Advances in Pain Research and Therapy.* New York, Raven Press, 1979; 3:601–606

92. Melzack R. Prolonged relief of pain by brief intense somatic stimulation. *Pain.* 1:357, 1975

93. Smith CM, Guralnick MS, Gelford MM, et al. The effects of transcutaneous electrical nerve stimulation in post-cesarean pain. *Pain.* 27:181, 1986

94. Wolf SL, Gersh MR, Rao VR. Examination of electrode placements and stimulating parameters in treating chronic pain with conventional transcutaneous electrical nerve stimulation (TENS). *Pain.* 11:37, 1981

95. Melzack R. The short form McGill pain questionnaire. *Pain* 30:191, 1987

96. Walsh TD, Leber B. Measurement of chronic pain: Visual analog scales and McGill-Melzack pain questionnaire compared. In: Bonica JJ, Lindblom U, Iggo A, eds. *Advances in Pain Research and Therapy.* New York, Raven Press, 1983; 5:897–899

97. Carley PJ, Wainpel SF. Electrotherapy for acceleration of wound healing: Low intensity direct current. *Arch Phys Med Rehabil.* 66:443, 1985

98. Kaada B. Promoted healing of chronic ulceration by transcutaneous nerve stimulation. *Vasa.* 12:262, 1983

99. Kahn J. Transcutaneous electrical nerve stimulation for nonunited fractures. *Phys Ther.* 62:840, 1982

100. Nordenstrom BEW. *Biologically Closed Electric Circuits: Clinical, Experimental and Theoretical Evidence for an Additional Circulatory System.* Stockholm, Nordic Medical Publications, 1983

101. Long DM. Stimulation of the peripheral nervous system for pain control. *Clin Neurosurg.* 31:323, 1984

102. Johansson F, Almay BG, Von Knorring L, et al. Predictors for the outcome of treatment with high frequency transcutaneous electrical nerve stimulation in patients with chronic pain. *Pain.* 9:55, 1980

103. Eriksson M, Schuller H, Sjolund B. Hazard from transcutaneous nerve stimulation in patients with pacemakers. *Lancet.* 1:1319, 1978

104. Shade SK. Use of transcutaneous electrical nerve stimulation for a patient with a cardiac pacemaker: A case report. *Phys Ther.* 65:206, 1985

105. Rasmussen MJ, Hayes DL, Vlietstra RE, et al. Can transcutaneous electrical nerve stimulation be safely used in patients with permanent cardiac pacemakers? *Mayo Clin Proc.* 63:443, 1988

106. Augustinsson LE, Bohlin P, Carlsson CA, et al. Pain relief during delivery by transcutaneous electrical nerve stimulation. *Pain.* 4:59, 1977

107. Vincenti E, Cervellin A, Mega M, et al. Comparative study between patients treated with transcutaneous electric stimulation and controls during labor. *Clin Exp Obstet Gynecol.* 9:95, 1982

108. Picaza JA, Cannon BW, Hunter SE, et al. Pain suppression by peripheral nerve stimulation, Part I: Observations with transcutaneous stimuli. *Surg Neurol.* 4:105, 1975

109. Klein J, Pariser D. Transcutaneous electrical nerve stimulation. In: Currier DP, Nelson RM, eds. *Clinical Electrotherapy.* Norwalk, CT, Appleton-Century-Crofts, 1987:209–230

110. Griffin JW, McClure M. Adverse responses to transcutaneous electrical nerve stimulation in a patient with rheumatoid arthritis. *Phys Ther.* 61:354, 1981

111. Linzer M, Long DM. Transcutaneous neural stimulation for relief of pain. *IEEE Trans Biomed Eng.* 23:341, 1976

112. Andersson SA. Pain control by sensory stimulation. In: Bonica JJ, Liebeskind JC, Albe-Fessard DG, eds. *Advances in Pain Research and Therapy.* New York, Raven Press, 1979; 3:569–585

113. Leo KC, Dostal WF, Bossen DG, et al. Effect of transcutaneous electrical nerve stimulation characteristics on clinical pain. *Phys Ther.* 66:200, 1986

114. Howson DC. Peripheral neural excitability: Implications for transcutaneous electrical nerve stimulation. *Phys Ther.* 58:1467, 1978

115. Janko M, Trontelj JV. Transcutaneous electrical nerve stimulation: A microneurographic and perceptual study. *Pain.* 9:219, 1980

116. Andersson SA, Hansson G, Holmgren E, et al Evaluation of the pain suppressive

effect of different frequencies of peripheral electrical stimulation in chronic pain conditions. *ACTA Ortho Scand.* 47:149, 1976

117. Benton LA, Baker LL, Bowman BR, et al. *Functional Electrical Stimulation: A Practical Clinical Guide,* 2nd ed. Downey, CA, Rancho Los Amigos Hospital, 1981

118. Fox EJ, Melzack R. Transcutaneous electrical stimulation and acupuncture: Comparison of treatment for low back pain. *Pain.* 2:141, 148, 1976

119. Leo K. Perceived comfort levels of modulated versus conventional TENS current. *Phys Ther.* 64:745, 1984 (abstract)

120. Miller BA, Smith KB, Real JL, et al. A comparison of modulated-rate and conventional TENS. *Phys Ther.* 64:744, 1984 (abstract)

121. Lein DH, Clelland JA, Knowles CJ, et al. Comparison of effects of transcutaneous electrical nerve stimulation of auricular, somatic, and the combination of auricular and somatic acupuncture points on experimental pain threshold. *Phys Ther.* 69:671, 1989

123. Santiesteban AJ. Comparison of electroacupuncture and selected physical therapy for acute spine pain. *Am J Acupunct.* 12:257, 1984

124. Gammon GD, Starr I. Studies on the relief of pain by counterirritation. *J Clin Invest.* 20:13, 1941

125. Inman VT, Saunders JB. Referred pain from skeletal structures. *J Nerv Ment Dis.* 99:660, 1944

126. Gunn CC. Motor points and motor lines. *Am J Acupunct.* 6:55, 1978

127. Walthard KM, Tchicaloff M. Motor points. In: Licht S, ed. *Electrodiagnosis and Electromyography,* 3rd ed. Baltimore, Waverly Press, 1971:153–170

128. Travel JG, Simons DG. *Myofascial Pain and Dysfunction. The Trigger Point Manual.* Baltimore, Williams & Wilkins, 1983

129. Mann F. *Acupuncture: The Ancient Chinese Art of Healing and How It Works Scientifically.* New York, Random House, 1971:27–34

130. Castel D, Castel JC. *Pain Management Desk Reference,* 3rd ed. Topeka, KS, Physiotechnology, 1987

131. Madill PV. Auriculotherapy (letter). *JAMA.* 252:1856, 1984

132. Melzack R, Katz J. Auriculotherapy fails to relieve chronic pain. *JAMA.* 251:1041, 1984

133. Melzack R, Katz J. Auriculotherapy (letter). *JAMA.* 252:1856, 1984

134. Nogier PFM. Auriculotherapy (letter). *JAMA.* 252:1855, 1984

135. Liu YK, Varela M, Oswald R. The correspondence between some motor points and acupuncture loci. *Am J Clin Med.* 3:347, 1975

136. Melzack R, Stillwell DM, Fox EJ. Trigger points and acupuncture points for pain: Correlations and implications. *Pain.* 3:3, 1977

137. Mannheimer JS. Electrode placements for transcutaneous electrical nerve stimulation. *Phys Ther.* 58:1455, 1978

138. Krause AW, Clelland JA, Knowles CJ, et al. Effects of unilateral and bilateral auricular transcutaneous electrical nerve stimulation on cutaneous pain threshold. *Phys Ther.* 67:507, 1987

139. Berlant S. Method of determining optimal stimulation sites for transcutaneous electrical nerve stimulation. *Phys Ther.* 64:924, 1984

140. Bishop B. Pain: Its physiology and rationale for management, part I: Neuroanatomical substrates of pain. *Phys Ther.* 60:13, 1980

141. Bishop B. Pain: Its physiology and rationale for management, part II: Analgesic systems of the CNS. *Phys Ther.* 60:21, 1980

142. Bishop B. Pain: Its physiology and rationale for management, part III: Consequences of current concepts of pain mechanisms related to pain management. *Phys Ther.* 60:24, 1980

143. Echternach JL, ed. *Pain. Clinics in Physical Therapy,* vol 12. New York, Churchill Livingstone, 1987

144. Mayer DJ, Price DD. The neurobiology of pain. In: Synder-Mackler L, Robinson A. *Clinical Electrophysiology. Electrotherapy and Electrophysiologic Testing.* Baltimore, Williams & Wilkins, 1989:141–201

145. Kaada B. Vasodilation induced by transcutaneous nerve stimulation in peripheral ischemia (Raynaud's phenomenon and diabetic polyneuropathy). *Eur Heart J.* 303, 1983

146. Currier D. Electrical stimulation for improving muscular strength and blood flow. In: Nelson RM, Currier DP. *Clinical Electrotherapy.* Norwalk, CT, Appleton & Lange, 1987: 141–164

147. Alon G, DeDomenico G. *High Voltage Stimulation: An Integrated Approach to Clinical Electrotherapy.* Chattanooga, TN, Chattanooga Corp, 1987

148. Taub A Campbell JN. Percutaneous local electrical analgesia: Peripheral mechanisms. In: Bonica JJ, ed. *Advances in Neurology.* New York, Raven Press, 1974; 4:727–733

149. Torebjörk HE, Hallin RG. Excitation failure in thin nerve fiber structures and accompanying hypalgesia during repetitive electric skin stimulation. In: Bonica JJ (ed). *Advances in Neurology.* New York, Raven Press, 1974; 4:733–735

150. Ignelzi RJ, Nyquist JK. Direct effect of electrical stimulation on peripheral nerve evoked activity: Implications in pain relief. *J Neurosurg.* 45:159, 1976

151. Devor M, Wall PD. The physiology of sensation after peripheral nerve injury, regeneration and neuroma formation. In Waxman SG, ed. *The Physiology and Pathobiology of Axons.* New York, Raven Press, 1978:377–388

152. Wall PD. The gate control theory of pain mechanisms. A re-examination and re-statement. *Brain.* 101:1, 1978

153. Jenkner FL, Schuhfried F. Transdermal transcutaneous electric nerve stimulation for pain: The search for an optimal waveform. *Appl Neurophysiol.* 44:330, 1981

154. Long DM, Hagfors N. Electrical stimulation in the nervous system: The current status of electrical stimulation of the nervous system for relief of pain. *Pain.* 1:109, 1975

155. Hoffert M. The gate control theory re-revisited. *J Pain Symptom Manage.* 1:39, 1986

156. Nathan PW, Rudge P. Testing the gate-control theory of pain in man. *J Neurol Neurosurg Psychiatr.* 37:1366, 1974

157. Nathan PW. The gate-control theory of pain: A critical review. *Brain.* 99:123, 1976

158. Langley GB, Sheppeard H, Johnson M, et al. The analgesic effects of transcutaneous electrical nerve stimulation and placebo in chronic pain patients. A double blind non-crossover comparison. *Rheumatol Int.* 4:119, 1984

159. Chan CWY, Tsang H. Inhibition of the human flexion reflex by low intensity, high frequency transcutaneous electrical nerve stimulation (TENS) has a gradual onset and offset. *Pain.* 28:239, 1987

160. Facchinetti F, Sandrini G, Petraglia F, et al. Concommitant increase in nociceptive flexion reflex threshold and plasma opioids following transcutaneous nerve stimulation. *Pain.* 19:295, 1984

161. Procacci P, Zoppi M, Maresca M, et al. Hypoalgesia induced by transcutaneous electrical stimulation. A physiological and clinical investigation. *J Neurosurg Sci.* 21:221, 1977

162. Lehmann TR, Russell DW, Spratt KF, et al. Efficacy of electroacupuncture and TENS in the rehabilitation of chronic low back pain patients. *Pain.* 26:277, 1986

163. Beecher HK. Nonspecific forces surrounding disease and the treatment of disease. *JAMA* 179:437, 1962

164. Beecher HK. The placebo effect as a nonspecific force surrounding disease and the treatment of disease. In: Janzen R, ed. *Pain: Basic Principles, Pharmacology, Therapy.* Baltimore, Williams & Wilkins, 1972: 175–180

165. Barr JO, Weissenbuehler SA, Bandstra EJ, et al. Effectiveness and comfort level of transcutaneous electrical nerve stimulation (TENS) in elderly with chronic pain. *Phys Ther.* 67:775, 1987 (abstract)

166. Andersson SA, Holmgren E. Analgesic effects of peripheral conditioning stimulation III. Effect of high frequency stimulation, segmental mechanisms interacting with pain. *Acupunct Electrother Res.* 3:22, 1978

167. Fordyce WE. *Behavioral Methods for Chronic Pain and Illness.* St. Louis, CV Mosby, 1976

168. Relman AS. Dealing with conflicts of interest (editorial). *N Engl J Med.* 313:749, 1985

169. Morgan S. Examining the ethics of electrotherapy. *Rx Home Care.* June 1986, pp 43–46

170. Paras T. Medical suppliers form alliance to address major TENS changes. *APTA Progress Report.* Feb 1986, p 9

171. Vander Ark GD, McGrath KA. Transcutaneous electrical stimulation in treatment of post operative pain. *Am J Surg.* 130:338, 1975

172. Long DM. Use of peripheral and spinal cord stimulation in the relief of chronic pain. In: Bonica JJ, Albe-Fessard DG, eds. *Advances in Pain Research and Therapy.* New York, Raven Press, 1976; 395–403

173. Stonnington HH, Stillwell GR, Ebersold MJ, et al. Transcutaneous electrical stimulation for chronic pain relief. A pilot study. *Minn Med.* 59:681, 1976

174. Long DM. External electrical stimulation as a treatment of chronic pain. *Minn Med.* 57:195, 1974

175. Loeser JD, Black RG, Christman A. Relief of pain by transcutaneous stimulation. *J of Neurosurg.* 42:308, 1975

176. Keravel Y, Sindou M. Anatomical conditions of efficiency of transcutaneous electrical neurostimulation in deafferention pain. In: Bonica JJ, Lindblom U, Iggo A, eds. *Advances in Pain Research and Therapy.* New York, Raven Press, 1983; 5:763–767

177. Doongaji DR, Vahia VN, Bharucha MPE. On placebos, placebo responses and placebo responders (a review of psychological, psychopharmacological and psychophysiological factors). II. Psychopharmacological and psychophysiological factors. *J Postgrad Med.* 24:147, 1978

178. Hamilton M. *Lectures on the Methodology of Clinical Research,* 2nd ed. Edinburgh, Churchill Livingston, 1974:119–121

179. Meyerson BA. Electrostimulation procedures: Effects, presumed rationale, and possible mechanisms. In: Bonica JJ, Lindbolm U, Iggo A, eds. *Advances in Pain Research and Therapy.* New York, Raven Press, 1983; 5:495–534

180. Thorsteinsson G, Stonnington HH, Stillwell GH, et al. The placebo effect of transcutaneous electrical stimulation. *Pain.* 5:31, 1978

181. Lewis D, Lewis B, Sturrock RD. Transcutaneous electrical nerve stimulation in osteoarthritis: A therapeutic alternative. *Am Rheum Dis.* 43:47, 1984

182. Abelson K, Langley GB, Sheppeard H, et al. Transcutaneous electrical nerve simulation in rheumatoid arthritis. *NZ Med J.* 96:156, 1983
183. Hargreaves A, Lander J. Use of transcutaneous electrical nerve stimulation for postoperative pain. *Nurs Res.* 38:159, 1989
184. Long DM, Campbell JN, Gucer G. Transcutaneous electrical stimulation for relief of chronic pain. In: Bonica JJ, Liebeskind JC, Albe-Fessard DG, eds. *Advances in Pain Research and Therapy.* New York, Raven Press, 1979; 3.
185. Ali J, Yaffe GS, Serrette C. The effect of transcutaneous electric nerve stimulation on postoperative pain and pulmonary function. *Surgery.* 89:507, 1981
186. Hansson P, Ekblom A. Transcutaneous electrical nerve stimulation (TENS) as compared to placebo TENS for the relief of acute oro-facial pain. *Pain.* 15:157, 1983
187. Finsen V, Persen L, Lovlien M, et al. Transcutaneous electrical nerve stimulation after major amputation. *JBJS.* 70B:109, 1988

CHAPTER *11*

Iontophoresis

John Cummings

Ion transfer, or *iontophoresis*, is the introduction of topically applied, physiologically active ions into the epidermis and mucous membranes of the body by the use of continuous direct current. Discovered by LeDuc in 1903, iontophoresis is based on the principle that an electrically charged electrode will repel a similarly charged ion.[1] Therefore, ions with a positive charge can be introduced into the tissues from the positive electrode, and negatively charged ions can be introduced by the negative pole. Although iontophoresis is not currently a widely used technique, it has been successfully used in the treatment of numerous conditions, including edema, ischemic skin ulcers, muscular pain, Peyronie's disease, hyperhidrosis, arthritis, fungus infections, bursitis, and tendonitis. This chapter discusses the theoretical basis for using iontophoresis and offers specific treatment methodologies of interest to physical therapists.

THEORETICAL BASIS OF IONTOPHORESIS

In its pure (distilled) state, water does not conduct an electrical current. However, when ionizable substances (such as acids, bases, salts, or alkaloids) are dissolved in water, the substances dissolve and dissociate into their component charged ions in a process called *ionization*. The resulting solutions, called *electrolytes*, are capable of conducting an electrical current by virtue of the migration of the dissociated ions. A current passes through an electrolyte because the electrically charged ions carry the electrical charge. When a continuous, unidirectional (galvanic) current (DC) is passed between two electrodes in an electrolytic solution, positive ions will be attracted toward the negative pole (cathode) and negative ions toward the positive pole (anode). This movement, or transfer, of ions is called *ion transfer*. The specific transfer of ions into the body for therapeutic purposes is called *iontophoresis*.

The force acting to move an ion through the surface of the body depends upon (1) the strength of the electric field and (2) the impedance of the tissues of the body to current flow. The therapist may compensate for skin impedance by altering the current amplitude as necessary to achieve the desired current density. It is the current density at the electrode–body-surface interface that is responsible for the velocity of the charged ions as they pass into the body. The current density may be increased either by decreasing the size of the electrode or by increasing the amplitude of the current. Since body tissues, especially the skin and mucous membranes, have a limited tolerance to the passage of an electrical current, the principal guide to a safe current density is the comfort of the patient. The physiological effects of direct current on the skin are well-known. The anode produces an acidic reaction in the underlying skin, has a hardening effect, and produces a mild heating effect secondary to vasodilation. The cathode produces an alkaline reaction in the underlying skin, has a softening effect, and (like the anode) produces a mild heating effect. These electro-chemical reactions under the electrodes may also be decreased by decreasing the current density under the cathode, either by increasing the size of the electrodes or by decreasing the amplitude of the current.

CONTINUOUS DIRECT CURRENT

Continuous, unidirectional (galvanic) current is the current of choice for ion-tophoresis, since this mode assures maximum ion transfer per unit of applied current.[2] Other current forms, such as conventional high-voltage pulsed, sine wave, and interferential currents, are not effective in iontophoresis.

One potential hazard inherent in the use of continuous unidirectional current for iontophoresis is the possible formation of an electrochemical burn on the skin underlying the electrodes. Normal, intact skin will not tolerate a current density greater than 1 mA/cm[2] when the applied current is continuous DC.[3] However, skin impedance is even lower in areas where the skin is abraded or lacerated, in areas of scarring, and in individuals with fair skin.

The alkaline reaction occurring under the cathode is much more caustic to the skin than is the acidic reaction occurring at the anode. To minimize the possibility of tissue destruction under the cathode while still maintaining an effective treatment, the physical therapist should selectively decrease the current density under the cathode. We know that if both electrodes are of equal size, the current density will be equal under each electrode; and that if the electrodes are of different sizes, the current density will always be greater under the smaller electrode. Therefore, the current density under either elec-trode may be selectively decreased by increasing the size of the electrode. By increasing the surface area of the cathode, we decrease the current density under the cathode. As the current density under the cathode decreases, the magnitude of the caustic alkaline reaction in the body tissue, which occurs as the continuous DC passes through the cathode, also decreases. One rule of thumb to follow when using iontophoresis is to keep the surface area of the cathode at least twice that of the anode at all times. This size relationship should be followed not only when the cathode is designated as the "active" electrode but also when the cathode is designated as the "dispersive" or "inactive" electrode.

One additional concern of the physical therapist is the anesthetic effect of continuous unidirectional current. Since continuous unidirectional current has an anesthetic effect on the skin underlying the electrodes, it is very likely that the patient may be totally unaware of the development of an electrical burn until after the conclusion of the treatment. Therefore, close monitoring of the skin underlying the electrodes is recommended during treatment. In addition, as a normal response to current flow, mild to moderate hyperemia (capillary dilation) is to be expected under both electrodes.

TRANSFER OF IONS

The effectiveness of a specific ion will depend upon (1) the number of ions transferred; (2) the depth of penetration; (3) whether the ions combine chemically with other substances in the skin and precipitates; and (4) whether the ions enter the capillaries and are carried away from the site of application by the blood. Histamine is one ion introduced into the body through iontophoresis that may have a systemic effect (flushing of the skin, headache, or both) if too much of the ion enters the vascular system.

The number of ions transferred into the body through iontophoresis is related to (1) the current density at the active electrode; (2) the duration of the current flow; and (3) the concentration of the ions in the solution. Although a body part might not absorb a specific ion when placed in an electrolytic solution, the ions in the solution may be driven into the skin if an electrical current is passed through the solution. The quantity of ions introduced across the body surface is directly proportional to the current density.[4] The amount of time that the current is allowed to flow also influences the number of ions transferred, since it is the current passing through the electrolytic solution that causes the ions to migrate according to their charge. The number of ions transferred is proportional to the cube root of the product of the current density and to the duration of its application.[5] Therefore, the longer a current is applied, the greater the number of ions that will be transferred. However, as the duration of the treatment increases, the skin impedance decreases, and the chance of an electrical burn increases.

The concentration of the ionic solution will also affect the number of ions transferred. Several investigators have demonstrated that medications at concentrations greater than 1 or 2 percent are not more advantageous than are medications of lower concentrations.[6,7]

Impedance to current flow and to ion transfer is primarily a function of the skin. However, certain dermal structures (such as hair follicles and sweat glands) represent areas of decreased skin impedance and provide gaps in the skin through which an electrical current (and ions) may readily flow.[8] In addition to these areas of decreased skin impedance, the overall impedance of the skin to current flow will generally fall somewhat during the treatment as the skin becomes more saturated with the electrolyte and the physiological reaction to the current flow results in an increased blood supply (vasodilation) to the area under the electrodes.[4]

Another factor inhibiting the transfer of ions is the tendency of some ions to form insoluble precipitates as they pass into the tissue.[9] Precipitates are formed with the transfer of heavy-metal ions, such as iron, silver, copper, and zinc. In a study on the penetration of the ferric ion ($FeCl_3$) into pig skin using iontophoresis, Gadsby concluded that the ferric ions only penetrated the skin to the depth of the dermis, since no ferric ions were found deep in the dermis.[10]

In another study Puttemans and colleagues studied the uptake of $I-$ by the tiered following iontophoresis of the potassium iodide. The fate of the absorbed iodine was investigated by measuring the total stable thyroidal iodine content by means of x-ray fluorescence before and after a series of ten iontophoretic treatments. They demonstrated that the average iodine content of the thyroid gland was increased by more than 30 percent following the series of 10 termagants.[11]

GENERAL METHODOLOGY

Prior to initiating treatment with iontophoresis, the therapist must

1. Be thoroughly knowledgeable about the presenting pathology.
2. Identify the appropriate ion for treating the pathology.
3. Identify the polarity of the ion of choice.
4. Select an electrical generator that delivers continuous, unidirectional current (continuous DC).
5. Determine whether the patient is allergic to the ion.
6. Inspect the body part to be treated to determine the presence of cuts, abrasions, scar tissue, new skin, or inflammation.
7. Check the patient's skin sensation in the area to be treated.
8. Gently clean the patient's skin in the area to be treated (to remove oils from the surface of the skin).
9. Fully explain the procedure to the patient.

Having selected the appropriate ion and electrodes, the solution or cream containing the ion is applied to the bare skin of the treatment area and is massaged into the superficial tissues. A warm towel (or several layers of gauze, a cloth diaper, or the like) moistened with warm tap water or with saline solution and folded smoothly (with no wrinkles), is then placed over the treatment area. Alternatively, the towel may be soaked with the solution containing the ion. The "active" pad electrode (precut block tin, aluminum foil, or commercial metal electrode), which is somewhat smaller than the towel and which has the same polarity as the ion, is placed on top of the towel in such a manner as to avoid overlapping the towel and touching the skin. This is very important, as contact between the electrode and the skin can cause a chemical burn. Good contact between electrode and towel, and between towel and skin, is essential in order to avoid "hot spots" resulting from areas of increased current density (such as folds in the towel).

A similar electrode (of opposite polarity and without the ion solution/cream), thoroughly moistened with tap water or saline solution, is used as the dispersive electrode, and is positioned ipsilaterally and conveniently at a distance (ie, at least 18 in) from the active electrode. The electrodes are kept in place using either rubber or webbed straps or sandbags. The pressure stabilizing the electrodes should be uniform to help ensure an even distribution of current. If either block tin or aluminum foil (folded into five to ten layers) are used as electrodes, they may be attached to the lead wires with alligator-type clips. The lead wires are then connected to the appropriate generator terminals.

Before connecting the lead wires to the generator, the therapist must make sure that both the generator and the amplitude control are turned off. The electrodes must never be placed or removed while the generator is turned on. Care must also be taken to ensure that electrodes used for ion transfer are not used for muscle stimulation. If the electrodes are later used for muscle stimulation, transfer of ions may inadvertently occur during stimulation of the muscle.

With the ionic solution or cream and moistened electrodes applied to the treatment area, the therapist is ready to initiate treatment. The generator is turned on, and the amplitude is slowly increased until the patient reports a prickly or tingling sensation. The patient is warned to notify the therapist immediately if there is any local pain or a burning sensation. The amplitude of the current is usually set so that the current density is between 0.1 and 0.5 mA/cm^2 of surface of the active electrode. The desired amplitude is maintained for the duration of the treatment, which is usually 15 min or less, provided that the patient remains comfortable and that there are no adverse systemic effects.[12] The patient must be checked every 3 to 5 min after treatment begins to ensure that the skin is not irritated. Often, as the treatment proceeds, the therapist will have to decrease the amplitude of the current in order to compensate for a progressive decrease in skin impedance to the current flow. Another point to remember is that the polarity of the electrodes should never be changed while the current is flowing. Although some clinicians suggest that the polarity of the current may be reversed for 1 min or so during treatment, the current must not be flowing when the polarity is reversed.[12]

When the treatment has been completed, the current amplitude is slowly reduced to zero, the generator turned off, and the electrodes removed. Kahn suggests that, following each treatment, an astringent gel be massaged into the skin under each electrode, followed by a light dusting of powder, in order to minimize skin irritation.[13]

SPECIFIC UTILIZATION OF IONTOPHORESIS

Numerous ions have been utilized in iontophoresis. Here, review will be made of those ions that are most commonly used by physical therapists and the conditions for which they are used.

Local Anesthetics

The successful use of iontophoresis to administer local anesthetics (in lieu of injection infiltration) has been reported in the dental, ear, nose, and throat, and ophthalmologic literature.[13–15] Gangarosa reports minimal patient discomfort during tooth extraction using iontophoresis for deep surface anesthesia.[14] Sisler reported using iontophoresis for local anesthesia in surgery of the conjunctiva and associated structures.[16] Iontophoresis is also used to anesthetize the external auditory canal and the tympanic membrane prior to minor surgery such as myringotomy or placement of ventilation tubes in patients with serous otitis media.[17–19]

A study by Russo and associates compared the duration and depth of anesthesia produced by lidocaine and physiological saline when administered by iontophoresis, subcutaneous infiltration, and topical application. To test for duration of anesthesia, either lidocaine or a placebo was administered by iontophoresis (anode as the active electrode), by subcutaneous infiltration, or by swabbing at each of three sites (3 cm apart) on the flexor surface of each forearm of 27 subjects. In the subjects receiving lidocaine iontophoresis, the current was slowly advanced from 0 to 2 mA during the first minute, to 4 mA during the second minute, and remained at that level for an additional 5 min. The maximum current density was 0.65 mA/cm^2. Sensation was tested by pressing the tip of a 21-gauge hypodermic needle on each application site every 5 min until feeling returned. Lidocaine iontophoresis produced local anesthesia of significantly longer duration ($P < 0.001$) than did either topical application of lidocaine or a placebo by any route of administration. However, the local anesthesia produced by lidocaine iontophoresis was of significantly shorter duration ($P < 0.001$) than was lidocaine infiltration. The results of this study showed that lidocaine iontophoresis is an effective method of producing local anesthesia for about 5 min without requiring the use of infiltration.[20]

Edema Reduction

Reduction of edema in acute and chronic conditions using hyaluronidase iontophoresis has been reported by Magistro, who dissolved one ampule of hyaluronidase (150 USP units) in 250 cc of 0.1 M acetate buffer solution (with a pH of 5.4). Using the anode as the active electrode, he passed between 1 and 2 mA of current per 2.5 cm^2 of active electrode for 20 to 40 min. In this study of 100 patients, the average total edema reduction was 0.6 to 1.9 cm (0.25 to 0.75 in), with no adverse reactions occurring in 362 treatments. Although the rate of edema reduction is quite rapid using this technique, in most instances in Magistro's study, the permanence of the reduction was difficult to maintain, as is true of other treatment methods. However, in terms of equipment, time required for treatment, and ease of application, edema reduction by hyaluronidase iontophoresis is advantageous.[21]

An additional study (by Schwartz) of five subjects attempted to determine a direct method of measuring the actual amount of hyaluronidase absorbed by the skin when administered by iontophoresis. This study demonstrated that intradermal wheals are dissipated more rapidly from areas treated with hyaluronidase iontophoresis than are similar wheals in areas treated by iontophoresis without hyaluronidase. Therefore, hyaluronidase administered by iontophoresis appears to cause increased absorption of fluid from both the skin and subcutaneous tissue.[22]

Inflammatory Conditions

Glass and associates have demonstrated, in a series of animal studies with rhesus monkeys, that radiolabeled dexamethasone sodium phosphate (Decadron) can be iontophoresed into the tissue surrounding the shoulder, elbow, hip, knee, and ankle joints. This study demonstrated that therapeutic dosages of the radiolabeled anti-inflammatory agent Decadron could be transferred iontophoretically into all tissue layers underlying the active electrode, including tendons and cartilage.[23]

Musculoskeletal inflammatory conditions in humans (eg, bursitis, tendonitis, ligamentous strain) have been successfully treated using dexamethasone sodium phosphate (Decadron) combined with Xylocaine iontophoresis. In a clinical study on the efficacy of Decadron and Xylocaine iontophoresis in the treatment of various musculoskeletal inflammatory conditions in 50 patients, Harris reports that 38 patients had excellent relief of pain and symptoms, 7 reported moderate relief, and 5 reported little or no change. Harris utilized a 1-cc solution containing 4 mg of Decadron combined with 2 cc of 4-percent Xylocaine, which was introduced into the positive electrode of a commercially available iontophoresis unit (Phoresor). The current was set at 1 mA and was increased by 1 mA each minute for 5 min, with the current remaining at 5 mA for an additional 15 min. Each patient received a maximum of three treatments within a 1-week period. When two or more treatments were administered, they were given every other day. Although this study indicates that iontophoresis is an effective mode of delivering ionized inflammatory drugs to inflamed tissues, Harris cautions that because of the well-publicized potential side effects of corticosteroids, these agents should be used with caution.[24]

In a similar study on the effect of the iontophoretic application of dexamethasone sodium phosphate and lidocaine hydrochloride on 53 individuals with tendonitis (supraspinatus, infraspinatus, and bicipital and lateral epicondylitis), Bertolucci concluded that patients younger than 45 years of age with shoulder dysfunction related to primary tendonitis respond well to steroids administered by iontophoresis. However, patients older than 45 years with a primary diagnosis of cervical degenerative change have less-significant pain relief in shoulder tendonitis, regardless of whether or not the steroids are administered by injection or by iontophoresis.[25]

In his handbook on low-voltage techniques, Kahn suggests that hydrocortisone iontophoresis (0.5 percent) accompany infrared, therapy massage, and rest in the treatment of epicondylitis. Kahn further reminds us that other therapeutic agents (exercise, massage, hydrotherapy, manipulation, and so on) should be used in conjunction with iontophoresis as part of a comprehensive physical therapy program.[26]

Skin Conditions

Iontophoresis has also been reported as successful in the treatment of numerous skin conditions, including idiopathic hyperhidrosis; small, open ulcers; and fungus infections. Idiopathic hyperhidrosis of the palms of the hands and the soles of the feet has been successfully treated using iontophoresis with either tap water or various drugs as the electrolyte.[26-33] the most commonly used electrolyte is ordinary tap water. Typically, the patient's hands or feet are placed in shallow pans, with the tap water deep enough to cover the hands or feet but not deep enough to reach the nail folds. Flat metal (tin or aluminum) electrodes are placed on the bottom of the pan. When using tap water, Kahn suggests alternating the polarity (15 min positive followed by 15 min negative) during treatment.[26] Levit, also using tap water as the electrolyte, and using a current amplitude of between 15 and 29 mA, used gradients lasting 10 to 15 min and given two to three times a week.[27] Both of these authors reported positive results in controlling moderate to severe hyperhidrosis.

The successful use of zinc-oxide iontophoresis in the management of small, open, ischemic ulcers has been reported in a case study by Cornwall, who suggests that zinc-oxide iontophoresis is most effective in lesions measuring less than 1 cm in diameter. Having filled the entire crater of the wound with a small amount of a 0.1-M zinc-oxide ointment, Cornwall placed two tap-water-soaked gauze pads over the area covered by the medication. A 6 by 6 cm anode made of pliable aluminum was placed over the moistened gauze and was anchored using a rubber bandage. Cornwall's method consisted of two 15-min treatments a day, 6 days a week, for a total of 20 days. Current amplitude was maintained between 4 and 5 mA for the duration of the treatment. Cornwall reports that the ulcers treated demonstrated a 98.7 to 99.5 percent closure after 20 days.[34]

In a more recent study Falcone and Spadaro studied the effective iontophoretic penetration of the silver ion, and its local antibacterial effect in vitro. Using tissue cultures of a variety of skin pathogens, they compared the bacteriocidal effect that a silver-coated fabric would have on the pathogens with the effect that a similar silver-coated fabric with a continuous, unidirectional current passing through it would have on the pathogens. Falcone and Spadaro demonstrated that the bacterial-free "clear zones" surrounding the electrically activated silver-coated fabric were significantly larger than those of the silver fabric without an electrical current. They concluded that the delivery of the free silver ion via iontophoresis may have clinical implications, such as that by making an open skin wound essentially bacteria-free, resurfacing by skin graft may be expedited or wound granulation enhanced.[35]

The successful use of 1-percent copper sulfate iontophoresis in the treatment of tinea pedia (athlete's foot) has been reported by Haggard and associates. They immersed the affected foot in a plastic foot tub containing a 1-percent copper sulfate solution, with a copper plate (acting as the anode) resting on the floor of the tub. A current of 10 mA was passed through the electrolyte for 15 min, two treatments a week. The authors reported that many of the patients showed marked improvement within 24 hr of receiving the initial treatment.[36]

Additional Applications

Although the most common ions used for iontophoresis have been discussed, many additional substances have been used effectively in iontophoresis. However, since invasive modes of application (such as injection) have provided for a more localized application and better dosage control, the popularity of iontophoresis as an effective technique for the administration of medications has decreased; along with the decreased use of the modality, many of the traditional ions used in iontophoresis have also lost their popularity. Although many ions previously proven effective in iontophoresis are not in widespread use today, the potential use of these substances in physical therapy should not be overlooked.

Histamine and mecholyl have been used to produce superficial vasodilation.[37] Harris has demonstrated an increase of over 100 percent in the superficial circulation of the skin, with no appreciable change in circulation in the underlying musculature (unless a systemic response occurred).[9] Such systemic responses to the application of either histamine or mecholyl may occur, especially if the patient is hypersensitive to the agent. The systemic response should be avoided and is characterized by a fall in blood pressure, an increase in pulse rate, sweating, and a flushing of the skin. However, histamine and mecholyl have traditionally been used as superficial vasodilators in the treatment of peripheral vascular disease, rheumatic arthritis, and varicose ulcers.[37]

Two additional ions of note are iodine and the acetate ion found in acetic acid. Iodine is a sclerolytic agent that is effective in reducing scar tissue.[26,38] The iodine increased the extensibility of the scar and may be used to increase the effectiveness of stretching scar tissue. The acetate ion is delivered through acetic acid iontophoresis; it is effective in reducing the size of calcium deposits (through absorption of the calcium) and may be used in the treatment of

TABLE 11–1. IONS CURRENTLY USED IN IONTOPHORESIS, INCLUDING THE MOST CONVENIENT SOURCE OF THE ION, IONIC POLARITY, AND INDICATIONS

Ion	Source	Polarity	Indications
Acetate	Acetic acid	Negative	Calcium deposits
Chloride	Sodium chloride	Negative	Soften scars and adhesions (sclerolytic agent)
Copper	Copper sulphate	Positive	Fungus infections (eg, athlete's foot)
Dexamethasone	Decadron	Positive	Musculoskeletal inflammation conditions (arthritis, bursitis); (anti-inflammatory agent)
Hyoluronidase	Wyadase	Positive	Edema reduction
Magnesium	Magnesium sulfate (Epsom Salts)	Positive	Muscle relaxant, vasodilation
Salicylate	Sodium salicylate	Positive	Edema reduction
Tap water		Alternating polarity	Hyperhydrosis
Xylocaine	Xylocaine	Positive	Bursitis, neuritis (analgesic agent)
Zinc	Zinc oxide	Positive	Dermal ulcers, slow-healing wounds

calcified tendonitis and to reduce muscle spasm.[26,39] A summary of these uses of iontophoresis is presented in Table 11–1.

CONTRAINDICATIONS

The contraindications to iontophoresis are few; however, several rules must be followed to ensure patients' safety:

1. Follow all general rules regarding electrical stimulation.
2. Never use an ion to which the patient is allergic.
3. Be certain that the patient's skin sensation is normal in the treatment areas; otherwise, the skin must be monitored more often during treatment.
4. Never apply the electrodes over denuded areas or over new scar tissue.
5. Metal electrodes must never come in contact with the skin.
6. Electrodes must be thoroughly and evenly soaked with tap water, saline, or the solution containing the ion.

7. Electrodes must make good contact with the skin and should be applied with a constant pressure.
8. The patient must thoroughly understand that he or she is to immediately report any burning or painful sensations to the therapist.
9. The therapist must use a DC generator that is reliable and that will enable the therapist to calculate the current density under each electrode.
10. The current must be increased slowly at the beginning, and decreased slowly at the conclusion, of the treatment.
11. Never remove or rearrange electrodes without first turning the unit off completely.

CONCLUSIONS

The interest in iontophoresis as an effective clinical agent is enjoying a slow, yet steady, renewal in this country. This is due in part to the increased clinical and commercial interest in electrotherapy and to an increase in well-designed studies that have provided additional evidence supporting the value of iontophoresis as a clinical agent. Although iontophoresis has met with some skepticism and criticism in the past, the technique has not been abandoned. The medical community is becoming more aware of the fact that iontophoresis has several advantages over injection as a delivery system for certain drugs. Specifically, iontophoresis is noninvasive, painless, and sterile; in addition, tissue damage due to needle penetration and subcutaneous injection is avoided. Physical therapists should continue to use iontophoresis as an effective agent in conjunction with other, more popular, treatment regimes.

REFERENCES

1. LeDuc S. *Electric Ions and Their Use in Medicine.* Liverpool, Rebman, 1903
2. Abramowitsch D, Neoussikine B. *Treatment by Ion Transfer.* New York, Grune & Stratton, 1946: 124
3. Shriber W. *A Manual of Electrotherapy,* 4th ed. Philadelphia, Lea & Febiger, 1975
4. Nightingale A. *Physics and Electronics in Physical Medicine.* London, F. Bell, 1959: 178
5. Trubatch J, Van Harreveld A. Spread of iontophoretically injected ions in a tissue. *J Theor Biol.* 36:355, 1972
6. O'Malley E, Oester Y. Influence of some physical chemical factors on iontophoresis using radio-isotopes. *Arch Phys Med Rehabil.* 36:310, 1955
7. Murray W, Levine LS, Seifter E. The iontophoresis of C_2 esterified glucocorticoids: Preliminary report. *Phys Ther.* 43:579, 1963
8. Johnson C, Shuster S. The patency of sweat ducts in normal looking skin. *Br J Dermatol.* 83:367, 1970

9. Harris R. Iontophoresis. In: Lucht S, ed. *Therapeutic Electricity and Ultraviolet Radiation.* Baltimore, Waverly, 1967

10. Gadsby PD. Visualization of the barrier layer through iontophoresis of ferric ions. *Med Instrum.* 13:281, 1979

11. Puttemans FJM, Gilles F, Lievens PC, Jonckeer M. Iontophoresis: Mechanism of action studied by potentiometry and x-ray fluorescence. *Arch Phys Med Rehabil.* 63:196, 1982

12. Stillwell GK. Electrotherapy. In: Kottke F, Stillwell G, Lehman J, eds. *Handbook of Physical Medical and Rehabilitation.* Philadelphia, W B Saunders, 1982: 370

13. Kahn J. A case report: Lithium iontophoresis for gouty arthritis. *J Orthop Sports Phys Ther.* 4:113, 1982

14. Gangarosa LP. Iontophoresis for surface local anesthesia. *J Am Dent Assoc.* 88:125, 1974

15. (Editorial) Iontophoresis—A major advancement. *Eye, Ear, Nose, Throat.* 55:13, 1976

16. Sisler HA. Iontophoresis local anesthesia for conjunctival surgery. Ann Ophthalmol 10:597, 1978

17. Comean M, Brummet R, Vernon SJ. Local anesthesia of the ear by iontophoresis. *Arch Otalaryngol.* 98: 114, 1973

18. Comean M, Brummett R: Anesthesia of the human tympanic membrane by iontophoresis of a local anesthetic. *Laryngoscope.* 88:277, 1978

19. Brumett A, Comean M. Local anesthesia of the tympanic membrane by iontophoresis. *Trans Am Acad Otolaryngol.* 78:453, 1974

20. Russo J, Lipman AG, Comstock TJ, et al. Lidocaine anesthesia: Comparison of iontophoresis injection and swabbing. *Am J Hosp Pharm.* 37:843, 1980

21. Magistro CM. Hyaluronidase by iontophoresis. *Phys Ther.* 44:169, 1964

22. Schwartz MS. The use of hyaluronidase by iontophoresis in the treatment of lymphedema. *Arch Intern Med.* 95:662, 1955

23. Glass JM, Stephen RL, Jacobsen SC. The quantity and distribution of radiolabeled depamethasone delivered to tissues by iontophoresis. *Int J Dermatol.* 19:519, 1980

24. Harris PR. Iontophoresis: Clinical research in musculoskeletal inflammatory conditions. *J Ortho Sports Phys Ther.*4:109, 1982

25. Bertolucci LE. Introduction of antiinflammatory drugs by iontophoresis: Double-blind study. *J Ortho Sports Phys Ther.* 4:103, 1982

26. Kahn J. *Clinical Electrotherapy.* Syosset, NY, Joseph Kahn, 1973

27. Levit F. Simple device for treatment of hyperhidrosis by iontophoresis. *Arch Dermatol.* 98:505, 1968

28. Shrivastava SN, Sing G. Tap water iontophoresis in palm and plantar hyperhidrosis. *Br J Dermatol.* 96:189, 1977

29. Grice K, Sattar H, Baker H. Treatment of idiopathic hyperhidrosis with iontophoresis of tap water and poldine methosulphate. *Br J Dermatol.* 86:72, 1972

30. Abdell E, Morgan K. Treatment of idiopathic hyperhydrosis by glycopyrronium bromide and tap water iontophoresis. *Br J Dermatol.* 91:87, 1974

31. Hill BHR. Poldine iontophoresis in the treatment of palmar and plantar hyperhidrosis. *Aust J Dermatol.* 17:92, 1976

32. Stolman LP. Treatment of excess sweating of the palms by iontophoresis. *Arch Dermatol.* 123:893, 1987

33. Akins DL, Meisenheimer JL, Dobson RL. Efficacy of the Drionic unit in the treatment of hyperhidrosis. *J Am Acad Dermatol.* 16: 828, 1987

34. Cornwall MW. Zinc iontophoresis to treat ischemic skin ulcers. *Phys Ther.* 61:359, 1981

35. Falcone AE, Spadaro JA. Inhibitory effects of electrically activated silver material on cutaneous wound bacteria. *Plast Reconstr Surg.* 77:455, 1986

36. Haggard HW, Strauss MJ, Greenberg LA. Fungous infections of hand and feet treated by copper iontophoresis. *JAMA.* 112:1229, 1939

37. Kovacs R. *Electrotherapy and Light Therapy.* Philadelphia, Lea & Febiger, 1949: 136

38. Tannenbaum M. Iodine iontophoresis in reducing scar tissue. *Phys Ther.* 60:792, 1980

39. Psaki C, Carol J. Acetic acid ionization: A study to determine the absorptive effects upon calcified tendinitis of the shoulder. *Phys Ther Rev.* 35:84, 1955

CHAPTER 12

Electrophysiological Evaluation: An Overview

Roger M. Nelson and David E. Nestor

The majority of the content of this book deals with the electrophysiological aspects of treatment; for example, the use of neuromuscular electrical stimulation (NMES) on innervated and denervated muscle, the use of high-voltage stimulation in the treatment of disease and injury, and the use of NMES to increase muscle strength. This chapter takes the electrophysiological process in a different direction; we now use the electrophysiological phenomena present in muscles and nerves to evaluate the functional integrity of the neuromuscular system. *Electrophysiological evaluation* may be defined (broadly) as encompassing the observation, recording, analysis, and interpretation of bioelectrical muscle and nerve potentials, detected by means of surface or needle electrodes, for the purpose of evaluating the integrity of the neuromusculoskeletal system.

Electrophysiological evaluation may be divided into two major components: evoked potentials and voluntary potentials. Major components of both are reviewed in this chapter. The objective of this chapter is to raise the reader's level of comprehension of the role that electrophysiological evaluation plays in the practice of physical therapy. Electrophysiological evaluation tests are often called diagnostic tests by some members of the health professions. Electrophysiological evaluation results do not give a clinical diagnosis of the patient's illness. There are no waveforms that are pathognomonic of specific disease entities. Electrophysiological evaluation aids in diagnosis insofar as the evidence of abnormality of the motor unit that it provides is or is not compatible with the clinical diagnosis under consideration. The electrophysiological evaluation results *must* be integrated with results of other tests, the clinical examination, and the history in arriving at the final diagnosis.

The referring physician must combine the results of the electrophysiological evaluation and the results of other tests in order to make a final diagnosis. Electrophysiological test results may be likened to the mosaic tiles that make up a mosaic picture. Without all of the mosaic tiles in place, a complete picture will not be evident. Similarly, the referring physician will need to use all of the tests to arrive at the final diagnosis.

This chapter begins with a description of evoked potentials and ends with a discussion of voluntary potentials. The intent of the chapter is not to make the reader proficient in the areas presented. Rather, an overview of the specialty field of electrophysiological evaluation is presented in order to make the reader aware of the use of this physical therapy practice area.

EVOKED POTENTIALS

The term *evoked* implies that some outside influence has caused a change in the excitable cell. (Recall Chapter 1 and the discussion of the excitable cell.) The cell discharges with an action potential when a critical threshold level is reached. In evoked potentials, the critical level of depolarization is used to evaluate the functional integrity of the neuromuscular system by externally controlling the discharge of the cell structure. The key ingredient in evoked potentials is the factor of control. The examiner has control over the amount, timing, and electrophysical parameters of the stimulation. The examiner allows only one physiological response to vary. For example, neural conduction is the response variable to nerve electrostimulation. Therefore, any abnormal calculated neural conduction value is assumed to be the result of a disease process or injury.

There are four major categories of evoked responses currently used in the clinical setting: (1) motor nerve conduction; (2) sensory nerve conduction; (3) electronic reflex testing; and (4) centrally recorded evoked responses. Motor nerve conduction studies use the information of the motor component of the peripheral nerve bundle. Sensory nerve studies use information from the large sensory fibers of the peripheral nerve bundles. These studies form the bulk of the evoked potential analysis used in the electrophysiological evaluation process. Electronic reflex testing uses information from the proximal portions of the peripheral nervous system. The distal portion of the peripheral nervous system is used as the carrier in determining conduction along the proximal portion of the nervous system. Centrally recorded evoked potentials use the distal, proximal, and central portions of the nervous system to record, transmit, and distribute the response to the brain.

Motor Nerve Conduction Velocity Studies
The peripheral nerve bundle conducts both afferent and efferent information. Afferent information travels from the periphery to the central nervous system for interpretation and processing; the afferent system is predominantly feed-

back. Efferent information begins in the central nervous system, eventually exiting the ventral root of the spinal cord and terminating on the peripheral components. The majority of efferent axons are from alpha motor neurons that innervate the peripheral components, such as voluntary striated skeletal muscle. Motor nerve conduction velocity (MNCV) studies seek to estimate the rate of movement of the induced impulse along the alpha motor neurons by an indirect method.

The method used to estimate conduction of motor nerve action potential impulses is indirect, because the alpha motor neuron impulses are not directly measured; rather, the response of alpha motor neurons to NMES is recorded from skeletal muscle. The result of alpha motor neuron response to stimulation is the evoked skeletal muscle action potential. The evoked response is recorded from a skeletal muscle innervated by that group of alpha motor neurons. It should be remembered that NMES of the peripheral nerve bundle causes depolarization and a subsequent synchronous volley of action potentials along both efferent and afferent nerve bundles. The selective recording of the motor response from the associated skeletal muscle allows an estimation of the impulse's rate of travel along the alpha motor axons, as well as an estimation of the number of motor units participating in the evoked muscle action potential.

The technique for performing motor nerve conduction studies includes the recording of the motor response from a superficially located skeletal muscle innervated by the peripheral nerve being studied. The muscle must be distal to the site of stimulation, innervated only by that particular nerve, and superficial. When the nerve is stimulated, an evoked muscle response is obtained. This response is called an evoked compound muscle action potential. When the nerve is electrically stimulated, a stimulus artifact is instantly introduced on the left-hand side of the oscilloscope (Fig. 12–1). The latency is expressed in milliseconds and represents the time delay from stimulus artifact to the beginning of the evoked muscle action potential. The latency reflects the amount of time that the impulse takes to move from the site of stimulation to the muscle.

Latency is commonly measured from the stimulus artifact to the beginning of the evoked muscle action potential. The measurement of latency reflects the conduction of the induced impulse along the largest and fastest motor axons in

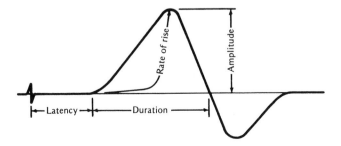

Figure *12–1.* Schematic rendition of an evoked muscle action potential resulting from supramaximal electrical stimulation.

the peripheral nerve. Terminal latency cannot be computed into a velocity segment for motor nerve conduction studies. Simply recording the latency is not sufficient to calculate *velocity*, which is a ratio of time divided by distance. The measurement of distance from the site of stimulation to the recording electrode on the muscle is inaccurate. Many physiological factors make such a measurement inappropriate. For example, as the action potential (impulses) reaches the terminal branch, the nerve starts to arborize, conduction slows as nerve diameter decreases, the actual distance of terminal branches is unknown, and the time for neurotransmitter activation is unknown.

A solution to the problem of terminal latency is to have an additional site at which to stimulate the nerve. If an additional site is available, the distal site latency may be subtracted from the more proximal latency, leaving the residual latency, which reflects conduction time along the nerve segment. Using the basic principle of two sites of stimulation along a nerve, the conduction of the motor portion of the peripheral nerve complex may be estimated (Fig. 12–2) for as many anatomic segments as the examined nerve allows.

Some important technical points to remember when performing motor-nerve conduction studies are to maintain (1) the same shape and negative

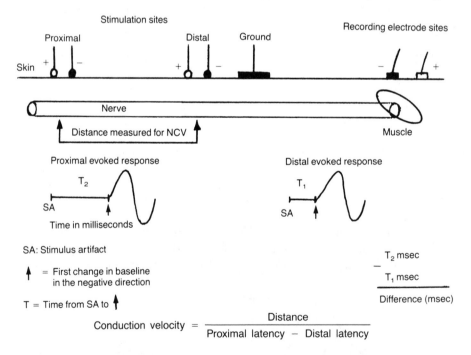

Figure 12–2. Calculation of motor conduction velocity. Conduction velocity (m/sec) of a nerve can be calculated by measuring the distance (mm) between two stimulation sites and dividing by the difference in latency (msec) from the more proximal stimulus and the latency (msec) of the distal stimulus.

phase amplitude of the evoked muscle action potential at all sites of stimulation; (2) close proximity of stimulating electrodes to the peripheral nerve bundle; and (3) a supramaximal evoked muscle action potential at all stimulation sites.

Most of the peripheral nerves in the human body that have a motor component have had motor nerve conduction velocities calculated and reported. An example of the technical procedures used to perform a motor nerve conduction study is shown in Table 12–1 and Figures 12–3 and 12–4. Evoked

TABLE 12–1. PROCEDURE FOR MEDIAN MOTOR NERVE CONDUCTION

Electromyograph Instrument Parameters

Filter settings/frequency response: 10–10,000 Hz
Sweep speed: 2–5 msec/div
Sensitivity/gain: 1000–5000 μV/div

Patient Position (Fig. 12–3)

The patient is positioned supine with arm abducted approximately 45 degrees. The forearm is fully supinated and the wrist is in a neutral position.

Electrode Placement (Fig. 12–3)

Active (recording) electrode: The active recording electrode is positioned directly over the anatomic center of the abductor pollicis brevis muscle. The electrode is placed one-half the distance between the metacarpophalangeal joint of the thumb and the midpoint of the distal wrist crease.

Reference electrode: The reference electrode is positioned *off* the abductor pollicis brevis muscle on the distal phalanx of the thumb over bone or tendon.

Ground electrode: The ground electrode should be firmly positioned on the dorsum of the hand between the recording and stimulating electrodes.

Electrostimulation (Fig. 12–4)

Transcutaneous electrostimulation is performed at the appropriate anatomic sites in the following order.

S1: Distal stimulation is performed at the wrist between the palmaris longus and flexor carpi radialis muscle tendons. The cathode (negative) pole of the stimulator should be placed proximal to the center of the active recording electrode over the abductor pollicis brevis muscle.

S2: Stimulation above the elbow is performed proximal and medial to the antecubital space and proximal to the elbow crease between the belly of the biceps muscle and the medial head of the triceps muscle. The stimulator should be positioned just lateral to the brachial artery to minimize the possibility of inadvertent electrostimulation of the ulnar nerve.

S3: Proximal stimulation is performed in the axilla at least 10 cm proximal to the above elbow site and immediately lateral and anterior to the brachial artery.

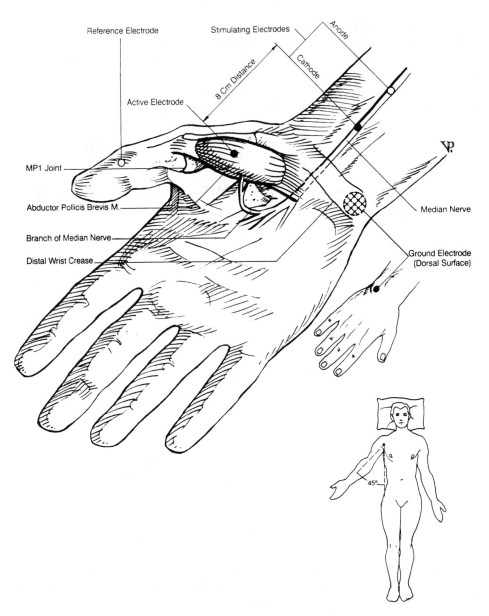

Figure 12–3. Body position of subject receiving median motor nerve conduction study showing location of recording and distal stimulating electrodes and ground.

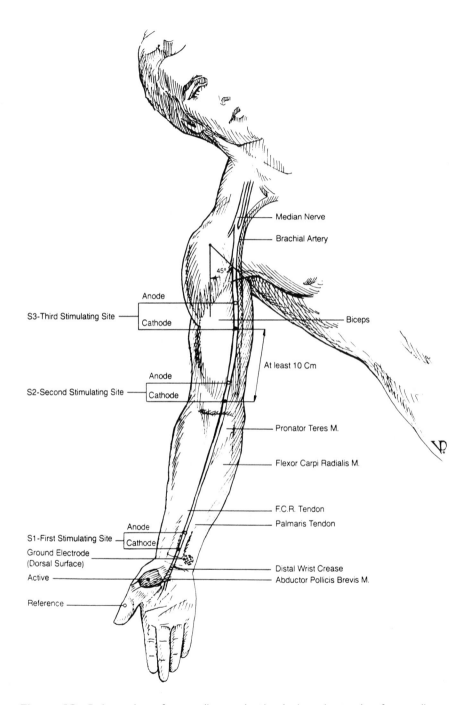

Median Nerve

Brachial Artery

45°

Anode

S3-Third Stimulating Site

Cathode

Biceps

At least 10 Cm

Anode

S2-Second Stimulating Site

Cathode

Pronator Teres M.

Flexor Carpi Radialis M.

F.C.R. Tendon

Palmaris Tendon

Anode

S1-First Stimulating Site

Cathode

Ground Electrode
(Dorsal Surface)

Active

Distal Wrist Crease

Abductor Pollicis Brevis M.

Reference

Figure 12–4. Location of recording and stimulating electrodes for median motor conduction study.

muscle action potential responses from all sites *should* be similar in waveform, amplitude, and duration of response.

Wrist site stimulation voltage, stimulus pulse duration, or both should be increased gradually and monitored carefully as a high-voltage, long-pulse-duration stimulation at the wrist may volume conduct to the adjacent ulnar nerve at the wrist, eliciting a short-latency volume-conducted ulnar response.

The clinical response should be carefully observed to avoid mistaking an ulnar for a median response. At the wrist, median stimulation elicits thumb palmar *AB*duction and opposition, while ulnar stimulation elicits thumb *AD*duction and metacarpal phalangeal flexion. At the above-elbow and axilla stimulation sites, median stimulation elicits wrist flexion in radial deviation involving the flexor carpi radialis muscle, while ulnar stimulation involves wrist flexion in ulnar deviation by contraction of the flexor carpi ulnaris muscle. Palpation of the tendons may help to distinguish the two contractions.

The wrist should be maintained in a standard position while measuring forearm distance. Wrist flexion decreases while wrist extension increases the distance. All distance measurements should be taken with a metal tape measure. The measurement of distance should approximate the anatomic course of the nerve being tested.

In clinical practice, the median, ulnar, common peroneal, and posterior tibial nerves are most often assessed. (Normal values are published in most textbooks; see the bibliography at the end of the chapter.)

Sensory Conduction

The estimation of conduction in the sensory segment of the peripheral nerve bundle follows the same basic paradigm as the motor component; with the sensory segment, however, the skin (dermis) and not the muscle becomes the effector organ. Unlike the muscle, the skin has the ability to be both effector and receptor. The two methods for sensory conduction are orthodromic and antidromic.

Orthodromic conduction refers to the normal way in which a physiological response travels. For example, the dermis of the skin is stimulated, thereby initiating a response by the cutaneous receptors of light touch, These receptors have endings in the dermis of the skin and conduct impulses to the central nervous system by way of the dorsal root. The impulse generated by dermal stimulation is recorded by surface electrodes over the peripheral nerve bundle at a superficial point. An example of the technical procedures used to perform an orthodromic sensory conduction study is shown in Table 12–2 and Figure 12–5. A low stimulation amplitude is usually adequate to elicit an orthodromic sensory response. The possibility of obtaining a spurious motor response is decreased using the orthodromic technique. Motor response and volume conduction effects may be lessened by decreasing NMES amplitude, decreasing pulse duration, or both, of the applied electrostimulation. *Special Concern:* Care must be taken to maintain a separation between the stimulating

TABLE 12–2. PROCEDURE FOR ORTHODROMIC MEDIAN SENSORY NERVE CONDUCTION

Electromyograph Instrument Parameters

Filter settings/frequency response: 20–2000 Hz
Sweep speed: 1–2 msec/div
Sensitivity/gain: 5–10 µV/div

Patient Position (Fig. 12–5)

The patient is positioned supine with arm abducted approximately 45 degrees. The forearm is fully supinated, the wrist is in a neutral position. The fingers may flex slightly when in a resting position.

Electrode Placement (Fig. 12–5)

Active (recording) electrode: The active recording electrode will be positioned directly over the cathode (distal) stimulating site used for evoking the median motor response at the wrist.

Reference electrode: The reference electrode will be positioned 2–3 cm proximal to the active electrode. This electrode will be positioned so that it is directly over the anode (proximal) stimulating site used for evoking the median motor response at the wrist.

Ground electrode: The ground electrode should be firmly positioned on the dorsum of the hand between the active and stimulating electrodes.

Electrostimulation (Fig. 12–5)

Transcutaneous electrostimulation is performed as follows. Stimulation is applied over the digital nerve via electrodes attached to the index finger. The cathode is positioned at the midpoint of the proximal phalanx of the index finger and the anode is positioned at or about the distal phalangeal joint line. A distance of no less than 10 cm, but not more than 14 cm, is maintained between the stimulating cathode on the index finger and the active electrode at the wrist.

cathode and anode on the index finger. Do not allow conducting gel to bridge this interelectrode space.

Antidromic conduction is the stimulation of the nerve bundle and subsequent recording of the distal impulse over the dermis of the skin. An example of the technical procedures used to perform an antidromic sensory conduction study is shown in Table 12–3 and Figure 12–6. A low stimulation amplitude is usually adequate to elicit the antidromic sensory response. Motor response and volume conduction effects may be lessened by decreasing electrostimulation amplitude, decreasing pulse duration, or both, of the applied electrostimulation. (NOTE: Motor responses from hand muscles and volume conduction are more of a technical problem when utilizing antidromic techniques than when using orthodromic techniques.) *Special Concern:* Care must be taken to main-

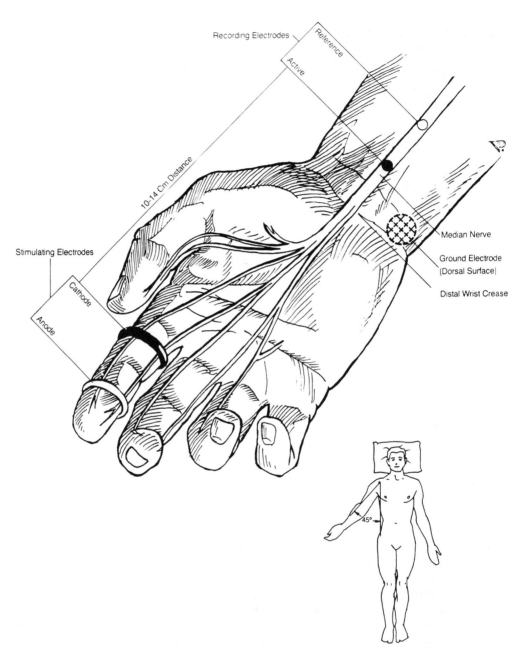

Recording Electrodes

Reference

Active

10-14 Cm Distance

Stimulating Electrodes

Cathode

Anode

Median Nerve

Ground Electrode
(Dorsal Surface)

Distal Wrist Crease

45°

Figure 12–5. Body position and location of recording, stimulating, and ground electrodes for orthodromic median sensory nerve conduction study.

TABLE 12-3. PROCEDURE FOR ANTIDROMIC MEDIAN SENSORY NERVE CONDUCTION

Electromyograph Instrument Parameters

Filter settings/frequency response: 20–2000 Hz
Sweep speed: 1–2 msec/div
Sensitivity/gain: 5–20 μV/div

Patient Position (Fig. 12–6)

The patient is positioned supine with arm abducted approximately 45 degrees. The forearm is fully supinated, the wrist is in a neutral position. The fingers may flex slightly when in a resting position.

Electrode Placement (Fig. 12–6)

Active (recording) electrode: The active recording electrode is attached to the index finger at the midpoint of the distance between the phalangeal flexion crease and the web space of the index finger so that a distance of at least 10 cm, but not more than 14 cm, is maintained between the stimulating electrode and the active electrode.

Reference electrode: The reference electrode is positioned at or about the distal interphalangeal flexion crease of the index finger so that a distance of at least 3 cm is maintained between the active and reference electrode.

Ground electrode: The ground electrode should be firmly positioned on the dorsum of the hand between the active and stimulating electrodes.

Electrostimulation (Fig. 12–6)

Transcutaneous electrostimulation is performed as follows. Stimulation is performed at the wrist between the palmaris longus and flexor carpi radialis muscle tendons proximal to the transverse carpal ligament.

---

tain a separation between the active and reference electrodes on the index finger. Do not allow conducting gel to bridge this interelectrode space.

Several differences exist between the sensory evoked action potential and the evoked muscle action potential. (1) Sensory potential is much smaller in amplitude than is muscle evoked potential. (2) Sensory potential has a single negative phase, whereas muscle evoked potential is biphasic. (3) Sensory potential is usually a single parameter that may be used to determine latency and, if desired, to compute a velocity. Recall that evoked muscle action potential includes components that involve terminal conduction and myoneural junctional delay. Sensory nerve endings have no junctional delay at the distal portions, because the sensory endings in the dermis are dendrites rather than terminal branches. (4) The last difference revolves about the physiological response; evoked potential results from the combined excitation of skeletal muscle fibers, whereas sensory potential represents the neural excitability of the low-threshold, large-diameter, cutaneous sensory neurons.

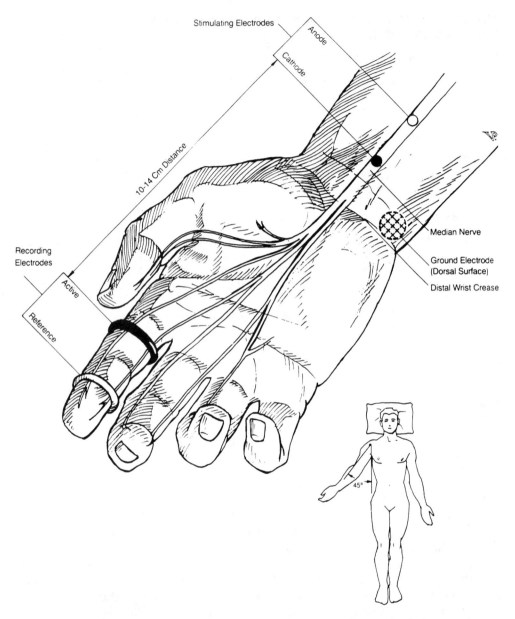

Stimulating Electrodes

Anode

Cathode

10-14 Cm Distance

Recording
Electrodes

Active

Reference

Median Nerve

Ground Electrode
(Dorsal Surface)

Distal Wrist Crease

45°

Figure 12–6. Body position and location of recording, stimulating, and ground electrodes for antidromic median sensory nerve conduction study.

Clinical Use of Motor and Sensory Conduction Studies

The ability to estimate the velocity of motor conduction helps to delineate a systemic problem from a local one. Velocity in systemic problems is generally decreased for all nerves tested. In disease and injury states, the lower-extremity nerves exhibit earlier changes in motor-nerve conduction than do those of the upper extremities. A local problem of decreased nerve conduction may be described by the example of a peripheral nerve sustaining a compressive force in an anatomic area where the nerve is bordered by uncompromising structures. When the nerve is bound between bone and connective tissue, the conduction of the induced stimulus is slower at the compressive site because of the increased internal resistance of the axis cylinder. The nerve may be compressed at any site, but certain anatomic areas have a predilection for compression.

For example, a common site for median-nerve compression is in the area of the wrist, as the median nerve passes through the carpal tunnel. When the nerve is compressed at a distal site, both motor and sensory distal latencies are prolonged. The computed velocity segments are unaltered. Compression tends to affect conduction along the sensory nerves prior to the motor nerve. Part of the physiological reason for earlier changes in sensory axons relates to the relative lack of myelin coating surrounding the sensory axons. Compressive alteration is more difficult to obtain in a motor axon because of the concentric rings of myelin coating surrounding it.

When a peripheral nerve bundle is damaged by disease, both motor and sensory nerve evoked components may illustrate physiological alterations in both computed velocity and evoked waveform characteristics. Each reported indicator of motor nerve conduction, such as amplitude, duration of the evoked muscle action potential, and latency of response, plays a part in the overall evaluation of the patient. The determination of the anatomic area, the degree of involvement, and the possible prognosis of the process may be estimated by using all of the elements listed above as common to the motor nerve conduction velocity segment. The differentiation of local versus systemic nerve involvement may be evaluated by sensory and motor nerve conduction techniques. For example, if the ulnar nerve is compressed at the elbow without metabolic compromise of the axon, the motor nerve conduction velocity computed for the segment below the elbow would be within normal limits. The computed velocity above the elbow, however, would be slower than for the segment below the elbow. In addition to the slower velocity component, a change in the evoked muscle action potential may also be evident. The potential's amplitude, resulting from stimulation above the elbow, would be diminished compared to the stimulation below the elbow.

The patient who has a systemic disease involving the peripheral nerves would tend to exhibit different findings in motor nerve conduction studies. For example, the individual who has diabetes may illustrate changes of slowing in motor nerve conduction velocity of approximately 20 percent, with an accompanied increase in negative phase duration for the evoked muscle action potential but with no decrease in negative-phase amplitude. The patient with chronic alcoholism illustrates little or no change in computed motor nerve conduction velocity but may exhibit changes in negative phase amplitude of the evoked muscle action potential.

Similarly, sensory evoked action potentials present information to the investigator about the functional integrity of the sensory component of the peripheral nerve complex. As mentioned earlier the sensory axons are more susceptible to focal-type compression and to systemic neuropathic changes than are motor axons. Therefore, focal compressive changes occur earlier in the sensory axons than in the motor axons. Recall that motor axons have concentric rings of myelin, whereas sensory axons have a disorganized myelin sheath. Compression or systemic disease (or both) that affects the myelin will influence the sensory axons prior to affecting the motor axons. Results of sensory conduction studies confirm the subjective description by the patient of earlier temporal involvement by illustrating the alterations in sensory conduction and sensory evoked potential parameters prior to changes in the motor nerve conduction components.

The major problem surrounding both motor and sensory nerve conduction studies remains the fact that both techniques measure only the distal component of the peripheral nerve. For example, the median nerve may be measured in motor and sensory conduction from the anterior cervical triangle to the wrist. Conduction proximal to the anterior cervical triangle is not possible with standard techniques. The following section amplifies upon the electrophysiological assessment technique used to evaluate the conduction of the evoked response through the proximal arc in the neural segment.

Electronic Reflex Testing
The reflex arcs that normally occur in the intact physiological state, the H reflex, F wave, and blink reflex, will now be reviewed. The F wave is not a reflex in the strict form of the definition. It is a recurrent response to NMES, but it has the ability to assess proximal conduction.

The term *evoked* implies that some control is exerted over the physiological situation. In electronic reflex testing, control is expressed by the NMES parameters used. The term *reflex* implies that a synapse is included in the arc and that some direct control over the physiological sequence is masked.

H Reflex. The "H" in H reflex is in honor of Hoffman, who originally described a monosynaptic, electrically induced equivalent of the tendon tap response. Hoffman reasoned that a tendon, when subjected to a brief and sudden stretch, produces a small, brief muscle contraction after an intervening time period. He hypothesized that NMES of the afferent peripheral nerve carrying neurons involved in the tendon tap response would cause the same type of response. He recorded a response both to tendon tap and to NMES of the nerve proximal to the muscle. The same small-muscle response was obtained with both stimuli.

The tendon tap causes a mechanical stretch of the muscle and of the associated, parallel-arranged muscle spindles. The stretch of the muscle spindles causes a volley of neural impulses up the afferent arc along the IA nerves, through the dorsal-root ganglia to the spinal cord, where the IA nerves synapse directly on the hononomous anterior horn cells. The excitation causes a twitch response of the extrafusal fibers associated with that spindle complex.

The electrically induced H reflex response bypasses the short spindle stretch and directly depolarizes the large IA fibers proximal to the muscle. For example, the soleus muscle in the lower extremity is innervated by the posterior tibial nerve. The posterior tibial nerve is stimulated in the popliteal fossa proximal to the soleus muscle. The afferent volley of impulses follows the same course as when the response is mechanically induced. The major difference between the tendon tap and NMES is the level of external control that the evaluator has over the physiologic response. The latter is controlled, with all parameters of stimulation chosen by the examiner. The response from the extrafusal fibers is synchronous and is recorded by surface electrodes over the soleus muscle. The time interval from stimulus delivery to response recording is approximately 30 msec.

Two components make up the H reflex arc: the afferent arc is along the IA fibers, while the efferent arc is along the alpha motor neurons. Because the H reflex indicates a response to IA nerve fibers, and because those nerve fibers are the afferent arc of muscle spindles, it follows that the H reflex is found only in those muscles that have an abundance of muscle spindles. Muscles that contain slow-twitch fibers have an abundance of spindles and commonly illustrate the appearance of an H reflex.

Clinical Use of H Reflex. The S_1 nerve root innervates the soleus muscle, which is composed predominantly of slow-twitch motor units. The proximal conduction of afferent impulses occurs along the IA fibers, through the dorsal root to the alpha motor neurons, which pass out of the S_1 foramen to innervate the soleus. The H reflex is used to assess proximal conduction; for example, the conduction of the impulse through the dorsal root into the dorsal portion of the spinal cord and then through the ventral root at S_1 to the muscle. Compression at the neural foramen will cause a concomitant slowing of the reflex latency. Assessing proximal conduction through the S_1 nerve root is thought to be possible with the H reflex.

F Wave. Unlike the H reflex, the F wave does not have separate afferent and efferent arcs. Rather, it has both afferent and efferent arcs in the same peripheral nerve. The alpha motor neuron serves both functions. The suspected physiological mechanism for the F wave is described as an afferent volley composed of antidromic stimuli followed by a reverberation of the impulse once it reaches the anterior horn cell. The alpha motor neuron is stimulated at a distal site, and the induced stimulus travels in an orthodromic fashion to the muscle. At the same time an antidromic impulse travels to the anterior horn cell of that nerve. It is thought that once the antidromic impulse reaches the axon hillock, it reverberates and causes an orthodromic volley of impulses back to the muscle. The time for the F wave is approximately 30 msec. Unlike the H reflex, the F wave is apparent upon maximal NMES. The F wave is inconsistent in its appearance and must be calculated on at least ten successive responses. The F wave is not a reflex, because no reflex arc is used. It is simply a reverberating response to supramaximal NMES of the alpha motor neurons.

Clinical Use of F Wave. The F wave, like the H reflex, is a measure of proximal conduction. The F wave may be obtained from most muscles upon appropriate neural stimulation. (Recall that the H reflex is present only in muscles with a high proportion of muscle spindles.) Those muscles that have a predominance of slow-twitch motor units have high spindle indexes. Since the F-wave response is possible from a variety of muscles and from muscles that have few or no spindles, the results of the F-wave test are useful in determining proximal conduction delays along many spinal segments. A comparison of proximal conduction components is useful when entrapment of the nerve at the foramen is expected. The latency of the F wave is also an important measure when comparing proximal conduction along a peripheral nerve to distal conduction along the same nerve. A comparison of proximal and distal conduction components is useful in ruling out polyneuropathic conductions, where distal segments of the nerve begin to die back before the proximal segments in the natural course of the disease process.

Blink Reflex. The blink reflex is a muscle response to stimulation of the supraorbital area. The stimulation may be a mechanical tap to the glabella or may be NMES of the supraorbital nerve. With both forms of stimulation, the observed response is the defensive reflex of eyelid closure by contraction of the orbicularis oculi. The mechanical tap cannot be controlled or sufficiently modulated; therefore, the use of NMES is preferred. Electrostimulation of the supraorbital nerve causes a reflex contraction of the orbicularis oculi. In bilateral recording from the orbicularis oculi, the observed response to NMES is composed of two distinct waveforms. The first component, or waveform, is called the Rl response. This response is always absent on the contralateral side when the nerve is electrostimulated.

The R2 component is the second evoked potential noted, and is less well organized than the R1 potential. The latency of the R2 potential is consistent, but the duration and amplitude tend to vary, indicating the need for an average value for amplitude on both the ipsilateral and contralateral sides of stimulation.

The blink reflex is unlike the H reflex and F wave. The difference lies in the fact that one electrostimulation causes two distinct responses of the orbicularis oculi. The first response (R1) represents the conduction along the trigeminal nerve. The second response (R2) represents the time of conduction along the trigeminal pontine relay and facial nerve. The presumed reason for the inconsistent response of R2 is the excitability of the interneuron pool at the pontine level, the axonal conduction of both the trigeminal and facial nerve, and the synaptic transmission throughout the reflex arc.

Clinical Use of Blink Reflex. The use of the blink reflex in the clinical setting provides the clinician with information about the afferent and efferent arcs of the trigeminal and facial nerves. An important portion is the efferent arc formed by the facial nerve. The proximal portion of the facial nerve may be examined with the blink reflex. Recall that the nerve-excitability test for facial nerve paralysis will only present information about the distal portion of the facial nerve. The proximal portion lies within the stylomastoid foramen. Since Bell's palsy is thought to involve the proximal portion of the facial nerve, the blink reflex may be the test of choice for evaluating the functional integrity of the nerve. The second component of the blink reflex (R2) represents proximal facial nerve conduction. Increased R2 delay, decreased amplitude of R2, or a lack of response of R2 may indicate facial nerve compromise.

Electronic reflex testing uses evoked responses to evaluate the proximal component of the peripheral nervous system. The principles of evoked responses, controlled by known parameters of NMES, allow for the evaluation of conduction of both afferent and efferent neural segments. A response, whether or not it is delayed in character, must be kept in perspective. The blink response is the result of a reflex action on the part of neurons, interneurons, and synapses. Since the response is a reflex and involves many possible sources of error, a negative result in one of these studies alone is not conclusive of a pathologic implication. Reflex testing should be considered one tile in the overall mosaic that is developed for that patient.

Centrally Recorded Evoked Potentials
Motor and sensory nerve conduction studies, and electronic reflex testing, form the majority of evoked potentials used by individuals in electrophysiological evaluation. Assessment of an integrated, functional, and complete nervous system includes the evaluation of *distal peripheral nerve conduction*, proximal conduction through reflex function and the central nervous system, through scalp-recorded evoked potentials.

There are three major types of centrally evoked responses currently used by clinicians in electrophysiological evaluation: somatosensory evoked potentials, brainstem auditory evoked potentials, and visual evoked potentials. All of the centrally recorded evoked potentials are useful in studying central nervous system dysfunction. The following discussion should be viewed as descriptive only and not as an in-depth or practical explication of this field.

Viewed in a historical perspective, central-scalp-recorded evoked potentials are a recent form of evoked potentials, when compared (for example) to motor and sensory nerve conduction studies or electronic reflex testing. The central scalp recording of evoked potentials is possible only through the use of the computer and the averaging abilities of the digital systems. The increased level of sophistication in electrical technology has enabled the development of centrally evoked potentials.

Somatosensory Evoked Potentials. When the distal portion of the peripheral nerve is electrostimulated at a minimal motor threshold, a volley of sensory impulses is known to be generated. The minimal motor threshold is used to standardize the excitation threshold of the sensory axons. (Recall that threshold-to-sensory stimulation is less than that of the motor threshold.)

The volley of orthodromic sensory potentials travels through the dorsal root ganglia into the spinal cord, where the sensory terminal branches form excitatory synapses with central nervous system dendrites, which (in turn) travel centrally and eventually terminate on the contralateral region of the postcentral gyrus of the sensory cortex. Using a specific configuration of surface electrodes placed on the contralateral scalp, the wave of depolarization may be recorded by averaging at least 1000 successive stimuli. A series of positive and negative waveforms is recorded, each described by its relative location from the beginning point.

Clinical Use of Somatosensory Evoked Potentials. Many disorders of the central nervous system do not result in symptoms in the early stages. Recorded somatosensory evoked potentials (SSEPs) often illustrate slowing in velocity segments at the central portion of the evoked waveforms. Monitoring spinal trauma cases in order to ascertain the degree of cord transection is another clinical use of SSEP. SSEP potentials are present even during the spinal shock stage, when reflex function is depressed. The qualitative role of SSEP is useful to the clinical neurologist when findings from other tests are inconclusive.

Brainstem Auditory Evoked Potentials. In the early 1970s, the ability to record auditory evoked responses from scalp-recording techniques was first reported. The use of a brief click was the source of auditory-nerve depolarization. The computer-averaging technique is the same for brainstem auditory evoked potentials (BAEPs) as with SSEPs, except that the stimulus source is a click of monaural quality applied to one ear, while the other ear receives a masking noise. The surface recording electrodes are placed on the ipsilateral vertex and are amplified up to 1 million times. An average of 1000 to 2000 click stimuli are used to obtain the desired signal from the brain. Since the gain of the amplifier is very high, the artifacts that might be produced by swallowing, moving, or any muscle contraction must be minimized. Therefore, BAEPs are often conducted as part of a sleep study.

Clinical Use of Brainstem Auditory Evoked Potentials. In clinical neurology, BAEPs are used to assess hearing loss that results from peripheral mechanisms. In patients in whom a progression of hearing loss is noted and in whom acoustic neuromas are expected, BAEPs are sensitive as an initial screening test. BAEPs are also used for patients who are suspected of suffering from a demyelinating disease. The ability to confirm a diagnosis of multiple sclerosis with just symptoms and signs is about 50-percent accurate. In those patients without symptoms and signs, the percentage drops dramatically (to 19 percent).

A valuable aspect of BAEPs is their ability to document those lesions that are unsuspected in the early stages of multiple sclerosis. Validation of the early changes of BAEPs with a diagnosis of multiple sclerosis continues by concurrent validation process. BAEPs have other uses in clinical neurology; for example, the evaluation of both the location and the extent of damage caused by intrinsic brainstem tumors, the evaluation of brain death, and the surgical monitoring of potentials during neurosurgical procedures in the region of the posterior fossa.

Visual Evoked Potentials. Visual evoked potentials (VEPs) are useful when the underlying process of damage and assessment of the neurologic area of a visual problem is difficult to determine. The ability to objectively evaluate the function of the visual pathway without conscious cooperation from the patient is helpful when patients present visual problems without a diagnosis. VEPs are also useful in detecting compromise of the optic nerve in the early stages of dysfunction. The objective nature of the test, along with the ability to perform VEPs without conscious cooperation on the part of the patient, make it possible to differentiate functional loss of sight from actual (organic) loss of sight. VEPs have been effective in determining early demyelinating disease, especially the early stage of multiple sclerosis.

The VEP technique requires all of the special hardware and software noted for other evoked potentials, and in addition requires an accurate, sharply focused visual stimulus in order to produce a synchronous volley of afferent visual stimuli. Unlike SSEPs and BAEPs, where 1000 to 2000 repetitive stimuli are needed, only 100 or 200 stimuli are required to obtain adequate VEPs. The VEP technique requires that the scalp-located surface electrodes be placed over the occipital area. The VEP response results from the type of original stimulus projected by the video display terminal. The examiner may record the response from stimulation of one eye independently or of both visual pathways at once. If separate responses for each eye are needed, careful attention must be given to maintenance of the same amplitude and latency parameters.

Clinical Use of Visual Evoked Potentials. VEPs are used in the clinical setting to test for demyelinating disease of the optic nerve. The predominant feature in demyelination of the optic nerve is a shift in the latency to the prolonged region of normal latency. VEPs are also used in patients with various central nervous system dysfunctions as an aid to early detection of the accompanying decline in visual impairment. Changes are noted in either the latencies or the characteristics of the waveforms.

VEPS are also useful in delineating the patient suffering from hysterical blindness. If VEPs are well-formed along the segment examined, and if the latencies are within the normal limits ascribed according to age and gender data limits in the presence of a visual acuity beyond 20/120, the blindness is not organic. Like other neurologic tests, the VEP test, if negative, indicates that an area within the central nervous system is in dysfunction.

VOLUNTARY POTENTIALS

Voluntary potential comes from muscle fiber membranes during a volitional contraction of a skeletal muscle. The potentials are recorded by a sterile needle

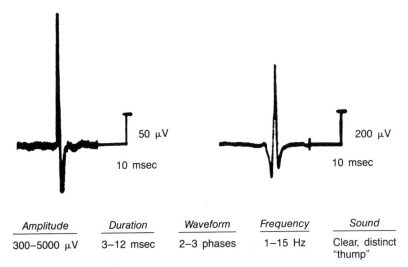

Amplitude	Duration	Waveform	Frequency	Sound
300–5000 μV	3–12 msec	2–3 phases	1–15 Hz	Clear, distinct "thump"

Figure 12–7. The motor unit consists of the anterior horn cell, its axon, neuromuscular junction, and all muscle fibers it innervates. A motor unit is the synchronous discharge of all muscle fibers innervated by the anterior horn cell. They occur during volitional activity. Initial deflection may be either positive or negative. The amplitude of the motor unit action potential is dependent upon the number of motor unit muscle fibers in close proximity to the recording electrode. The rate of rise time of the motor unit action potential is dependent upon the closeness of the recording electrode to the active muscle fibers. The motor unit action potential duration is dependent upon the relative density of the muscle fibers in the recording area. Duration of motor unit action potentials increases as intramuscular temperature decreases. Duration of motor unit action potentials also increases with age. The percentage of polyphasic motor unit action potentials increases with a decrease in temperature and with muscle fatigue.

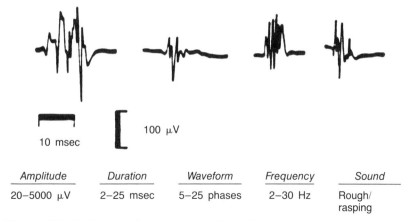

Amplitude	Duration	Waveform	Frequency	Sound
20–5000 μV	2–25 msec	5–25 phases	2–30 Hz	Rough/ rasping

Figure 12–8. Polyphasic potentials. Complex motor unit action potential with multiple phases; probably results from the asynchronous discharge of muscle fibers in the motor unit; represents the electrical expression of a motor unit undergoing reorganization. Polyphasics are observed in partial compressive neuropathies and in muscular dystrophy. Initial deflection may be either positive or negative. They occur during volitional activity. High amplitude long duration (HALD) polyphasic potentials are usually seen in long-standing, chronic neuropathies.

electrode inserted in the muscle. The use of a needle electrode is essential to the proper recording and subsequent display of the action potentials. The needle electrode enables the examiner to move throughout a muscle in order to sample action potentials from all aspects of the muscle. (Recall that the motor unit distribution in a muscle is in a mosaic-like pattern.) The muscle fibers of the motor unit are distributed throughout a relatively large portion of the muscle. The needle electrode allows the movement of the recording electrode to approximate the source of the action potential.

The action potential recorded from a motor unit within a muscle that is actively contracting has certain morphometric characteristics. The structural component of the voluntary motor unit action potential depends upon the size of the motor unit, the histological type of muscle fiber, and the density of the motor unit structure within the muscle (Figs. 12–7 and 12–8). The size of the motor unit depends on the function of the muscle. For example, a muscle that has one joint to act on, that performs postural, sustained contractions, and that has few strength components, will have fewer muscle fibers per motor unit than will a muscle with the opposite functional need characteristics.

The decreased size of the small motor unit will yield a small amplitude recorded action potential. The type of muscle fiber will also yield an action potential with a particular size. A fast motor unit will have muscle fiber membranes that are larger and that conduct the action potential along the muscle fiber membrane faster than the membranes of a slow motor unit. The larger muscle fiber membranes will yield a larger amplitude, a faster rise-time response, and a shorter-duration action potential than a slow motor unit. The relative density of motor units within a muscle will also affect the recorded morphometric parameters of the muscle action potential. Because of the high specificity of the muscle function, a muscle with motor units that are closely spaced will have recorded action potentials of short durations and of relatively low amplitudes.

Several factors must be accounted for when analyzing the shape, size, and duration of the recorded voluntary muscle action potentials. The major consideration is the relative proximity of the recording electrode to the active muscle fibers. The rise time of the action potential decreases in an exponential fashion when distance from the active muscle fiber increases by 10 percent from the recording electrode. The rise time is crucial in the estimation of the overall shape of the waveform. A slow rise time will both increase the duration and decrease the amplitude. A short rise time in the recorded muscle action potential is indicated by the crispness in sound heard from the speaker.

ELECTROMYOGRAPHY

The term *voluntary* implies the use of some conscious effort on the part of the subject to perform a function. In that subcategory of electrophysiological evaluation called electromyography, the patient is asked to move a particular muscle so that voluntary potentials in the form of motor units might be recorded, displayed, and subsequently analyzed. Strictly defined, the term *electromyography* involves both the recording of action potentials from muscle fibers under conditions of voluntary movement and the observance of those spontaneous action potentials recorded from muscle fibers in a state of neural dysfunction.

A typical electromyographic evaluation of a skeletal muscle by a needle electrode includes the use of four distinct and separate processes: electrode insertion, oscilloscope observation during rest, oscilloscope observation of voluntary motor unit action potentials during minimal contraction, and oscilloscope observation during a level of muscle contractions graded from weak to strong. An example of the technical procedures used to perform clinical electromyography (EMG) is shown in Table 12–4.

Initially, the evaluator must choose a series of skeletal muscles to test. The muscles are chosen on the basis of nerve root and by peripheral nerve innervation. Once a muscle is chosen, the area of skin overlying that muscle is cleansed by rubbing it with a sterile pad containing a 70-percent isopropyl alcohol solution. The needle is inserted into the muscle, and the oscilloscope is observed while the muscle is at rest and while the needle is moved about. A muscle that is in a state of irritability will react to the movement of a needle electrode by having an increased time period of injury potentials during the needle's movement. The insertional activity or injury potentials are in the form of a burst of short-duration potentials that persist for less than a few millisec-

TABLE 12–4. PROCEDURE FOR CLINICAL EMG

Introduction

1. Decide on distribution of:
   - Nerve root
   - Plexus
   - Peripheral nerve.
2. Know location of the anatomic structures in no. 1, above.
3. Decide on representative muscles in decision of no. 1, above.
4. Know the action and function of the muscle.
5. Know the specificity of muscle function.
6. Know the cross-sectional anatomy of the muscle.
7. Know the relative mass of the muscle.
8. NOTE:
   - Use latex gloves and protective eyewear for all routine electromyographic studies.
   - Use latex gloves, protective eyewear, and gown for all electromyographic studies performed on HIV patients.

Motor Unit Observation

Machine settings:
   Gain   = 100–200 µV/div
   Filter = 10,000 Hz high, 10 Hz low
   Sweep = 10–20 msec/div

Patient preparation:
1. Cleanse the skin overlying the muscle with a sterile alcohol pad.
2. While cleaning the skin, feel the consistency of the target muscle.
3. Insert the sterile needle electrode through the skin to a point just under the dermal layer.
4. Switch the preamplifier to the "ON" position.
5. Move the needle into the muscle using a brisk, probing movement.
6. While moving the needle, observe the relative presence and the amount of spontaneous, insertional activity.
7. Stop electrode movement and observe (sight and sound) for other spontaneous activity.
8. Ask the patient to perform a minimal voluntary isometric muscle contraction (keep in mind the muscle testing position and muscle function).
9. While under minimal voluntary isometric contraction, observe the motor units which are in close proximity to the recording electrode:
   - A rapid rise time and resultant high frequency "click" is heard when a motor unit is close to the recording electrode.
   - The amplitude of the voluntary motor unit potential is measured from the largest negative peak to the largest positive peak of the motor unit being observed when the recording electrode is near that motor unit.
10. Observe the voluntary motor unit action potential for its shape (phases), amplitude, and duration.

continued

TABLE 12–4. (Continued)

11. Observe and measure (according to no. 10, above) two or three voluntary motor units in each area of the muscle being tested.
12. Move the needle further into the muscle and repeat steps 6 through 11.
13. Sample additional sites in the muscle by using the quadrant position technique and evaluate 4 to 8 levels and sites in each muscle being tested.

Recruitment and Interference Evaluation

EMG machine settings:
   Gain   = 500–1000 μV/div
   Filter = 10,000 Hz high, 10 Hz low
   Sweep = 20–50 msec/div
Patient preparation:
   1. Move the needle electrode to the anatomic cross-sectional center of the muscle.
   2. Request the patient to gradually increase the force of voluntary isometric muscle activity until maximum effort is accomplished.
   3. Observe the voluntary motor unit action potentials for:
      • Motor unit recruitment pattern, small to large (poor-fair-good).
      • Interference pattern—decreased number of motor units firing rapidly: incomplete, decreased, full.

onds. If a muscle is irritable because of some injury to the neural supply system, the length of time of insertional activity increases as the needle is moved in the muscle. Insertional activity is a subjective measure, however; because it lacks an objective scale, it should not be used by itself to evaluate muscle health.

When voluntary contraction at low levels of force takes place, the action potentials that result are evaluated for shape, size, and duration. The shape of the voluntary motor unit should be two or three phases. The investigator must know the morphometric and histochemical constituents of the muscle being examined. The size or amplitude of the muscle action potential is related to muscle size, histological type, and expected motor unit density. At least 10 to 15 voluntary motor units should be examined for their duration, amplitude, and phase number in at least eight different anatomic areas of the skeletal muscle.

Recruitment of motor units and judgment of the interference pattern is the last area that the examiner assesses in the electromyographic assessment of the skeletal muscle. The examiner requests that the patient voluntarily contract the skeletal muscle in an isometric manner; that is, with a progressively increasing level of muscle tension without limb movement. The motor units that begin to discharge as the tension levels become progressively greater should be of higher and higher amplitude. This results from the recruitment of larger motor units, with progressively increasing amplitudes, as tension requirements increase. In addition to increasing the amplitude of motor unit discharge, the active units should also increase in their firing rate. Recruitment pattern is a qualitative or quantitative description or both of the sequence of appearance of motor unit action potentials with increasing strength of voluntary muscle contraction. *Interference pattern* is a term used to identify the relative firing frequency of discharging motor units.

The normal sequence of events that occurs in response to the gradual increase in muscle tension involves motor units discharging and gradually increasing in their discharge rate. The rate of discharge increase is fixed; when a motor unit cannot discharge faster, a fusion frequency is reached, so another physiological method is used to increase tension: new and larger motor units are recruited. The larger motor units will discharge at their preferred frequency, with the smaller units continuing to discharge at their fusion frequency. The result of the old, quickly discharging motor units and the new, larger motor units is a gradual disappearance of the electronic baseline. The electromyographer observes increases in amplitude and in the interference pattern. The gradual increase in amplitude (due to motor unit recruitment) and the increase in the baseline disruption (due to an increase in the discharge frequency) account for the proper physiological sequencing of available motor units in normal muscle.

Spontaneous Activity (Figs. 12–9 to 12–12)

Electrical silence is noted when a needle electrode is placed in a healthy muscle that is not actively contracting. At rest, healthy muscle will not yield

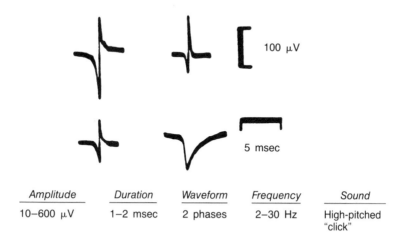

Amplitude	Duration	Waveform	Frequency	Sound
10–600 μV	1–2 msec	2 phases	2–30 Hz	High-pitched "click"

Figure 12–9. Fibrillation potentials. Represents spontaneous, repetitive discharge of a single muscle fiber. *Initial deflection is positive.* It indicates altered muscle membrane excitability and an unstable muscle membrane that depolarizes in a variety of circumstances, and may result from denervation (separation of muscle from nerve), metabolic dysfunction (altered electrolyte state), inflammatory diseases (polymyositis), trauma (injection sites), or lack of trophic influence (stroke or spinal cord injury).

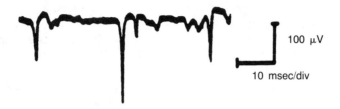

100 μV

10 msec/div

Amplitude	Duration	Waveform	Frequency	Sound
30–4000 μV	2–10 msec	2 phases	2–100 Hz	Dull "thud"

Figure 12–10. Positive sharp wave potentials. Positive sharp waves may represent asynchronous discharge of a number of denervated muscle fibers. They reflect an altered muscle membrane excitability. *Initial deflection is positive.* Its shape is the most constant of all EMG potentials. They appear spontaneously at rest and are not predictable. They are seen in both neuropathies and myopathies.

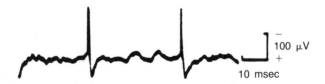

−
100 μV
+

10 msec

Amplitude	Duration	Waveform	Frequency	Sound
20–250 μV	1–4 msec	2 phases	30–150 Hz	High-pitched noise

Figure 12–11. End Plate Potentials. End plate potentials are produced when the EMG needle electrode comes into contact with nerve fibrils within the muscle. Patients complain of increased pain when these potentials are present. Slight needle movement should relieve the pain, eliminate the end plate "noise," and clear the screen display of these potentials. *Initial deflection is negative.*

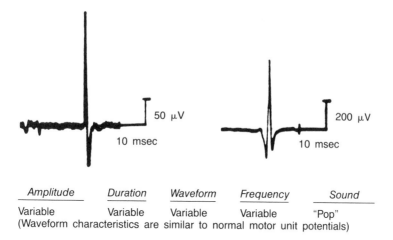

Amplitude	Duration	Waveform	Frequency	Sound
Variable	Variable	Variable	Variable	"Pop"

(Waveform characteristics are similar to normal motor unit potentials)

Figure 12–12. Fasciculation potentials. Fasciculations are seen in patients with and without neuromuscular disease. Fasciculation potentials may be either benign or pathological. Pathological significance is best determined by the coexistence of fibrillation and positive sharp waves in the same muscle. Waveform configuration is the same as the normal motor unit action potential. Initial deflection may be either positive or negative.

any form of electrical membrane potentials. If a muscle loses its innervation in a rapid fashion, such as with a ligation or a significant and rapid compression of the peripheral nerve supply, the muscle is without neuronal supply and, after 14 to 21 days, begins to fibrillate continuously.

The fibrillation occurs because the muscle membrane becomes increasingly sensitive to acetylcholine. The receptor sites along the muscle membrane, normally dormant in the innervated state, become active and highly sensitive to minute amounts of acetylcholine. The electrical membrane potentials spontaneously released by the muscle membranes are of short duration and low amplitude; they are called *fibrillation potentials*. Denervation fibrillation potentials occur in a muscle that is at rest. Upon attempts at voluntary muscle contraction, no active motor units are observed.

There are other forms of spontaneous activity in muscle that are indicative of neural dysfunction. All types of activity remain spontaneous, in that they occur without volitional effort. (The reader is referred to the references at the end of this chapter for a complete description of each of the spontaneous forms of activity, along with their pathologic implications.)

ELECTROPHYSIOLOGICAL EVALUATION

The preceding material has provided the elements involved in electrophysiological evaluation of the patient with a suspected neurological disorder but has not discussed the actual evaluation process. Specific tests must be correctly chosen, and the proper nerves and muscles must be selected for study, in order to optimize the results and their ultimate interpretation. The evaluation process begins with a physical examination to determine the possible site or sites of neural injury. The choice of nerves and muscles examined may change as the electrophysiological evaluation proceeds.

Usually, motor nerve conduction (latency, velocity, amplitude) studies are performed first, followed by sensory nerve studies (latency, amplitude). Which muscles are tested depends upon the peripheral nerve innervation and the root level of the muscles. The addition of reflex testing and evoked potential analysis depends upon the pathologic findings of the earlier electrophysiological procedures. The use of centrally recorded evoked potentials depends upon the pathologic results of peripheral nerve conduction studies and electric reflex testing.

A hierarchy is established that allows for the development of procedures to answer the question: What is wrong with this patient? The electrophysiological evaluation must answer the question. The physician must be given the results of all of the tiles of the mosaic, so as to allow him or her to develop the full disease picture.

REFERENCES

Aminoff M. *Electromyography in Clinical Practice.* Menlo Park, CA, Addison-Wesley, 1978

Aminoff M. *Electrodiagnosis in Clinical Neurology.* New York, Churchill Livingstone, 1980:589

Ashbury A, Johnson P. *Pathology of the Peripheral Nerve.* Philadelphia, WB Saunders, 1978

Bradley W. *Disorders of Peripheral Nerves.* Oxford, Blackwell, 1975

Brooke, M. *A Clinician's View of Neuromuscular Diseases.* Baltimore, Williams & Wilkins, 1977

Brown W. *The Physiological and the Technical Basis of Electromyography.* New York, Churchill Livingstone, 1985

Chu-Andrews J. *Electrodiagnosis, An Anatomic and Clinical Approach.* Philadelphia, JB Lippincott, 1986

Cohen H, Brumlik J. *A Manual of Electroneuromyography,* 2nd ed. New York, Harper & Row, 1976

Dawson D, Hallett M, Millender L. *Entrapment Neuropathies.* Boston, Little, Brown, 1983

Delagi EF, Perotto A, Iazetti J, Morrison D. *Anatomic Guide for the Electromyographer,* Springfield, MO, Charles C Thomas, 1980

DeLisa J, Mackenzie K, Baran E. *Manual of Nerve Conduction Velocity and Somatosensory Evoked Potentials,* New York, Raven Press, 1982

Desmedt J, ed. *New Developments in Electromyography and Clinical Neurophysiology.* London, Basel S, Karger, 1973; 1, 2, 3

Desmedt J, ed. *Clinical Uses of Cerebral, Brainstem and Spinal Somatosensory EP's.* London, Basel S, Karger, 1979

Dyck PJ, Thomas JE, Lambert EH, eds. *Peripheral Neuropathy.* Philadelphia, WB Saunders, 1975; 1, 2

Electromyography: International Journal of Electromyography Abstracts. Louvain, Belgium, Nauwelaerts Publishing House, 1989

Goodgold J. *Anatomical Correlates of Clinical Electromyography.* Baltimore, Williams & Wilkins, 1974

Goodgold J, Eberstein A. *Electrodiagnosis of Neuromuscular Disease,* Baltimore, Williams & Wilkins, 1983

Hammer K. *Nerve Conduction Studies.* Springfield, MO, Charles C Thomas, 1982

Hoppenfeld S. *Physical Examination of the Spine and Extremities.* New York, Appleton-Century-Crofts, 1976

Hoppenfeld S. *Orthopaedic Neurology.* Philadelphia, JB Lippincott, 1977

Jabre J, Hackett E. *EMG Manual.* Springfield, MO, Charles C Thomas, 1983

Johnson E. *Practical Electromyography,* 2nd ed. Baltimore, Williams & Wilkins, 1988

Kimura J. *Electrodiagnosis in Disease of Nerve and Muscle,* 2nd ed. Philadelphia, FA Davis, 1989

Kopell H, Thompson W. *Peripheral Entrapment Neuropathies.* Huntington, NY, Robert E Krieger, 1976

Leffert R. *Brachial Plexus Injuries.* New York, Churchill Livingstone, 1985

Lenman J, Richie A. *Clinical Electromyography,* 2nd ed. Philadelphia, JB Lippincott, 1978

Liveson J, Spielholtz N. *Peripheral Neurology.* Philadelphia, FA Davis, 1979

Loeb G, Gans C. *Electromyography for Experimentalists.* Chicago, University Press, 1986

Ludin H. *Electromyography.* New York, Thieme-Stratton, 1980

Ma D, Liveson J. *Nerve Conduction Handbook.* Philadelphia, FA Davis, 1983

McComas A. *Neuromuscular Function and Disorders.* London, Butterworths, 1977

Mayo Clinic and Mayo Clinic Foundation. *Clinical Examinations in Neurology,* 4th ed. Philadelphia, WB Saunders, 1971

Oh S. *Clinical Electromyography, Nerve Conduction Studies.* Baltimore, University Park Press, 1984

Oh S. *Electromyography: Neuromuscular Transmission Studies.* Baltimore, Williams & Wilkins, 1988

Patten J. *Neurological Differential Diagnosis.* New York, Springer-Verlag, 1977

Rosenfalck P. *Electromyography: Sensory and Motor Conduction Findings in Normal Subjects.* Copenhagen, Laboratory of Clinical Neurophysiology Rigshospitalet, 1975

Schaumburg H, Spencer P. *The Neurology and Neuropathology of the Occupational Neuropathies. J Occup Med.* 18:789, 1976

Schaumburg H, Spencer P, Thomas P. *Disorders of Peripheral Nerves.* Philadelphia, FA Davis, 1983

Smorto M, Basmajian J. *Electrodiagnosis, A. Handbook for Neurologist.* Hagerstown, MD, Harper & Row, 1977

Snyder-Mackler L, Robinson A. *Clinical Electrophysiology: Electrotherapy and Electrophysiologic Testing.* Baltimore, Williams & Wilkins, 1989

Spinner M. *Injuries to the Major Branches of Peripheral Nerves of the Forearm.* Philadelphia, WB Saunders, 1978

Stalberg E, Young R, eds. *Neurology Clinical Neurophysiology*. Boston, Butterworths International Medical Reviews, 1981

Sumner A. *The Physiology of Peripheral Nerve Disease*. Philadelphia, WB Saunders, 1980

Sunderland S. *Nerves and Nerve Injuries*. Edinburgh, E & S Livingston, 1968

Vinken P, Bruyn G. *Diseases of Nerves: Handbook of Clinical Neurology, Part 7*. Amsterdam, North Holland Publishing Co, 1970

Weller R, Cervos-Navarro J. *Pathology of Peripheral Nerves*. London, Butterworths, 1977

Wolf S. *Electrotherapy*. New York, Churchill Livingstone, 1981

CHAPTER *13*

Electromyographic Biofeedback: An Overview

Steven L. Wolf

There is little question that modern technology has provided the medical community with new and highly sophisticated devices. In fact, any instrument that will facilitate restoration of function in a cost-effective manner is capable of attracting attention from clinicians. Within the context of rehabilitation, electronic devices designed to ameliorate pain, facilitate muscle contractility, or enhance purposeful movement have become plentiful, as new or existing manufacturers within the United States and abroad have expanded product ventures. Biofeedback instruments have a potentially unique place in the realm of technological advances because of their unique purposes and features. This chapter is designed to review the principles of electromyographic biofeedback, including the electronics, rehabilitation applications, and training strategies in both orthopedic and neurological conditions, and the limitations specific to the utility of such devices.

In 1969, a group of physicians, psychologists, and scientists met in Monterey, California, to discuss a common interest. These individuals believed that, given an appropriate interface, patients could control one or more physiological processes. For example, blood pressure, heart rate, or even skin conductance could be self-regulated if the content of information about such physiological processes, and the speed with which this content could be transmitted to the patient, were provided in a timely manner. At the time, implicit in these beliefs was the heretical notion that autonomic (or involuntary) physiological processes could be brought under voluntary control. This conglomeration of individuals founded the Biofeedback Research Society. This later became the Biofeedback Society of America; which has since contemporized its name to the Association of Applied Psychophysiology and Biofeedback and includes clinicians and scientists representing more than 15 disciplines.

The most significant event to occur at this early meeting was the development of the term *biofeedback,* which came to be defined as "the use of appropriate instrumentation to bring covert physiological processes to the conscious awareness of one or more individuals."[1,2] The creation and expansion of this term should not suggest that its utility was original at that time. As early as 1960, Marinacci and Horande had demonstrated that patients could be trained to change muscle output by increasing or decreasing activity (as seen on a clinical electromyograph).[3] The notion that individuals could inherently control physiological processes actually had its development many years earlier within the basis of cybernetic theory.[4] In modern-day parlance, biofeedback generally means the transduction of a physiological event into auditory and visual signals that are proportional in magnitude to the event. If appropriate criteria are used to present such signals to the patient, his or her responsiveness could be "shaped" to enhance or improve homeostatic mechanisms or to restore lost function. Indeed, appropriate biofeedback instrumentation exists to help patients control heart rate, electroencephalographic voltages, skin conductance, peripheral blood flow, skin temperature, anal or urinary sphincter contraction, force, joint motion, or muscle activity.[5-7]

PRINCIPLES OF ELECTROMYOGRAPHIC BIOFEEDBACK

The term *electromyographic (EMG) biofeedback* refers to the use of appropriate instrumentation to transduce muscle potentials into auditory or visual cues for the purpose of increasing or decreasing voluntary activity. Imagine, for a moment, a typical interaction between a physical therapist and his or her patient. Most clinicians in physical therapy treat primarily through observation and palpation ("the laying on of hands"). We generally tend to provide instruction to the patient, observe the patient's response to our instruction, and then serve as a feedback interface to the patient after we have assessed his or her performance. At best, this interaction takes several seconds. Such a time differential between command and feedback is exceptionally long, especially if the patient is attempting to modify subsequent motor activity. Furthermore, the response to the patient is usually very nonspecific. Such feedback statements as "try harder" or "relax more" are difficult for most patients to grade in terms of acceptable criteria. If biofeedback is to be a viable modality to be interfaced within any therapeutic plan, its success rests upon both the speed at which feedback is provided and the specificity of the content of such feedback. You need only envision your own ability to learn a new skill or sport. In keeping with the basic tenets of motor learning, timely and relevant knowledge of performance will enhance skill acquisition.

Electromyographic biofeedback provides instantaneous and ongoing information as a visual or auditory cue that is strictly contingent upon resting or contractile muscle states. The specificity of the feedback is defined by the location and interelectrode distance of the pickup sensors (electrodes).

Typically, surface electrodes applied to the skin overlying a given muscle or muscle group will sense small voltage changes (muscle action potentials) and will lead such potentials from the silver–silver chloride recording area of the electrode to an amplifier. The electromyographic activity is then amplified from the microvolt range and is processed by the instrumentation. This process consists of filtering appropriate frequency components of the electromyographic response, rectifying the bidirectional waves of depolarization and repolarization that are the muscle signals, and integrating these rectified responses over time. During the process of integration, the rectified voltage or analog signals are converted to a digital value. It is this digital value that is displayed to the patient in the form of a dial moving across the face of the meter, as a sequence of lights that are progressively activated or deactivated, or as a change in a tracing crossing an oscilloscope-like screen. At the same time, an audio amplifier is activated so that increases in muscle activity are displayed as an increase in pitch or as a repetition rate of a specific sound. The electronic components, as well as the physiology underlying the basis for electronic processing of muscle signals, require further discussion and elaboration. It is important to remember that these visual displays, particularly a line that changes its relative height as it crosses a screen, are not EMG levels themselves but rather represent visual cues proportional to such levels.

The Genesis of Muscle Activity

Electromyographic biofeedback instruments provide visual or auditory displays that are proportional to the amount of resting or voluntarily induced muscle activity. This activity is the result of depolarization and repolarization of muscle fibers. Numerous texts addressing muscle physiology discuss, in great detail, the voltage changes resulting from transient alterations in muscle cell membrane permeability.[8–11] These muscle fibers are activated in response to motor-axon innervation. Each alpha motor neuron and its terminal arborations, which innervate multiple muscle fibers, are referred to together as a *motor unit*. Motor units are heterogeneously dispersed within muscle, and each has specific histological and electrophysiological properties.[12–14] Typically, motor units are activated asynchronously, leading to a smooth contraction or relaxation of muscle. An example of how axon terminals from a motor neuron can innervate muscle fibers is depicted in Figure 13–1. More recently, neurophysiologists have scrutinized the properties of muscle fibers innervated by a single motor neuron. These *muscle units* are usually not adjacent to one another.[15] Studies of cats, for example, indicate that the average density of muscle units is from two to five fibers per 100 and that the territory subsumed for the entire muscle unit may be between 20 and 33 percent of the mean cross-sectional area of a muscle.[16] Of course, this geometry and muscle-unit representation will vary among species and according to the size (number of muscle fibers)

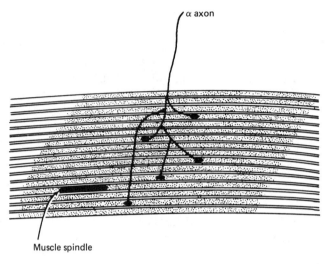

Figure 13—1. Illustrative representation of terminal innervation to muscle fibers from axonal branching of a motor neuron. This total complement is referred to as a *motor unit, while the aggregate of innervated muscle fibers is called a muscle unit.*

α axon

Muscle spindle

within any given muscle. Like the motor units that innervate them, muscle units have specific physiological and histochemical properties.

During voluntary contractions, or when a hyperactive muscle is suddenly perturbed (stretched), the resultant muscle activity (recorded from either indwelling or surface electrodes) is the result of temporal and spatial summation from various motor units that are activated. Generally, the more motor units activated, or the greater the frequency of discharge from motor units, the more muscle activity generated (and subsequently recorded). Conversely, activation of fewer motor units with lower frequency discharges will result in less muscle activity. At any given moment, the pictorial representation on a biofeedback unit is a function of the overall recorded muscle activity.

Electrodes. Electrodes serve as sensors for muscle activity. Typically, two types of electrodes are used. Percutaneous, or indwelling, electrodes may be placed within a specific muscle by manual insertion. Usually, fine-wire electrodes or monopolar needle electrodes serve this purpose (Fig. 13—2). Fine-wire electrodes consist of insulated wire, usually less than 75 μm in diameter. The ends of these wires have had their insulation removed and thus provide a recording surface. The hypodermic needle through which they are threaded enters the muscle and, when withdrawn, enables the fine wires to remain anchored within the muscle. The length of the hypodermic needle being used in this insertion procedure depends upon the depth at which the particular muscle resides from the skin surface. (In selecting the shaft length of a hypodermic needle, such factors as subcutaneous fat and muscle thickness must also be considered.) The benefit underlying the use of percutaneous electrodes is the specificity and localization of pickup, usually confined to one specific muscle. This form of recording is advisable when "deep" muscles are to be explored or when patients have considerable subcutaneous fat. (Fat serves as

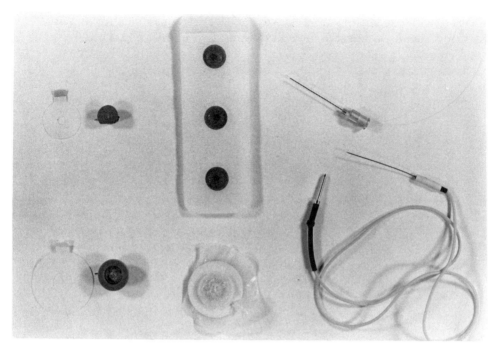

Figure 13–2. Examples of recording electrodes. Left, monopolar and fine-wire electrodes for percutaneous placement. Center, disposal surface electrodes: Right, different-sized, permanent surface electrodes, with their adhesive collars lying adjacent.

an attenuator of generated muscle signals and may result in low-level or poor-quality recordings if surface EMG is used.) Percutaneous electrode placements are often beyond the purview of allied health professionals. Therefore, physical therapists use surface electrodes even for situations in which indwelling electrode recordings might be more appropriate.

There are numerous types of surface electrodes (Fig. 13–2). Disposable electrodes are designed to be used once and often come pregelled; that is, with adequate conducting medium already placed on a sponge overlying the recording surface of the electrode. Other disposable electrodes require application of a gel. Still other karaya-based electrodes can be reused several times. Nondisposable, or permanent, electrodes require the application of a collar or adhesive around the periphery of the electrode prior to filling the electrode proper with a conducting medium. Once this procedure has been undertaken, the collar overlying the adhesive is removed and the electrode is gently tacked to the skin, which has been previously prepared by a brisk alcohol rub (which reduces skin impedance by removing oil and superficial epithelia). The recording surface of these permanent electrodes varies, and selection of the appropriate recording diameter is based upon the size of the muscles from which the recordings are to be made. For example, small, permanent surface electrodes are used when recording from facial muscles, whereas electrodes with large recording diameters (greater than 1 cm) are often employed when limb muscle groups are the targets of choice.[1] The recording surface of all cutaneous electrodes is made of a silver–silver chloride base or a gold base. These metals have been selected because of the ease with which they can "pick up" muscle potentials. The conducting medium should have a high salt concentration, because salt is an excellent conductor of generated muscle activity.

The electrodes that record muscle activity must be "referenced" to a common ground electrode. Because of the excellent quality of input amplifiers, the rule that reference electrodes be equidistant from the ground is no longer applicable. Of concern, however, is the interelectrode spacing between active electrodes. When training patients to relax hyperactive muscles or to reduce EMG (as part of a process to minimize stress or physiological arousal), widely spaced electrodes are appropriate. Wide spacing permits a sampling of many muscles, thereby providing a better indication of overall muscle activity during the relaxation process. During neuromuscular re-education, when selectivity of muscle activity becomes an important consideration, closely spaced electrodes that record from a limited volume of muscle should be employed. By closely spacing electrodes, one has a greater chance of specificity of recording from muscles underlying the skin surface. A major disadvantage of surface EMG (in general) and during EMG biofeedback training (in specific) is that one is never sure precisely from where the recorded activity is generated.

The activity that is recorded at the skin–electrode interface must be conducted to an amplification system. This process is usually accomplished by electrode leads to an input cable. Often, these leads are not shielded. (Shielding of leads involves a covering or wrapping made of a metallic substance, designed to minimize the possibility of pickup from stray electromotive forces generated elsewhere in the environment.) A good clinical procedure to follow is to tape electrode leads to the skin surface. By so doing, one minimizes the possibility of *movement artifact*. This concept refers to the generation of transient activity along the cable line when a cable is suddenly moved or disturbed. This transient is led to the biofeedback processing system and is subsequently integrated and presented to the patient. The concern for movement artifact is heightened when biofeedback is integrated within a therapeutic exercise plan. Under this circumstance, the clinician often prefers that the patient undergo dynamic movement involving the limb segment at which the surface electrodes are placed. Gently taping electrode leads to the skin surface will minimize the possibility of creating transient nonbiologic activity that will be processed by the unit as the patient moves. Similarly, the clinician must be sure that electrodes are not touched or manipulated during limb movements. Just a little advanced thinking on hand placements during feedback-assisted exercise will easily circumvent this potential problem.

Processing the Electromyographic Signal
Electromyographic activity arriving at the biofeedback unit is first *amplified* (Fig. 13–3). Generally, the amplification factor is 1000, so that EMG levels that

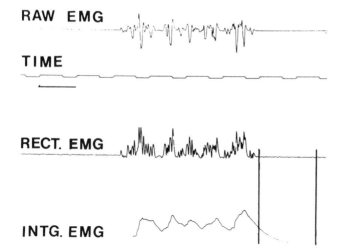

Figure 13–3. Processing of the EMG signal generated by a brief contraction of the right forearm flexor mass. Upper trace, raw amplified (×1000) EMG; second trace, time markers every 100 msec; third trace, rectified raw amplified signal; fourth trace, integrated EMG (time constant of integrator = 100 msec).

are often within the microvolt range are elevated to the millivolt range. Because muscle signals are bidirectional (depolarization and repolarization), the activity is next *rectified*. Rectification means the inversion of one phase of a muscle potential so that the entire potential now appears unidirectional; that is, appears on one side of the baseline. Signals can be either *half-wave rectified* (removal of one direction of the voltage change) or *full-wave rectified* (one direction of the voltage change is "flipped" so all voltages are retained and are unidirectional). Finally, the rectified EMG undergoes a process of *integration*. Integration means examining the area under a curve per unit of time. Essentially, the unidirectional rectified EMG forms an envelope that consumes an area defined by the EMG peaks and by a reference baseline. Integrators used in EMG feedback devices tend to sample the EMG ten times a second (every 100 msec) and provide a quantified value proportional to the area defined within that 100-msec band. The process by which this *analog*, or rectified voltage signal, is given a numeric equivalent is referred to as *analog-to-digital conversion*. In fact, it is this numeric that is sometimes displayed as visual feedback to the patient. Thus, a dial moving across a meter will point to a number that is equivalent to the integrated value at that moment in time.

One additional component within most feedback devices is a *level detector, goal,* or *threshold*. A level detector is essentially a scanner that can be changed on the feedback machine by the clinician in order to determine where the integral of EMG is, with respect to the placement of the scanner. For example, if the integral of EMG is greater than the level of the scanner, then an audio amplifier may be activated. Activation of the audio amplifier then provides audio feedback to the patient when his or her level of EMG exceeds the threshold previously set. This procedure would be appropriate if patients were being trained to increase muscle output. By gradually raising the level detector, the patient is required to generate a greater magnitude of muscle activity in order to activate the audio amplifier. Conversely, if the threshold level is contingent upon activity generated below the integral of EMG, then the audio amplifier would be activated (or, perhaps, turned off) when the integrated muscle activity is less (lower than) the threshold detector level. This procedure might be appropriate to use when training a patient to reduce muscle activity; for example, in reduction of resting levels of EMG from spastic muscle. Moving the level detector to coincide with the training procedures developed by the physical therapist is referred to as *shaping*. Thus, we can shape a patient's responses *up* when recruitment of muscle is an appropriate training strategy or *down* when relaxation of muscle is our desired goal.

Unfortunately, the electronics underlying these processes are not so simple. A reasonable question involves the time lapse between the generated muscle activity and the actual feedback of that activity. The delays in this process are a function of the *time constant* of the integrator. Time constant is the product of the resistors and capacitors in an integrated circuit network or, in real time, represents that time required to produce approximately a two-thirds change in a previous voltage level. Most integrators of EMG biofeedback equipment have time constants that vary between 0.1 and 0.5 sec (100 and 500 msec). The faster the time constant, the more quickly the visual display will respond to changes in patient muscle activity. Conversely, the slower the time constant, the longer the time between changes in muscle activity and visual feedback. This latter consideration is appropriate when undertaking general relaxation training. In this situation we are examining relatively small amounts of change in muscle activity. Therefore, the immediacy of change in the feedback signal is not exceptionally important. If we are having the patient perform dynamic contractions involving changes in excess of 100 μV of muscle activity, then a faster time constant is appropriate. Under this condition, if the time constant were too slow during a dynamic movement, the patient might already be engaged in subsequent muscle activities prior to receiving visual feedback from a previous muscle movement. Most contemporary feedback devices provide the clinician with an opportunity to change the time constant of the integrator so that the speed of visual feedback is appropriate for the type of training.

All muscle activity comprises wave forms that possess varying *frequency components*. The frequency components of an EMG signal are determined by the duration of a signal and by the rate of rise (depolarization) and fall (repolarization) of the muscle signal. Typically, most of the energy within EMG signals falls between 80 and 250 cycles per second (cps, or Hz). Volume-conducted EMG from distant muscles, with respect to surface electrode placements, may have slower frequency components. To help us specify the frequency component of EMG that we wish to have processed, feedback devices employ *filtering* of the EMG signal. The incorporation of filters enables us to screen out unwanted signals whose frequencies are too high or too low. By employing a high-pass filter, for example, we can eliminate lower frequencies that might contain 60-Hz noise interference. (Recall that 60 Hz is the inherent frequency of most currents used to operate equipment.) In addition, many feedback devices are battery-operated rather than based upon a common current source. Use of battery-operated machines and optical isolation help to minimize interference, or 60-Hz pickup.

APPLICATIONS (Table 13–1)

Muscle Relaxation

Electromyographic feedback is often used to reduce elevated levels of muscle activity. Most frequently, these elevations occur among individuals who have hyperarousal of physiological systems, with or without the presence of pain, and among individuals with neural disruption leading to hypertonus of select muscle groups. Traditionally, EMG feedback for stress reduction involved equidistant active-lead active-electrode placements on the frontalis muscle. [17,18] It was believed that overall body stress was reflected by tension or hyperactivity in this muscle of facial expression. The notion was to integrate EMG feedback with progressive relaxation training (or autogenic relaxation exercises). Reductions in frontalis-integrated EMG activity would be associated with a reduction of arousal in other physiological systems (such as heart rate, skin conductance, or peripheral blood flow). What clinicians neglected to observe was the anatomic location of the frontalis muscle with respect to surrounding structures. Because this muscle is in relative isolation, activity from other muscle groups could be volume-conducted and picked up by electrodes overlying the frontalis. Such activities as gentle eye closure, swallowing, approximation of maxilla and mandible, and upper respiratory movement could result in elevated levels of frontalis activity that would be undetected by the clinician. As a result, we now refer to EMG activity recorded from these placements as *frontal* muscle

TABLE 13–1. OVERVIEW OF CLINICAL CONDITIONS AMENABLE TO EMG BIOFEEDBACK INTERVENTIONS

Goal	Conditions
Recruitment	Peripheral nerve injury
	Muscle weakness
	Immobilization
	Joint surgery
	Deconditioning (atrophy)
	Pain
	Antagonists to spastic muscles
	Muscle transfers
Relaxation	Stress-related hyperarousal
	Pain
	Spasticity
	Rigidity
	Torticollis

activity, and clinicians recognize that recordings obtained from this area reflect more than simply the direct underlying muscle activity. Alternatively, many physicians have used forearm musculature placements during relaxation training. By using limb placements, the issue of volume conduction becomes less prominent. Nonetheless, clinicians must recognize that, even in a relatively quiet resting posture, distant limb movements may have an effect upon the target EMG recordings. For example, simply pressing the back of the leg into a recliner seat will affect forearm extensor electromyography.[19]

Paraspinal placements of active electrodes about the lumbar vertebral column are often employed when attempting to train patients with chronic lower-back pain to reduce resting EMG activity.[20,21] The notion underlying this paradigm is that paraspinal muscle activity will be elevated as a result of the patient's discomfort. By training patients to reduce this muscle activity, concomitant levels of anxiety and tension would be alleviated, also. Although the premise underlying this procedure would appear to be appropriate, training in static postures in order to achieve this goal does not necessarily carry over into the ways in which individuals would use paraspinal musculature during more dynamic movements.[23] During dynamic movements of the trunk, paraspinal back musculature can be viewed as acting to control sagittal and rotatory trunk movements in concert with abdominal musculature. These erector spinae muscles are anatomical mirror images separated by a vertebral column. The examination of how activity relates in these muscles during motion and under normal circumstances helps to appreciate activity under abnormal conditions precipitated by musculoskeletal pathology. By using EMG feedback to train abnormal response patterns towards normal, non-discogenic lower-back pain can be alleviated. Cram[24] has developed a scanning procedure to help clinicians identify resting differences in bilateral paraspinal EMG as a basis for electrode placement sites in biofeedback retraining.

Among patients with spasticity, muscle relaxation becomes a paramount issue. Although some degree of spasticity may be appropriate, hyperactive stretch reflexes often impede purposeful movement. Often, clinicians attempt to train patients in relaxation with electrode placements overlying spastic muscle. If spasticity is present at rest, clinicians will attempt to shape resting levels downward using threshold feedback that would require the patient to produce levels of integrated EMG below the threshold. More commonly, however, patients will be trained to reduce activity in spastic muscle following slow or quick prolonged stretch. Here, voluntary effort through feedback is based upon conscientious efforts to "damp" hyperactive stretch reflex responses.[25,26] The primary goal is to train patients to show a lower reflex response to stretch and to reduce the time required to return EMG to a prestretch baseline level as the muscle is maintained in the lengthened position. As will be noted below, this form of relaxation training plays an integral role in feedback strategies among neurological patients undergoing rehabilitation for the development of purposeful movement.

Muscle Recruitment

The application of EMG feedback to patients with musculoskeletal disorders is relatively straightforward. Because appreciation of muscle length changes (proprioception) and sensory status is not compromised, the task of the patient is simply to recruit more motor units and to discharge them more frequently (spatial and temporal summation). The strategy employed is to shape patient responses upward. This procedure implies that the patient must generate more activity in order to reach a threshold level that is continuously moved upward by the clinician. With respect to electrode placements, one must consider the specific pathology that is being treated. For example, in the case of a weak quadriceps femoris muscle mechanism following meniscus surgery, electrodes would be widely spaced across the muscle's mass, and the sensitivity (or setting) for feedback would be extremely high. This situation means that little activity would be required to provide meaningful feedback. As the patient recruited more muscle activity, the sensitivity scales on a feedback machine would be lowered, thereby requiring the patient to generate more activity in order to receive appropriate visual or auditory feedback. As the muscle group strengthened, selective areas or specific members of the quadriceps femoris muscle mass might be preferentially weak. In this situation, active electrodes would be moved closer together so as to overlie the area of weakness, thereby providing more specific feedback from that muscle segment. Under the condition of more closely spaced electrodes, the clinician would repeat the training procedure, starting with high sensitivity scales and moving toward lower sensitivity, thus making the patient work harder to achieve the appropriate feedback signal.

Among neurological patients who may possess varying degrees of dyskinesia, more caution must be exercised in using feedback for the purpose of muscle recruitment. Most often, we wish to train patients to increase activity in muscles antagonistic to the hyperactive or spastic groups. Typically, electrode placements must be very closely spaced under this circumstance, in order to minimize the possibility of volume-conducted pickup to the muscle group being recruited from the spastic muscles. Wide spacing over weak antagonist muscles may result in erroneous feedback through volume conduction from the antagonist muscle group if the movement effort causes contraction or if activity emanates predominantly from the hyperactive group.

Patients with peripheral nerve injury represent the one neurological group for whom this treatment strategy is inappropriate. To use biofeedback as an assist to muscle retraining for these patients, one must have documented evidence of re-innervation to those muscles governed by the affected nerve. Such evidence is usually obtained by percutaneous EMG recordings in response to voluntary efforts. With re-innervation present, the biofeedback training strategy for these patients is identical to the situation discussed earlier for orthopedic patients with muscle weakness. In short, these patients are treated as though they possess muscle weakness rather than a neural deficit. The training strategy, then, would consist of wide electrode placements and feedback at a very high sensitivity setting, followed (over time) by progressively narrowing the interelectrode distance between active electrodes and by lowering the sensitivity of the feedback machine. This strategy would require the patient to generate more muscle activity. Caution must be exercised when using feedback among these patients so as to avoid fatigue.

TRAINING STRATEGIES FOR NEUROLOGICAL PATIENTS

Whether we are dealing with stroke, closed head injury, spinal cord injury, or cerebral palsy, the premises underlying training strategies are basically identical: treatment of the extremity progresses from a proximal to a distal manner.[27,28] Whether the feedback application is to the upper or lower extremity, the proximal-to-distal training strategies usually begin with the patient in a comfortable (supine) posture and progress toward the patient sitting, standing and, finally, making functional use of the involved extremity; that is, manipulation of the environment for the upper extremity and ambulation for the lower extremity.[25,27] All of the training strategies that are brought to bear during static postures, when feedback is presented to specific muscles acting on joints, are also utilized during functional activities. Tables 13–2 and 13–3 summarize the training strategies for neurological patients in treatment of the

TABLE 13–2. EMG BIOFEEDBACK TRAINING STRATEGIES FOR NEUROLOGICAL PATIENTS—UPPER EXTREMITY

Joint	Movement	Muscle(s)	Goal
Shoulder	Flexion	Upper trapezius	Relax
		Anterior deltoid	Recruit
Shoulder	Abduction	Pectoralis major (sternal head)	Relax
		Middle deltoid	Recruit
Elbow	Extension	Wrist flexor mass	Relax
		Wrist extensor mass	Recruit
Forearm	Supination	Biceps brachii	Recruit (without elbow flexion)[a]
Finger	Extension	Finger flexors (distal volar aspect)	Relax
		Finger extensors (digital dorsal aspect)	Recruit
		First dorsal interosseous	Recruit
Thumb	Extension Abduction	Extensor pollicis longus (dorsum of wrist joint)	Recruit
Thumb	Flexion	Flexor pollicis brevis	Relax or recruit[b]

[a] When voluntary supination not present or incomplete.
[b] Dependent upon presence of thumb flexor spasticity.

TABLE 13–3. EMG BIOFEEDBACK TRAINING STRATEGIES FOR NEUROLOGIC PATIENTS—LOWER EXTREMITY

Joint	Movement	Muscle(s)	Goal
Hip	Extension	Gluteus maximus	Recruit
Hip	Flexion	Sartorius (near anterior iliac spine)	Recruit
Hip	Abduction	Adductor mass	Relax
		Gluteus medius	Recruit
Knee	Flexion	Quadriceps	Relax
		Hamstrings	Recruit
Ankle	Dorsiflexion	Gastroc-soleus	Relax
		Tibialis anterior	Recruit
Ankle	Eversion	Extensor digitorum brevis	Recruit

upper and lower extremities, respectively. Training begins with efforts to relax hyperactive musculature at rest and during passive stretch. Once the patient is able to reduce hyperactive stretch responses, recruitment of antagonist muscles follows. It is beneficial to monitor the spastic muscle, as well as the weakened antagonist, during these efforts. Under this circumstance, the spastic muscle may be undergoing a lengthening contraction as the antagonist shortens. If the patient has learned to reduce passive stretch responses of hyperactive musculature, then he or she should be able to maintain lower levels of EMG when the antagonist muscle is actively contracting. By proceeding in a proximal distal manner, the patient should develop controlled efforts over proximal joints as activity in distal joints is assessed.

The list of items that appears in Table 13–3 fails to address electrode placement for scapular stabilization. Recording scapular musculature (for example, levator scapulae or rhomboideus) is difficult because activity generated from these muscles is contaminated by the concomitant pickup of intercostal musculature and heartbeat. The most appropriate location for providing feedback from scapular musculature is at the inferior angle of the scapula, directly over the insertion of the serratus anterior. This muscle is comparatively thick at this level. Consequently prospects for recording respiratory or heart musculature activity are reduced.

Recently Tries[29] has noted that isolated EMG can be recorded and consequently "fed back" from the infraspinatus by closely spaced electrodes along the lateral (vertebral) middle one third of the scapula, at which location this muscle is no longer covered by the middle trapezius. This insight now allows us to work toward shoulder external rotation, a much-needed movement, particularly among neurological patients with typical upper extremity flexion synergies.

One must train reduction of substitute movements from upper trapezius muscle during efforts at shoulder flexion. Attempts to record from a more appropriate muscle, the supraspinatus, are hindered by the fact that upper trapezius overlies this muscle. Therefore, anterior deltoid is the primary muscle for recruitment in shoulder flexion efforts. Also note that considerable variation exists for the control of pronation of supination at the forearm. For patients who cannot voluntarily supinate, the biceps is the muscle of choice for training. Because this muscle may be hyperactive, efforts must be made to recruit the biceps brachii as a supinator without inducing elbow flexion. The supinator is a very difficult muscle to isolate with surface electrode placements. In attempting to recruit the pronator teres, closely spaced miniature electrodes must be used, because this muscle rests closely beside the wrist flexor mass. To train for finger extension or flexion, electrode placements must be at the distal forearm in order to minimize the possibility of pickup from wrist musculature. At this level, the flexors and extensors of the wrist have become tendonous, while muscle fibers are still present in those muscles governing finger movements.

Of particular concern in feedback applications to the lower extremity is control over knee flexion efforts. Particular attention must be paid to reducing activity in the quadriceps femoris muscle at heel strike and to the initiation of knee flexion activity at toe off. By addressing these issues within ambulation efforts, the possibility of minimizing recurvatum is enhanced. Most literature has addressed the issue of controlled ankle dorsiflexion during the swing phase of gate.[30,31] It was believed that, by reducing hyperactive plantar flexion activity recruiting the tibialis anterior muscle, "drop foot" could be alleviated, Although this notion is correct, past research has failed to address control over the ankle joint during the swing phase of gait. Most patients will tend to invert the ankle, even during efforts at dorsiflexion. Therefore, recording activity from the extensor digitorum brevis muscle during the swing phase of gait may be beneficial. If patients can be trained to recruit this muscle, the possibility of adding an eversion component during ankle movements is enhanced. The peroneal musculature is most difficult to isolate with surface electromyography because of the thin intramuscular septum between the lateral and posterior compartments of the leg. With peroneal electrode placement, volume-conducted activity from triceps surae often contaminates recordings, causing the patient to receive false feedback during efforts at eversion.

Whether one is treating patients with musculoskeletal or neuromuscular disorders, the strategies discussed thus far are typically referred to as *targeted muscle training*. Targeted training refers to the monitoring of muscle activity from one or more specific muscles within a limb segment. There are, however, alternatives to targeted muscle training. Several years ago, the notion was advanced that homologous muscles with similar functions could be monitored simultaneously.[32] In no case is this possibility more obvious than in the utilization of EMG feedback to train for symmetric facial expression among patients with facial nerve palsy. Because we usually use facial muscles symmetrically, it was suggested that bilateral placements over an appropriate muscle could enable the patient to match the activity in the unaffected muscle with output of activity from the involved muscle. This approach would require a dual-channel unit or two separate single-channel units, In essence, then, EMG generated from the uninvolved muscle would serve as a template (or standard) against which output from the involved muscle could be measured. Rather than using a level detector, an effort to produce symmetric quantified EMG would enable the patient to voluntarily control output from the uninvolved muscle as a basis for the genesis of output from the involved musculature.

Recently, we have expanded this notion to incorporate efforts at training function in the upper extremity of neurological patients.[33] Specifically, by using a dual-channel feedback unit, homologous muscle groups could be monitored in an effort to achieve functional restitution. For example, in training for elbow extension, bilateral movements would be attempted, and the patient would match the EMG of the involved triceps brachii to that of the uninvolved muscle. The obvious benefit derived from this approach is prospect of patients engaging in self-training so that clinicians would not need to constantly attend to client efforts. The notion of "motor copy" with EMG feedback has proven to be effective in treatment of the upper extremities of neurological patients who had some degree of isolated wrist or finger extension. Like patients subjected to targeted feedback training where attention is directed totally to the involved upper extremity, motor copy patients made similar gains but over a more protracted time course, almost as though it took longer to retrain the nervous system to achieve similar functional goals.

BIOFEEDBACK INTEGRATED WTHIN A THERAPEUTIC EXERCISE PLAN

When one reviews the literature on biofeedback applications for any neuromuscular disorder, it becomes apparent that feedback training has been employed in an isolated fashion.[34–39] The reason for application of EMG biofeedback independent of other therapeutic measures is to assess the efficacy of this modality without possible contaminating influences. Apparently, what has emerged from the absorption of these publications is the erroneous belief that EMG biofeedback should be used independently of other therapeutic plans. Obviously, the integration of feedback during a therapeutic regimen, whether it be a neuromuscular re-education technique or progressive resistance exercise, can be of benefit to both patient and clinician. The patient who is given feedback is aware of how a specific muscle or muscle group is performing with respect to the therapeutic task and may reorient his or her voluntary efforts at recruitment or relaxation accordingly (or in light of suggestions offered by the clinician). From a different perspective, the feedback may be of value to the clinician even without the patient observing visual or auditory cues of muscle performance. For example, in using neuromuscular re-education procedures (such as those advocated by Brunstromm, Bobath, or others), the clinician would have ongoing and immediate information about whether postural or movement manipulations have an effect upon muscle tone within specific muscles. The awareness of the presence or absence of such changes would not necessarily suggest a fallacy or inadequacy of a neuromuscular technique; rather, this information would help the clinician adjust, change, or modify such a procedure so as to produce the desired results.

Recently this notion has been expanded to permit not only on-line use of feedback during any therapeutic intervention in rehabilitation but also the capability of quantifying the response at the conclusion of the specific exercise, movement, or task. This approach is referred to as concurrent assessment of muscle activity (CAMA).[40] In this way the clinician may be able to relate exact changes in muscle activity to the treatment approach. This capability will assume growing importance because more emphasis is being placed upon demonstrable proof that treatment interventions produce both measurable physiological and task-oriented changes. Thus, for example, the belief that a precise change in trunk to pelvis orientation can yield changes in muscle "tonus" can be readily and easily documented through EMG acquisition. One must remember that the intent here is not to prove or disprove any particular therapeutic approach, but rather to help clinicians find appropriate commands, hand placements or resistive patterns to assure maximal correct responses in a time-effective manner.

There are limitations to the use of EMG feedback, regardless of whether the information generated is for the purpose of assisting the patient, the clinician, or both. Unquestionably, the process of "setting up" a patient is time-consuming. For most clinicians who have minimal experience in the use of biofeedback instrumentation, 2 to 3 min are usually required to prepare a patient for dual-channel recording. This setup time includes skin preparation, electrode preparation, placement of electrodes, and securing of leads to the input cable. When one considers that the contact time for patient treatment is limited, perhaps the period required for preparing the patient and finally disassembling the electrodes after treatment might appear inappropriate. In reality, the time element is considerably short, in light of what can be gained by the patient's use of such a device.

A second concern to many clinicians is the cost of feedback equipment. Yet, such costs are comparable to other electrical instruments and are, in many cases, considerably cheaper. Most important, however, is the realization that what can be gained from the integration of feedback within therapeutic exercise plans is based solely upon the clinicians' knowledge of anatomy and kinesiology. Inadequate skin preparation or electrode placement is one issue. Lack of adequate knowledge about where to place electrodes is another. For clinicians who are unfamiliar with anatomy and with the relationship of muscles to skin surface during movement, feedback will be inappropriate. For those clinicians who base any neuromuscular re-education procedure upon such knowledge, this concern would not be an issue.

DOCUMENTATION

Like any therapeutic intervention, adequate documentation of treatment plans and outcome measures is imperative. In an age where cost-effectiveness and

DAILY TREATMENT RECORD

Name: _____   Date: _____

| Device | Muscle or Group | Type of Electrode | Electrode Site | Patient Position | Strategy | ROM | | | EMG | | | | |
						Active	Passive	Resting	Peak Value Voluntary	Peak Value Involuntary	Relax. Time	Muscle Grade

Comments: _____

Figure 13–4. Example of elements that might be recorded during a biofeedback training session.

Name: _____ Ankle: _____

GASTROC.	Passive*						Active*					
		Stretch (PF→DF)					P. Flexion			D. Flexion		
	EMG Resting	Slow		Fast			Range	EMG	Relax Time	Range	EMG	Relax Time
		EMG	Relax Time	EMG	Relax Time							
1	μv	μv	M / S	μv	M / S		°	μv	M / S	°	μv	M / S
2	μv	μv	M / S	μv	M / S		°	μv	M / S	°	μv	M / S
3	μv	μv	M / S	μv	M / S		°	μv	M / S	°	μv	M / S

Electrode placement (measured distal from the popliteal fossa line): _____ cm (medial) _____ cm (distal): _____ cm
(between lateral and medial electrodes)

Comments:

ANT. TIBIALIS	Passive*	Active*							
		D. Flexion				P. Flexion			
	EMG Resting	Range	EMG	Relax Time		Range	EMG	Relax Time	
1	μV	°	μV	M S		°	μV	M S	
2	μV	°	μV	M S		°	μV	M S	
3	μV	°	μV	M S		°	μV	M S	

Electrode placement (measured distal from the patella): _____ cm and _____ cm

Comments: _____

*Sitting with hips and knees flexed = 90°; feet suspended.

Figure 13–5. A specific example of components that could be recorded during a training session for ankle musculature. Note that documentation includes passive and active movement, range of motion, and EMG.

demonstrable efficacy are paramount, such concerns are very real. Figure 13–4 provides an example of how daily records can be kept. Contained on the treatment sheet is information that would facilitate both adequate documentation and replication of the treatment strategy with biofeedback. A location for comments could include anatomic landmarks for electrode placements, so that other clinicians could carry out treatments in the absence of the primary therapist.

A more specific example of documentation is provided in Figure 13–5 for the gastrocnemius and anterior tibialis muscles. Notice that information is replicated three times, using the output from an EMG machine to record resting and peak levels of electromyographic activity. Documentation is undertaken during both passive and active efforts on the part of the patient. Also recorded is the time in minutes and seconds for specific movements of these muscles.

Clinicians should be encouraged to develop their own documentation schema. Documentation forms should be simple, clear, and easily replicable or modified.

With the total integration of microprocessor capability to evaluate physiological responses instantaneously, establishing data bases for the processing, recording, and storing of EMG data from feedback machines is now commonplace. The need to create individual forms such as the one shown in Figure 13–5 is being replaced by computer-generated formats. Depending upon available clinic computer facilities, many existing microprocessors can indeed be used in conjunction with biofeedback hardware for data storage, with each patient having his or her own disk or disk space on a hard disk drive. The benefits of this approach are savings in space and time while insuring permanent records that are easily retrievable. Contemporary data acquisition will use increasingly more sophisticated computer software. Clearly the rehabilitation clinician should become an informed user of these tools to document treatment efficacy.

A LOOK TOWARD THE FUTURE

Muscle biofeedback will not continue to operate in a vacuum independent of other therapeutic modalities. Lecraw[41] has highlighted the ways in which biofeedback can be used with other modalities. Clinical reports have already appeared that combine electrical stimulation contingent upon self-initiated levels of EMG.[42] The future holds prospects for expanding this approach so that not only will electrical stimulation be contingent upon heightened or reduced levels of muscle activity, but the mode of stimulation may be radiometrically delivered in any one of several options, including linear ratio, logarithmic, and exponential. We will have to be prepared to determine the most feasible clinical applicants for an increasingly sophisticated technology.

In addition more portable feedback units containing microprocessors will be produced. These units will be used in the home to reinforce clinic-generated treatment goals and to modify muscle behaviors at the work site. Once again it will behoove clinicians to be prepared to apply this technology.

SUMMARY

This chapter has reviewed principles of EMG feedback so as to make the clinician more comfortable with these instruments. An ability to adequately prepare a patient to use a feedback device is mandatory prior to executing any therapeutic intervention or strategy. The use of EMG feedback for stress reduction and spasticity has been discussed, and various orthopedic and neurological conditions for which feedback can be employed have been presented.

An overview of training strategies and basic principles underlying the sequencing of treatment with biofeedback was reviewed. Finally, apparent advantages, limitations, and methods of documentation were provided.

Clinicians are encouraged to use this and other forms of "high tech" within their practice, lest individuals in other disciplines usurp the utility of this therapeutic tool. Electromyographic feedback devices should be used to inform clinicians about the efficacy of their treatment plans with respect to changes in muscle activity or to assist patients in achieving desirable therapeutic goals. These considerations are paramount in an age where audits and cost-effective clinical services will determine reimbursement.

REFERENCES

1. Wolf SL. Essential considerations in the use of EMG biofeedback. *Phys Ther.* 58:25, 1978
2. Bilodeau IMcD, ed. Information Feedback. In: Bilodeau IMcD and Bilodeau AM, eds. *Principles of Skill Acquisition*, 5th ed. New York, Academic Press, 1969
3. Marinacci AA, Horande M. Electromyogram in neuromuscular re-education. *Bull Los Angeles Neurol.* 25:57, 1960
4. Weiner H. *Cybernetics: Or Control and Communication in the Animal and the Machine.* New York, Wiley, 1948
5. Basmajian JV, ed. *Biofeedback: Principles and Practice for Clinicians*, 2nd ed. Baltimore, Williams & Wilkins, 1989
6. Schwartz MS, ed. *Biofeedback: A Practitioner's Guide.* New York, Guilford Press, 1987
7. Hatch JP, Fisher JD, Rugh JD. *Biofeedback: Studies in Clinical Efficacy.* New York, Plenum Press, 1987
8. Cohen DH, Sherman SM. Spinal organization of motor function. In: Berney RM, Levy MN, eds. *Physiology*, 2nd ed. St. Louis, CV Mosby, 1986:196–214
9. Kirchberger MA, Schwartz IL. Excitation and contraction of skeletal muscle. In: Best JB, ed. *Physiological Basis of Medical Practice*, 11th ed. Baltimore, Williams & Wilkins, 1985:58–100

10. Guyton AC. Contraction of skeletal muscle. In: Guyton AC. *Textbook of Medical Physiology*, 7th ed. Philadelphia, WB Saunders, 1988:120–134

11. Vander AJ, Sherman JH, Luciano DS. *Human Physiology: The Mechanisms of Body Function*, 3rd ed. New York, McGraw-Hill, 1980:211–249

12. Person RS, Kudina LP. Discharge frequency and discharge pattern of human motor units during voluntary contraction of muscle. *Electroenceph Clin Neurophysiol*. 32:471, 1972

13. Belanger AY, McComas AJ. Extent of motor unit activation during effort. *J Appl Physiol*. 51:1131, 1981

14. English AW, Wolf SL. The motor unit: Anatomy and physiology. *Phys Ther*. 62:1763, 1982

15. Stuart DG, Enoka RM. Motoneurons, motor units, and the size principle. In: Rosenberg RN, ed. *The Clinical Neurosciences*, New York, Churchill-Livingstone, 1983; 5: 471–517

16. Burke RE. Motor Units: Anatomy, physiology and functional organization. In: Brooks VB, ed. *Handbook of Physiology*, vol 2. *The Nervous System: Motor Control*. Bethesda, American Physiological Society, 1981:61–84

17. Budzynski TH, Stoyva JM, Adler CS, et al. EMG biofeedback and tension headache: A controlled outcome study. *Psychosomat Med*. 6:509, 1973

18. Stoyva JM. Guidelines in cultivating general relaxation: Biofeedback and autogenic training combined. In: Basmajian JV, ed. *Biofeedback: Principles and Practice for Clinicians*, 2nd ed. Baltimore, Williams & Wilkins, 1983:149–169

19. Fair PL. Biofeedback-assisted relaxation strategies in psychotherapy. In Basmajian JV, ed. *Biofeedback: Principles and Practice for Clinicians*, 2nd ed. Baltimore, Williams & Wilkins, 1983:170–191

20. Swanson DM, Maruta T, Swenson WM. Results of behavior modification in the treatment of chronic pain. *Psychosom Med*. 41:55, 1979

21. Turner JA, Chapman CR. Psychological interventions for chronic pain: A critical review, I. Relaxation training and biofeedback. *Pain*. 12:1, 1982

22. Wolf SL, Nacht M, Kelly JL. EMG feedback training during dynamic movement for low back pain patients. *Behav Ther*. 13:395, 1982

23. Wolf SL, Wolf LB, Segal RL. The relationship of extraneous movements to lumbar paraspinal muscle activity: Implications for EMG biofeedback training to low back pain patients. *Biofeed Self-Reg*. 14:63, 1989

24. Cram JR. Surface EMG recordings and pain-related disorders: A diagnostic framework. *Biofeed Self-Reg*. 13:123, 1988

25. Baker M, Regenos E, Wolf SL, et al. Developing strategies for biofeedback: Applications in neurologically handicapped patients. *Phys Ther*. 157:402, 1977

26. Wolf SL, Baker MP, Kelly JL. EMG biofeedback in stroke: Effects of patient characteristics. *Arch Phys Med Rehabil*. 60:96, 1979

27. Kelly JL, Baker MP, Wolf SL. Procedures for EMG biofeedback training in involved upper extremities of hemiplegic patients. *Phys Ther*. 59:1500, 1979

28. Binder SA, Moll CB, Wolf SL. Evaluation of electromyographic biofeedback as an adjunct to therapeutic exercise in treating the lower extremities of hemiplegic patients. *Phys Ther*. 61:886, 1981

29. Tries J. Emg biofeedback for the treatment of upper extremity dysfunction: Can it be effective? *Biofeed Self-Reg*. 14:21, 1989

30. Shiavi RG, Champion SA, Freeman FR, et al. Efficacy of myofeedback therapy in

regaining control of lower extremity musculature following stroke. *Am J Phys Med.* 58:185, 1979

31. Basmajian JV, Kukulka CG, Narayan MG, et al. Biofeedback treatment of foot-drop after stroke compared with standard rehabilitation technique: Effects on voluntary control and strength. *Arch Phys Med Rehabil.* 56:231, 1975

32. Booker HE, Rubow RT, Coleman PJ. Simplified feedback in neuromuscular retraining: An automated approach using electromyographic signals. *Arch Phys Med Rehabil.* 50:621, 1969

33. Wolf SL, Lecraw DE, Barton LA. A comparison of motor copy and targeted feedback training techniques for restitution of upper extremity function among neurologic patients. *Phys Ther.* 69:625, 1989

34. Mroczek N, Halpern D, McHugh R. Electromyographic feedback and physical therapy for neuromuscular retraining in hemiplegia. *Arch Phys Med Rehabil.* 59:258, 1978

35. Prevo AJH, Visser SL, Vogelaar TW. Effect of EMG feedback on paretic muscles and abnormal co-contraction in the hemiplegic arm, compared with conventional physical therapy. *Scand J Rehabil Med.* 14:121, 1982

36. Burnside IG, Tobias S, Bursill D. Electromyographic feedback in the remobilization of stroke patients: A controlled trial. *Arch Phys Med Rehabil.* 63:217, 1982

37. Basmajian JV. Conscious control and training of motor units and motor neurons. In: Basmajian JV, ed. *Muscles Alive: Their Functions Revealed by Electromyography*, 4th ed. Baltimore, Williams & Wilkins, 1978:115–129

38. Wolf SL, Binder-Macleod SA. Electromyographic biofeedback applications to the hemiplegic patient: Changes in upper extremity neuromuscular and functional status. *Phys Ther.* 63:1393, 1983

39. Wolf SL, Binder-Macleod SA. Electromyographic biofeedback applications to the hemiplegic patient: Changes in the lower extremity neuromuscular and functional status. *Phys Ther.* 63:1404, 1983

40. Wolf SL, Edwards DI, Shutter LA. Concurrent assessment of muscle activity (CAMA): A procedural approach to treatment goals. *Phys Ther.* 66:218, 1986

41. Lecraw DE. Biofeedback in stroke rehabilitation. In: Basmajian JV, ed. *Biofeedback: Principles and Practice for Clinicians*, 3rd ed. Baltimore, Williams & Wilkins, 1989:105–117

42. Fields RW. Electromyographically triggered electrical muscle stimulation for chronic hemiplegia. *Arch Phys Med Rehabil.* 68:407, 1987

CHAPTER 14

Magnetotherapy: Potential Clinical and Therapeutic Applications

Robert Kellogg

The term *magnetotherapy* as defined by *Dorland's Illustrated Medical Dictionary* means "the treatment of disease by magnets or magnetism."[1] The purpose of this chapter is to introduce the reader to the uses of magnetics in medicine along with discussing the present and potential applications of magnetically induced current flow. In order to provide a well-rounded appreciation for the subject of magnetotherapy, this chapter is organized into five sections: (1) historical perspective of magnetics in medicine; (2) basic physics concerning magnetics and magnetically induced currents; (3) biomagnetic fields and magnetic stimulation as diagnostic aids; (4) magnetotherapy in tissue healing and pain management; and (5) potential applications for magnetically induced current flow in muscle stimulation.

HISTORICAL PERSPECTIVE

Magnetics as it relates to medicine enjoys a long and colorful history that closely parallels the history of conventional electrical stimulation. As early as the sixth century BC, lodestones, a type of rock, were known to possess the ability to attract pieces of iron and related rocks.[2] This phenomenon was initially thought to be supernatural in origin, leading to the use of lodestones in spiritual and medicinal ceremonies. In the 17th and 18th centuries the use of magnets in medicine was well publicized and the focus of much controversy.[3] In 1778, Franz Mesmer claimed that an invisible magnetic fluid permeates the universe and that the human body contained poles similar to a magnet. He further claimed that if the body's poles were not aligned with the normal universal magnetic flow illness could result. In order to counter these "malalignment" illnesses, Mesmer would use a form of hypnotism (*mesmerism*) in addition to the surface application of magnets to realign the body's magnetic poles. During this same time frame, Maximilian Hell, a Jesuit priest and noted astronomer, also developed the use of magnets into therapeutic tools, hotly contesting Mesmer's claims.[4] Because of the high degree of controversy a royal commission that included Benjamin Franklin was appointed to investigate the therapeutic claims of magnetic therapy. This commission concluded that no physical evidence existed to support the therapeutic claims.[3]

Practical uses of magnets were developed, such as the removal of metallic foreign bodies from the eye. The continued discoveries by Galvani, Volta, Tesla, and Oersted concerning the physics of electricity, magnetics, and similar properties continued to fuel their use in medicine.[2,3] In 1893, d'Arsonval reported the magnetophosphene visual effect when subjects were exposed to a magnetic field oscillating up to 100 Hz.[5] A phosphene response is described as a faint flickering visual sensation generated by sources other than light. A magnetophosphene response is the result of retinal excitation when the retina is exposed to electromagnetic stimulation.[6] D'Arsonval's findings were readily replicated and provided measurable evidence that magnetic fields can and do cause a physiological response.

In the early 1900s magnetic therapy continued to be used for the treatment of anaemia, arteriosclerosis, chorea, convulsions, hysteria, insomnia, migraine, neuralgia, neurasthenia, neuritis, and rheumatisim,[7] The influence of magnetic exposure on pain was reported by Hansen in 1938. He reported that pain subsided after the application of a strong electromagnet over the site of pain.[8]

Kolin and co-workers, in 1958, were the first to stimulate a peripheral nerve experimental model with an alternating magnetic field.[9] In their experiment they used a frog sciatic nerve preparation with the attached gastrocnemius muscle. This preparation was wrapped around a magnet that was activated by time changing fields of 60 and 1000 Hz. The resulting nerve activation and muscular contraction was attributed to the formation of eddy currents induced in the conductive tissues. In 1965, Bickford and Fremming expanded upon the idea of animal peripheral nerve stimulation and developed a magnetic stimulator capable of excitation of the human peripheral nerves. Bickford and Fremming also recognized the potential application of magnetic stimulation as a tool to stimulate and study the central nervous system.[10] It was not until 1985 that technology allowed the techniques of Barker, Jalinous, and Freeston to successfully stimulate the human cortex with a pulsed magnetic field and record the subsequent evoked peripheral motor response.[11]

In contrast to the use of magnetic fields to influence the human body other scientific disciplines have studied the process of biomagnetism. *Biomagnetism* is the phenomenon where biological material produces an external magnetic field.[12] The first solid measurements of the biologically generated magnetic fields of the heart (magnetocardiograms) were made in 1963 by Baule and McFee using a gradiometer. The technical difficulties in obtaining these measurements are immense when one considers that the biologically generated magnetic fields are one million to one billion times *weaker* than the earth's magnetic field.[3] The development of shielded rooms and point contact SQUIDs (superconducting quantum interference devices) enabled Cohen, in 1969, to record brain (magnetoencephalogram), muscle, and organ biomagnetic fields.[12] With further technological development these biomagnetic recording devices are proving to be useful tools in the study of cellular, cardiac, and brain function.[3]

PHYSICS

Electric and magnetic phenomena are virtually inseparable. The Dutch physicist Hans Oersted discovered that a compass needle is deflected when exposed to a wire carrying electrical current.[2] The deflection is an indication that the magnetized needle is being repulsed by the magnetic field created by the flow of current in the wire. A straight wire carrying an electrical current will produce a magnetic field (following the right hand rule of direction) whose amplitude is proportional to the current of the straight wire and inversely related to the distance from the wire (Fig. 14–1). For a circular wire (loop) with current flowing, the magnetic field will follow the right-hand rule of direction, at an amplitude proportional to the current of the wire and inversely related to the radius of the loop (Fig. 14–2).

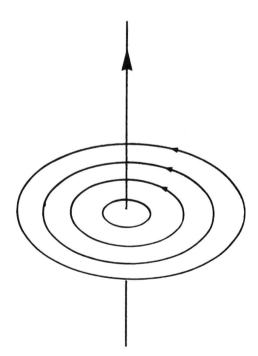

Figure 14–1. Generation of a magnetic field (circular loops) in response to current flowing along a straight wire.

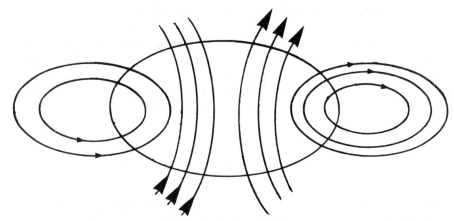

Figure 14–2. Illustration of the magnetic field pattern generated when a current flows through a circular loop.

The generation of a magnetic field in response to current flowing through a wire is well established. The reverse is equally well established. A current will be generated in a wire if exposed to a changing magnetic field or if the wire is moved through a constant magnetic field. In 1831, both Michael Faraday and Joseph Henry performed experiments that confirmed that changing magnetic fields can induce electrical currents in conductive substances.[3] Faraday's law of induction states that the induced voltage depends upon the time rate of change of the magnetic flux. A current flowing through a circular loop (Fig. 14–3) produces a magnetic field. As the current flow is started and stopped the magnetic field changes. This changing magnetic field induces current flow in the nearby wire loop. To stimulate neural tissue in the human body the concept of current flow is induced magnetically.

A magnetic field as described above is generated in response to the flow of current through a wire. The resultant magnetic field can be measured as an amplitude (Hz) in amperes per meter (A/m). More commonly the magnetic field is described in terms of flux density with the units gauss or tesla, where 10,000 gauss equal 1 tesla (T).[6] In order to give the above units some frame of reference the earth provides a magnetic field with a flux density of 30 to 70 μT. The magnetic flux densities of a magnetic resonance imaging (MRI) device are on the order of 1 to 2 T.[13]

The basic design of a clinical instrument used to generate a pulsed magnetic field can be illustrated by examining the Cadwell MES-10 stimulator. The components of this magnetic stimulator requires an energy supply, an energy storage site (capacitors), an on/off switch, and a stimulator coil (Fig. 14–4). When the switch is closed an electrical current flows through the coil wire. A magnetic field is generated by this flow of current, which is also capable of inducing a current flow in nearby conductive tissue. If the original current is pulsed or alternated, the induced currents in the conductive tissue can reach a

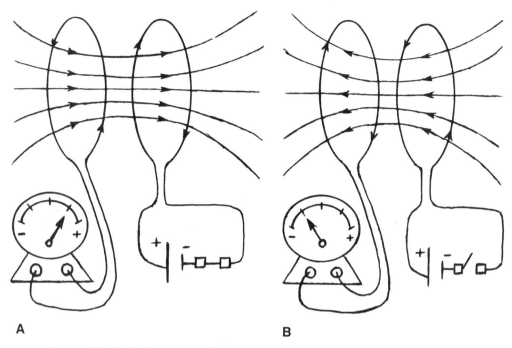

Figure 14–3. A. As current flow starts within the loop, a magnetic field is generated that induces current flow in the nearby loop. **B.** As current flow is stopped by opening the switch, the generated magnetic field decreases, causing reversal of the current flow in the nearby loop. (*Adapted from Wilson JD, with permission.²*)

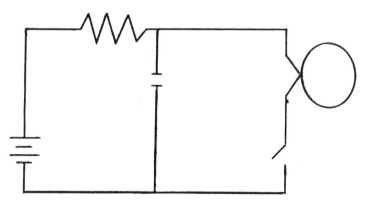

Figure 14–4. Representation of a magnetic pulse stimulator. Left side represents energy source, central portion represents energy storage site capacitors, and right side represents coil stimulator head.

level that will cause depolarization of neural tissue. Figure 14–5 illustrates a coil placed over a thigh with a representation of the induced current flow within the thigh tissue. Please note three facts: (1) the current flow within the tissue is *opposite* in direction to the current flow within the coil; (2) the current amplitude is greatest just beneath the coil edges; and (3) the induced current flow is not related to intervening tissue but is related to the distance from the coil.

The fact that the depth of magnetic field is not hampered by the impedance offered by the skin or bone gives it some special characteristics. Magnetic stimulation (1) is relatively painless; (2) is useful for stimulating deep-lying neural structures; and (3) has no need for direct contact between the stimulator and skin.[14] Magnetically induced currents bypass the sensory pain receptors. The current produced at the skin surface is not great enough to cause the pain receptors to depolarize, while the more sensitive large-diameter motor neurous are depolarized to a threshold level, resulting in a motor response. Deeply located structures such as the sciatic nerve or brachial plexus

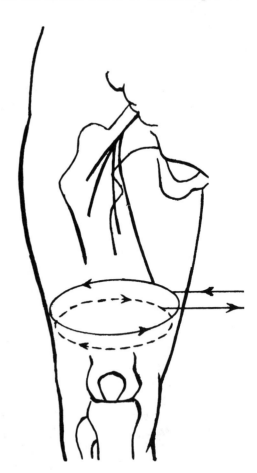

Figure 14–5. A charged coil is placed over the anterior thigh. The resulting pulsed magnetic field induces current flow in conductive tissue within the thigh. Note that the current flowing in the thigh is opposite in direction to the current flowing in the coil.

a͞e easy to stimulate with a magnetic field because the stimulating event is not attenuated by intervening tissue. Magnetically induced currents can produce a motor threshold depolarization in deep structures without producing intolerably high currents at the skin level.

The third characteristic, no essential skin to stimulator contact, is easy to visualize with the help of Figure 14–6. Conventional neuromuscular electrical stimulation (NMES) requires that the skin be coupled with the stimulating electrodes to provide a path for current to flow. Magnetically induced current flow is not dependent upon direct contact with the stimulator, but requires only that the target tissue be within the magnetic field. In fact the magnetic stimulating coil should be well-insulated from the surface tissue to prevent injury from the heat within the coil.

There are several important points to be kept in mind when considering the use of magnetically induced current flow as a method of stimulation: (1) the magnetic field has to be pulsed or time varied, as a static magnetic field will not cause neural tissue depolarization; (2) the induced current flow is proportional to the magnetic field rate of change,[15] and the induced current

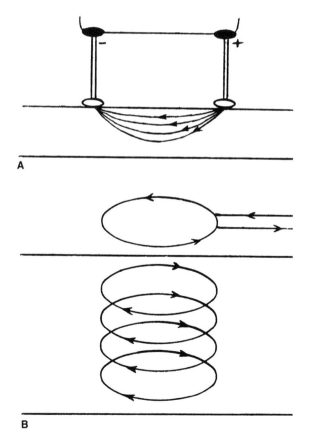

A

B

Figure 14–6. A. Depiction of the need for direct skin-to-stimulator contact with conventional NMES, with the resultant attenuation of current amplitude as it passes through the layers of impedance between the stimulator and the target tissue. **B.** The current flow is induced in the most conductive tissue without requiring skin-to-stimulator contact, with no attenuation because of intervening tissues.

takes on characteristics of the magnetic pulse rate; and (3) the term "magnetic stimulation" is misleading in that the depolarizing stimulus is *not* a direct result of the magnetic pulse. The bioelectrical currents occurring within the conductive tissues cause neural depolarization. As suggested by Geddes, the term "electrodeless electrical stimulation" may be a better descriptive term.[16]

Recording Magnetic Fields

The recording of biologically generated magnetic fields is in its infancy in terms of technology and application. The recording of biomagnetic fields is technologically demanding and therefore largely limited to the research laboratory. Extremely sensitive SQUID devices are used in conjunction with detection coils, developed along the concepts of first- and second-order gradiometers, to record biomagnetic fields.[3,12] These biomagnetic fields are the result of bioelectrical activity generated by conducting cells. The magnetic fields of these activated cells can be recorded and studied based upon temporal sequencing, amplitude, and spatial organization. A schematic representation of the biomagnetic field generated in the sensory cortex in response to stimulation of the right hand is presented in Figure 14–7.

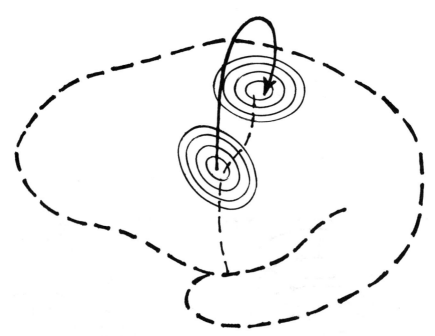

Figure 14–7. Biomagnetic fields generated by the cerebral cortex in response to sensory stimulation. These biomagnetic fields can be recorded from specific portions of the cortex depending upon body part involved and sensory modality being stimulated.

MAGNETIC FIELDS USED AS DIAGNOSTIC AIDS

The modern use of magnetic fields in medicine currently focuses on magnetic stimulation and biomagnetic recordings as assistive devices in diagnostics. The most commonly recognized and validated diagnostic use of magnetic fields is in the area of (MRI). A discussion of MRI theory, physics, instrumentation, and application is beyond the scope of this text. For readers who are interested in this technique, some fascinating and informative books are available.[17,18] The emphasis in this section will be on the use of magnetic stimulation in electrophysiological evaluation and the potential use of biomagnetic field recordings.

While Bickford and Fremming[10] are credited with first conceptualizing the use of magnetic stimulation as an adjunct to conventional electrophysiological evaluation, Barker and co-workers published the first paper on its use in a clinical setting.[19] Barker and associates magnetically stimulated the cerebral cortex, cervical spine, and lumbar spine in healthy people, people with multiple sclerosis, and people with motor neuron disease. The people with multiple sclerosis showed increased cortex-to-spine latencies, while the central latencies of the people with motor neuron disease were found to be normal.[19] These results were confirmed by Hess and co-workers in a study that compared healthy subjects with people who had multiple sclerosis.[20] In studying the effects of cortical magnetic stimulation on the distal evoked muscle action potential (MAP), Hess and associates found that if the stimulus was generated over a mild background of volitional activity the evoked MAP amplitude was greatly enhanced and the distal latency decreased by 3 msec.[21]

Bickford and co-workers sustained the augmented effect of combined magnetic and conventional electrical stimulation on evoked MAP response amplitude. In their study the ulnar nerve was stimulated at the elbow, and the evoked MAP recorded from a hypothenar muscle. The amplitude of the electrical and the magnetic stimulus was adjusted to a threshold motor level contraction. Next, the two stimulators (electric and magnetic) were triggered simultaneously, which resulted in an evoked MAP amplitude two to four times greater than the amplitudes of the independent stimulators. The combined stimuli may cause an augmentation of neural depolarization by an increased ability for the electric current to flow through the neural tissues.[22]

Several reports have been presented that compare magnetically induced facial nerve stimulation to conventional electrical stimulation. The two techniques provide similar latency measurements, with magnetic stimulation having the advantage of being both less painful and capable of stimulating the facial nerve deep within the temporal bone.[23,24] Magnetic stimulation on proximal nerves and spinal nerve roots lacks an accurate site of marking the point of depolarization on the anatomic structure. Confidence that stimulation is occurring proximal to the site of the lesion is another problem.[25–27] Two articles specifically present the use of magnetic stimulators in routine electrophysiological studies. Evans and associates studied the stimulation of the median nerve at the wrist and found that they were unable to achieve supramaximal stimulation without stimulating the ulnar nerve simultaneously. They also found it difficult to determine the exact point of nerve depolarization, thus making it impossible to obtain accurate length measurements.[28] Amassian and co-workers determined that the best orientation of the stimulator coil to the nerve is orthogonal–longitudinal (Fig. 14–8), which decreased the chance for spread of stimulus to other conductive tissues. They also determined that the magnetically induced effective cathode and anode lay within a few millimeters of each other.[29]

Biomagnetic field research is currently being conducted in the areas of cardiology, neurology, and other subspecialties of physiology. Recording biomagnetic fields in cardiology is experimental. It is not clear if the magneto-cardiogram will provide information that is significantly better than that currently collected by the electrocardiogram. Potential areas of application include (1) actual spatial discrimination of cardiac muscle dysfunction and (2) localization of conduction block without resorting to cardiac catheterization.[12]

Recording the magnetoencephalogram is an exciting new tool for mapping the cerebral cortex. Magnetoencephalograms provide information similar to that provided with the conventional electroencephalogram. Biomagnetic field studies support the term *tonotopic* representation over the auditory cortex.

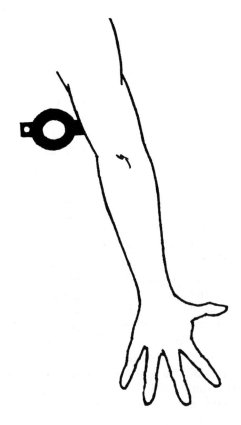

Figure 14–8. The orthogonal–longitudinal orientation of the coil stimulator Amassian found to provide the best stimulation of the ulnar nerve with the least amount of volume conduction to other tissues.

Other biomagnetic fields of experimentation include the localization of epileptic seizure activity and the objective measurement of pain responses.[3,12]

The final area of intensive research for biomagnetic fields as diagnostic aids has to do with improving the understanding of cellular physiology. Areas of particular interest include (1) liver metabolism and iron storage; (2) lung function and clearance of foreign particles; and (3) nerve and muscle cell membrane action potential examination.[3,12]

TISSUE HEALING AND PAIN MANAGEMENT

The healing of nonunion fractures remains the most publicized use of magnetic stimulation. Bassett was the first to apply the inductive electrical stimulation technique using a pulsed magnetic field to stimulate nonunion fracture sites.[30] The first pulsed electromagnetic fields were generated by a single external coil. In an effort to improve the magnetic field's uniformity,[31] later stimulators used quasi-Helmholtz coils. The field flux densities used in these bone stimulators varies from 1 to 30 mT.[13] The efficacy of pulsed magnetic stimulation in the care of patients with nonunions, failed fusions, congenital pseudarthrosis, and avascular necrosis has been reported.[31,32] Critics of this technique point out that part of the treatment regime consists of prolonged periods of immobilization and therefore it is not the magnetic stimulation influencing the healing.[33] In a double-blind study control group used sham stimulators and illustrated an increased number of successful unions of previously ununited fractures.[33] The authors attribute success in the sham group to the extended periods of immobilization associated with the pulsed magnetic stimulation treatment. The true clinical utility of magnetic stimulation as an adjunct to fracture healing remains in doubt.[33]

Soft tissue injury response to static magnetic fields has been studied by Leapers and associates.[34,35] In these model studies a magnetic coil was used over experimentally induced wounds. No significant differences were noted between the control and experimental animals at 3, 7, 10, and 14 days postwound. The healing effects of electromagnetic stimulation on rabbit ligaments was reported by Frank and co-workers, who used a pulsed magnetic field with a flux density of 25 mT.[36] Histological and biochemical evidence of increased wound maturity was noted at 21 and 42 days postinjury for the stimulated group compared to the control group.[36] Rotator cuff tendonitis has been reported to respond successfully to pulsed magnetic stimulation.[31,37] In both reports a large percentage of patients with rotator cuff tendonitis showed marked improvement within 4 weeks of starting the therapy.[31,37]

The study by Binder and associates included a control group and an experimental group in a double-blind design. The control and experimental groups differed significantly at 2 and 4 weeks of therapy. The control group was switched to receiving true stimulation at the 4-week point. By week 6 of the study both groups were equally improved.[37]

Trentin and Visentin conducted a study on the effects of low-amplitude magnetic stimulation on patient populations with rheumatoid arthritis and degenerative arthritis.[38] Using a visual analogue scale to evaluate pain as well as active range of motion measurements, each group was treated with low-amplitude (30 to 80 mT) pulsed magnetic stimuation. After an average of 15 to 19 treatments the improvement in the rheumatoid arthritis group was poor, while the short-term improvement in the degenerative arthritis group was considered good. Improvement was limited to less than 4 months in duration in the degenerative arthritis group.[38]

In an effort to explain the pain relief benefits of low-amplitude pulsed magnetic stimulation, Warnke states that three factors may be involved: (1) the active widening of blood vessel diameters secondarily to changes in autonomic nerve activity; (2) the increase in oxygen partial pressure in terminal tissue; and (3) the change in local perfusion and velocity of capillary blood flow.[39] Adey's article on physiological signalling across cell membranes indicates the effect of low-frequency electromagnetic fields occurs at the cellular membrane level. This interaction may indicate an amplification process of weak triggers associated with the normal binding of hormones, antibodies, and neurotransmitters to their specific binding sites.[40]

In an effort to document changes in blood flow and tissue oxygenation, Railton and Newman studied these parameters in a double-blind experiment. In response to pulsed magnetic stimulation with a flux density of 100 G, no significant changes were noted in skin temperature or transcutaneous oxygen tension measurements.[41] Ueno and associates examined the change in skin capillary blood flow using a laser Doppler flowmeter in response to pulsed magnetic field exposure as produced by an induction heater. In this study the magnetic field flux densities were 16, 32, and 48 mT. The frequency of stimulation was 3.8 KHz, as compared to 25 Hz in the Railton and associates study.[41,42] The results of this investigation indicate that skin capillary blood flow decreases in response to high-frequency, low-amplitude pulsed magnetic stimulation. This change in blood flow is thought to represent an increase in vasoconstrictor tone.[42]

MAGNETICALLY INDUCED SKELETAL MUSCLE STIMULATION

A natural progression of magnetically induced electrical stimulation has developed into its use as a muscle skeletal stimulator. Bickford and co-workers recognized its potential use as a rehabilitation tool for patients with central nervous system dysfunction.[22] Cadwell Laboratories has developed a prototype magnetic stimulator for investigational use as a muscle stimulator. The MES-10 unit has been modified to provide a stimulus rate of 60 pps, with a peak magnetic field flux density of 1.5 T (15000 G). Pulse waveform and duration are illustrated in Figure 14–9. Several pilot studies are being conducted at the physical therapy education program, University of Kentucky, to investigate this

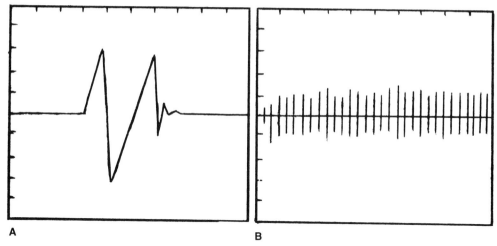

A   B

Figure 14–9. **A.** Cosine pulse waveform (1 V/div, 100 msec/div). **B.** A train of magnetically induced electrical pulses at 60 Hz from the Cadwell modified MES-10 (time scale of 50 msec/div).

unit's potential usefulness in generating high levels of muscle contraction, altering blood flow, and preventing muscular atrophy in orthopedically injured patients.

An initial pilot study was designed to evaluate the magnetic stimulator's ability to induce a contraction of the quadriceps femoris muscle. Twenty volunteer, healthy subjects (13 women and 7 men) with ages ranging from 20 to 37 years were stabilized in an isokinetic device with their hip and knees flexed at 60 degrees. All subjects were tested isometrically. No subject generated any muscle torque when the stimulator was triggered at an amplitude less than .5 T (5000 G). All subjects were able to tolerate maximal magnetic stimulator output (1.5 T), which produced torque values from 11 to 120 ft-lb (14.9 to 162.7 N.m [Newton meters]), with a mean value of 59 ft-lb (79.9 N.m). As a percentage of their maximal volitional contraction (MVC) the range was 8 to 82 percent MVC, with an average of 40.6 percent MVC.[43]

In an effort to better understand the relation between stimulator coil size and muscle response, 11 volunteer subjects were exposed to peak pulsed magnetic stimulation of the quadriceps femoris muscle with two different-size coils (17 and 26 cm diameter). Each subject had the quadriceps femoris muscle stimulated isometrically while secured to an isokinetic dynamometer. In all subjects the larger coil (26-cm diameter) generated a stronger muscle contraction. This contraction was on the average 38 percent greater than the torque generated by stimulation with the small coil. This result between coils of different diameters relates to the principle expressed by the formula:

$$E = \frac{\delta B}{\delta t} \times \frac{r}{2}$$

where

- E is the amplitude of the magnetic field,
- $\delta B/\delta t$ is the rate of change of the magnetic field, and
- r is the radius of the circular coil.[44]

To determine if an augmentation phenomenon occurs with muscle torque measurements with combined magnetic and electrical stimulation, 10 subjects volunteered for simultaneous quadriceps femoris muscle stimulation. Each subject was secured to an isokinetic dynamometer set in the isometric mode. The subjects had a conventional neuromuscular stimulator of 2.500 Hz modulated at 50 bursts per second connected to their thigh with surface electrodes over the quadriceps femoris muscle. The magnetic stimulator coil was placed over the conventional NMES electrodes. The subjects tolerated a conventional electrically induced contraction equalling an average of 51 percent of their MVC. The average contraction generated by the magnetic stimulator was 44 percent of the MVC value. When the two types of stimulation were applied simultaneously the average contraction was 65 percent of the MVC value. Of major importance is that the subjects all reported that the simultaneously generated contraction was less painful than the electrically generated contraction.

A blood flow study evaluating the effect of magnetic stimulation on skin capillary blood flow was done using a laser Doppler capillary blood flow meter. The subjects were stabilized to the isokinetic dynamometer set in the isometric mode. The coil electrode was centered over the midanterior thigh, with the Doppler sensor located in the center of the coil. Each subject was magnetically stimulated to a contraction level of 10 to 20 percent of their MVC value. Stimulation was maintained for 10 sec "on," 20 sec "off," for a total of 5 min. Blood flow readings were taken continuously for 5 min prior to stimulation, during stimulation, and for 5 min after stimulation. All subjects showed an increase in their total skin capillary blood flow after stimulation. The values are expressed as a percentage increase over baseline prestimulation readings. The range of blood flow increase was 5.7 to 51.6% percent, with a mean value of 23.3 percent and a standard deviation of $\pm$ 15.1 percent.[43]

Another pilot study was conducted by combining the simultaneous use of conventional NMES and magnetic stimulation to prevent muscle weakness and wasting in patients during the first 6 weeks after reconstructive surgery of the anterior cruciate ligament. Sixteen patients having knee surgery received control (no induced contractions, n = 3), neuromuscular electrical stimulation only (NMES, n = 7), and MES (n = 7) treatments. Before surgery all NMES and magnetic stimuli treatment patients were measured for MVC by a dynamometer system and for thigh girth. Two NMES-only and all magnetically stimulated patients were also measured for MVC (torque) 6 weeks after surgery. Using MVC, the current amplitudes of NMES and magnetic stimuli to produce the equivalency of 50 percent of MVC for treatment purposes over 6 weeks after surgery were determined. Patients receiving magnetic stimulation also rated both NMES and magnetic stimulation modes of treatment for pain. All patients received progressive physical therapy over the first 6 weeks after surgery. Results revealed that the two NMES-only patients gained 24.7 percent in torque, while MES patients lost 13.2 percent torque compared with a mean 49.6 percent loss reported in the literature.[45,46] The mean percent of thigh girth lost during the 6 weeks after surgery was 8.3 for controls, 0.5 for NMES only, and 2.3 for magnetically stimulated patients. Magnetically stimulated patients rated the MES treatments as being 50 percent more tolerable than the conventional NMES-only treatments.[47] These results are encouraging for the use of magnetic stimulation and hold promise for future use in physical therapy.

SUMMARY

The use of magnetic fields in medicine is experiencing a new surge of interest as technological advances allow for more sophisticated applications of magnetic theory. Currently the use of magnetic fields is blossoming in research institutions. Of special importance is the study of these fields and their biologic activity in the realm of biophysics and physiology, particularly at the cellular level. As a clinical tool there are already several popular applications in the field of electrophysiology. From a therapeutic standpoint magnetotherapy has yet to be illustrated as an efficacious modality. Continued development of its potential in the laboratory and evaluation of its uses in well-controlled clinical studies will be required prior to magnetotherapy having a respected place in the field of rehabilitation.

REFERENCES

1. *Dorland's Illustrated Medical Dictionary*, 27th ed. Philadelphia, WB Saunders, 1988: 972
2. Wilson JD. *Physics: Concepts and Applications.* Lexington, MA, DC Heath, 1977: 545–605
3. Williamson SJ, Kaufman L. In: Weinberg H, Stronik G, Katila T, eds. *Biomagnetism Applications and Theory: Frontiers in the New Science of Biomagnetism.* New York, Pergamon Press, 1985: 471–489
4. Smith CW. In: Frohlich H, ed. *Biological Coherence and Response to External Stimuli: Electromagnetic Effects in Humans.* Berlin, Springer-Verlag, 1988: 205–232
5. Adey WR. Tissue interactions with nonionizing electromagnetic fields. *Physiol Rev.* 61: 435, 1981
6. Mild KH, Oberg PA. In: Buser PA, Cobb WA, Okuma T, eds. Kyoto Symposia (EEG suppl 36): *Neurophysiological Effects of Electromagnetic Fields: A Critical Review.* Amsterdam, Elsevier Biomedical Press, 1982: 715–729
7. Matijaca A. *Principles of Electro-Medicine, Electro-Surgery and Radiology.* Butler, Benedict Lust, 1917: 68
8. Hansen KM. Some observations with view to possible influence of magnetism upon the human organism. *Acta Med Scand.* 97:339, 1938

9. Kolin A, Brill NQ, Broberg PJ. Stimulation of irritable tissues by means of an alternating magnetic field. *Proc Soc Exp Biol Med.* 102:251, 1959

10. Bickford RG, Fremming BD. Neural stimulation by pulsed magnetic fields in animals and man. Digest of the 6th International Conference on Medical Electronics and Biological Engineering, Tokyo, 1965

11. Barker AT, Jalinous R, Freeston IL. The design, construction and performance of a magnetic nerve stimulator. IEEE International Conference on Electric and Magnetic Fields in Medicine and Biology, December 1985, pp 59–63

12. Cohen D. In: Weinber H, Stronik G, Katila T, eds. *Biomagnetism Applications and Theory: Introduction. A Perspective of Biomagnetism.* New York, Pergamon Press, 1985: 4–8

13. Stuchly MA. Human exposure to static and time-varying magnetic fields. *Health Phys.* 51:215, 1986

14. Barker AT, Freeston IL, Jalinous DR, Jarratt JA. Magnetic stimulation of the human brain and peripheral nervous system: An introduction and the results of an initial clinical evaluation. *Neurosurgery.* 20:100, 1987

15. Cadwell J, Cadwell C. *The Theory of Magnetic Stimulation and Its Clinical Applications* (videotape). Kennewick, WA, Cadwell Laboratories, 1989

16. Geddes IA. Optimal stimulus duration for extracranial cortical stimulation. *Neurosurgery.* 1:94, 1987

17. Elster AD. *Cranial Magnetic Resonance Imaging.* New York, Churchill Livingstone, 1988: 1–16

18. Stark DD, Bradley WG. *Magnetic Resonance Imaging.* St. Louis CV Mosby, 1988

19. Barker AT, Freeston IL, Jalinous R, Jarratt JA. Magnetic stimulation of the human brain and peripheral nervous system an introduction and the results of an initial clinical evaluation. Motor evoked potential conference abstract, Purdue University, 1986

20. Hess CW, Mills KR, Murray NMF. Measurement of central motor conduction in multiple sclerosis by magnetic brain stimulation. *Lancet.* August 16:355, 1986

21. Hess CW, Mills KR, Murry NMF. Responses in small hand muscles from magnetic stimulation of the human cortex. *J Physiol.* 388:397, 1987

22. Bickford RG, Guidi M, Fortesque P, Swenson M. Magnetic stimulation of human peripheral nerve and brain: response enhancement by combined magnetoelectrical technique. *Neurosurgery.* 20:110, 1987

23. Estrem SA, Conway RR, Platt W, et al. Magnetic stimulation for facial nerve electroneurography. *Muscle Nerve.* Sept.: 994, 1988 (abstract)

24. Windmill IM, Shields CB, Martinez SA, Edmonds HL. Assessment of facial nerve injuries using transcranial magnetically evoked motor potentials (abstract). *Muscle Nerve.* 11:994, 1988

25. Smith SJM, Murray NMF. Electrical and magnetic stimulation of lower-limb nerves and roots. *Muscle Nerve.* 11:652, 1986 (abstract)

26. Conway RR, Hof J, Buckelew S. Lower cervical magnetic stimulation: Comparison with CB needle root stimulation and supraclavicular stimulation. *Muscle Nerve.* 11:997, 1988 (abstract)

27. Evans BA, Daube JR, Litchy WJ. Comparison of magnetic and electric stimulation of spinal nerves (abstract). *Muscle Nerve.* 11:997, 1988

28. Evans BA, Lichy WJ, Daube JR. The utility of magnetic stimulation for routine peripheral nerve conduction studies. *Muscle Nerve.* 11:1074, 1988

29. Amassian VE, Maccabee PJ, Cracco RQ. Focal stimulation of human peripheral

nerve with the magnetic coil: A comparison with electrical stimulation. *Exp Neurol.* 103:282, 1989

30. Brighton CT. Present and future of electrically induced osteogenesis. In: Straub LR, Wilson PD, eds. *Clinical Trends in Orthopaedics.* New York, Thieme-Stratton, 1982:1–15

31. Bassett CAL, Jackson SF. A critique of medical uses of weak pulsing electromagnetic fields. In Chiabrera A, Nicolini C, Schwan HP, eds. *Interactions Between Electromagnetic Fields and Cells.* New York, Plenum Press, 1985:569–579

32. De Hass WG, Beaupre A, Cameron H, English E. The Canadian experience with pulsed magnetic fields in the treatment of ununited tibial fractures. *Clin Orthop.* 208:55, 1986

33. Barker AT, Dixon RA, Sharrard WJW, Sutcliffe ML. Pulsed magnetic field therapy for tibial non-union, interim results of a double blind trial. *Lancet.* 8384: 994, 1984

34. Leaper DJ, Foster ME, Brennan SS, Davies PW. Do magnetic fields influence soft tissue wound healing? A preliminary communication. *Equine Vet J.* 17:178, 1985

35. Leaper DJ, Foster ME, Brennan SS, Davies PW. An experimental study of the influence of magnetic fields on soft-tissue wound healing. *J. Trauma.* 25:1083, 1985

36. Frank C, Schachar N, Dittrich D, et al. Electromagnetic stimulation of ligament healing in rabbits. *Clin Orthop* 175:263, 1983

37. Binder A, Park G, Hazleman B, Fitton-Jackson S. Pulsed electromagnetic field therapy of persistent rotator cuff tendinitis a double-blind controlled assessment. *Lancet* March 31:695, 1984

38. Trentin L, Visentin M. The use of pulsating magnetic fields in cervical and upper arm pain. In: Ruzzi R, Visentin M, eds. *Pain.* Italy, Piccin/Butterworths, 1983:163–166

39. Warnke U. The possible role of pulsating magnetic fields in the reduction of pain. In: Ruzzi R, Visentin M, eds. *Pain.* Italy, Piccin/Butterworths, 1983:229–238

40. Adey WR. Physiological signalling across cell membranes and cooperative influences of extremely low frequency electromagnetic fields. In: Frohlich H, ed. *Biological Coherence and Response to External Stimuli.* Berlin, Springer-Verlag, 1988:164–167

41. Railton R, Newman PP. Magnetic field therapy—Does it affect soft tissue? *Orthop Sports Phys Ther.* 4:241, 246, 1983

42. Ueno S, Lovsund P, Oberg PA. Effects of alternating magnetic fields and low frequency electric currents on human skin blood flow. *Med Biol Eng Comput.* 24:57, 1986

43. Currier DP, Kellogg RM, Nitz A. Pulsed magnetic stimulation: Effects upon quadriceps torque and blood flow. *Phys Ther.* 69:395, 1989 (abstract)

44. Barker AT, Jalinous R, Freeston IL. Non-invasive magnetic stimulation of the human motor cortex. *Lancet.* 1:1106, 1985

45. Morrissey MC, Brewster CE, Shields CL, et al. The effects of electrical stimulation on the quadriceps during postoperative knee immobilization. *Am J Sports Med.* 13:40, 1985

46. Wigerstad-Lossing I, Grimby G, Jonsson T, et al. Effects of electrical muscle stimulation combined with voluntary contractions after knee ligament surgery. *Med Sci Sports Experc.* 20:93, 1988

47. Currier DP, Ray JM, Nyland J, et al. Magnetoelectrical stimulation in the prevention of muscle wasting and weakness after reconstructive surgery of the anterior cruciate ligament. (In preparation)

Algorithm for Steps in Electrotesting/Therapy Strategies

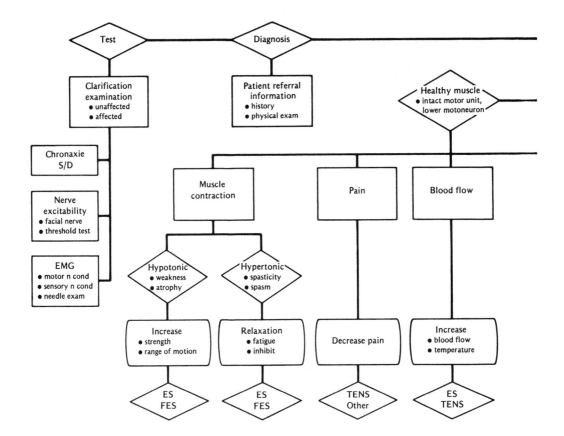

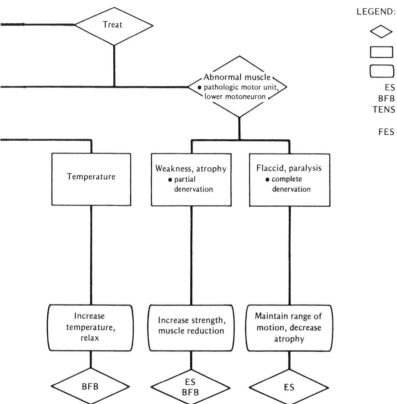

LEGEND:

◇ = Decision

▢ = Function

▢ = Goal

ES = Electrical stimulation
BFB = Biofeedback
TENS = Transcutaneous Electrical
Nerve Stimulation
FES = Functional Electrical
Stimulation

Uses of Pulsed Electrical Stimulation and Suggested Conditions

USES OF PULSED ELECTRICAL STIMULATION AND SUGGESTED CONDITIONS

Use	Ramp	Pulse Duration	Frequency (pps)	Amplitude	Wave Form	Miscellaneous
Muscle contraction	Slow on (1–5 sec)	0.1	50–90	High (50% of MVC)	Monophasic Biphasic Polyphasic	1:5 on–off ratio 8 contractions 2 × wk × 10 sessions
Relaxation	Slow on (1–5 sec)	0.1	35–90	Tolerance	Monophasic Biphasic Polyphasic	1:1 on–off ratio 10–20 contractions as needed
Re-education	—	0.05–0.3	1 per sec	Moderate	Monophasic	Manually control
Spasticity	Slow on	0.05–0.3	50–90	Moderate	Monophasic Biphasic Polyphasic	1:1 on/off ratio 20–30 min prior to treatment (exercise)
Range of motion	Slow on–off	0.05–0.1	50–90	Strong	Monophasic Biphasic Polyphasic	10–20 contractions 30 min/day × 3 wk or more

Pain						
Reduce pain, TENS						
High (acute)	—	0.05–0.1	10–100	Low sensory	Monophasic Biphasic Polyphasic	2–4 hr/day 2–3 wk
Low (chronic)	—	0.05–0.1	1–10	Weak muscle contraction	Monophasic Biphasic Polyphasic	2–4 hr/day 4–8 wk
Blood flow						
Increase muscle	—	0.1–0.3	4–32	Moderate	Monophasic Biphasic Polyphasic	10 min as needed
Nerve conduction	Rapid rise	0.1–0.5	1 per sec	Supramaximum	Monophasic	As needed
Denervation	Rapid rise	1–5	1–20	Moderate	Monophasic	5–10 sec on, 10 min rest 1/hr/24 hr
Wound healing	—	0.05–0.3	0(DC– and +) 80–105	Low	Monophasic	45 min/day as needed

Index